NUTRITION FOR DEVELOPING COUNTRIES

WITH SPECIAL REFERENCE TO THE MAIZE, CASSAVA AND MILLET AREAS OF AFRICA

MAURICE H. KING

M.D. CANTAB., F.R.C.P. LOND.
WHO Staff Member, the Lembaga Kesehatan Nasional, Surabaya, Indonesia
Formerly Professor of Social Medicine
in the University of Zambia

FELICITY M. A. KING

B.M. OXON., M.R.C.P. LOND.
Formerly Nuffield Research Fellow in Community Paediatrics
in the University of Zambia

DAVID C. MORLEY

M.D. CANTAB., M.R.C.P., D.C.H. LOND.
Reader in Tropical Child Health
in the University of London

H. J. LESLIE BURGESS

M.B.CH.B. ST.AND., D.P.H. LOND., D.T.M. & H. LIVERPOOL, M.P.H. HARVARD
Formerly WHO Area Nutrition Adviser, Malawi

ANN P. BURGESS

B.SC. NUTRITION
Queen Elizabeth College, London

Nairobi Oxford
OXFORD UNIVERSITY PRESS
Dar es Salaam

Oxford University Press

OXFORD LONDON GLASGOW
NEW YORK TORONTO MELBOURNE WELLINGTON
NAIROBI DAR ES SALAAM CAPE TOWN
KUALA LUMPUR SINGAPORE JAKARTA HONG KONG TOKYO
DELHI BOMBAY CALCUTTA MADRAS KARACHI

Oxford University Press, P.O. Box 72532, Nairobi, Kenya

ISBN 0 19 572244 2

© OXFORD UNIVERSITY PRESS 1972
Reprinted 1973

Reprinted with minor corrections 1975, 1976, 1979

MADE IN EAST AFRICA

The costs of producing this volume
have been most generously subsidized,
in equal amounts,
by
WAR ON WANT
and by a private donation
in memory of Talivaldis 'Tali' Grant
a British volunteer who was killed in a car accident
in November 1971 whilst in the service of
the National Food and Nutrition Commission of Zambia

THIS BOOK IS DEDICATED TO THE UNDERWEIGHT CHILD

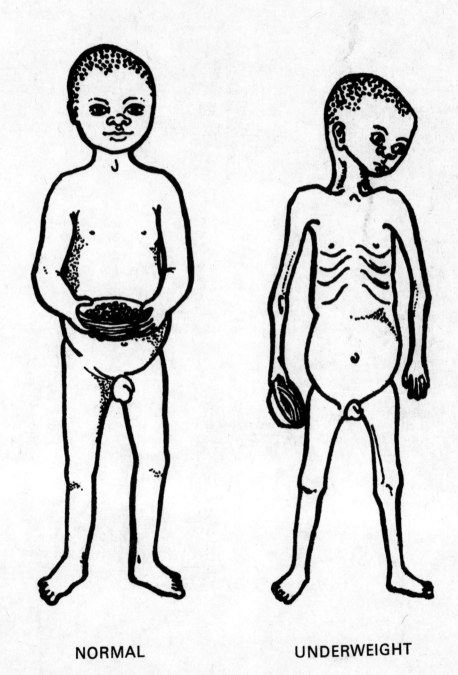

NORMAL   UNDERWEIGHT

A note on the second and third reprint 1975

Preface

There are said to be between ten and twenty million malnourished children in the world, as well as many more who are less seriously affected. Much of this malnutrition, with all its tragic consequences, could be prevented if only families would feed their children with the foods that are already available, or could be grown in the country. The knowledge necessary to achieve this already exists, and must now be applied on the widest scale. Such is the purpose of this book, which hopes to show the reader how to feed his own children, how to teach other people to do the same, how to make the community diagnosis of malnutrition in his district, how to initiate community health action, and how to supervise the growth of children using a weight chart.

Food patterns vary greatly and nutrition teaching has to be adapted to particular times and places. This book has been written for the 'maize, millet and cassava areas of Africa', most examples being taken from Zambia. It will inevitably be less applicable elsewhere, and adaptations to other countries and languages are likely to be needed. At the time of going to press a Swahili version is, for example, already in preparation. Because of the widespread need for a text of this kind, and because adaptation promises to be less laborious than writing from scratch, the authors and the publishers will welcome any attempts that nutritionists in other parts of the world may make to adapt its material to their own needs and languages, so making local versions for their particular countries.* Several chapters, the first and second for example, will need almost no change for other areas, and it may be possible to adapt most of the material with little change, keeping the same section headings and most of the pictures. It is probable that less adaptation will be necessary than might appear at first sight. Thus the second experimental edition which preceded this version was, for example, considered suitable for medical assistants in New Guinea when used in conjunction with duplicated notes to adapt it to the very different nutritional patterns of that country. The book's length may seem a disadvantage, and a reader's guide may help the less experienced student to select what he needs; a suggestion that has recently been made in Zambia, where its use is being considered for a correspondence course in nutrition at the junior secondary level.

In accordance with recent international decisions, joules have replaced calories throughout. The writers were kindly allowed to see the draft of FAO's 1972 revised recommendations for protein and joule requirements which have been incorporated in the text. Great care has been taken in dissecting what is useful for the reader to know from the vast corpus of available knowledge. A radical approach has been taken; much conventional material has been omitted, especially in respect of the vitamins, while greater emphasis than usual has been placed on the proteins and on protein-energy malnutrition. Because the purpose of applied nutrition is to achieve effective action, great attention has been paid to the practical aspects of nutrition teaching, which have been described as 'things to do' at the end of each chapter. Most of the book is written in simple English using a strictly limited vocabulary and syntax. (A count of 5,000 words taken from sections randomly distributed through the book showed that only 440 different ones had been used, including many that only occurred once or twice.) Only this Preface and Sections 11.24b, 11.24c and 12.3 are in ordinary, or standard, English.

If a book such as this is to succeed in its purpose, it must live and develop, casting out old material and incorporating new ideas as one edition succeeds another. This calls for a partnership between the writers and their readers in the interests of those they try to help. So we look forward to hearing where our labours have succeeded and where they have not, and to including in a subsequent edition any suggestions that you may have to offer.

*Any such enquiries for translation or adaptation must be referred, in the first instance, to the publishers of this edition (Oxford University Press, P.O. Box 72532, Nairobi, Kenya) who will consult the authors. However, such permission will not be unreasonably withheld subject to the necessary formalities being complied with.

A note on the occasion of the first reprint, 1975

The widespread demand for this book during the two years that it has been available has shown the great need for a work of this kind, and we are pleased to find that adaptations to several other languages and food cultures are being prepared. We have taken the opportunity of this impression to substitute the term protein energy malnutrition (PEM) for protein joule malnutrition (PJM). On the advice of Dr and Mrs Braun, we have inserted a new 'block in the food-path'—emotional deprivation or 'lack of love'.

Meanwhile, we have completed the experimental edition of a manual of health centre paediatrics which is cross referenced both to this book and to *A Medical Laboratory for Developing Countries* (M. H. King, Oxford University Press, London), the three books being intended as a trilogy for workers in the basic health services.

Introduction

Many children do not get enough of the right foods to eat. They do not grow well, they become ill, many die, and they do not grow up as clever, as healthy, or as tall as they should be. We say that they are malnourished, or that they are suffering from **malnutrition. Nutrition** is the study of food and the way our bodies use food. 'Mal' means bad. Malnutrition therefore, means bad nutrition. There are many reasons why children are malnourished. One of them is that people do not know enough about nutrition or how to feed children. This is why we have written this book. Some of the people who might want to read it have not been long in school, so we have tried to write it in easy English with as few new words as possible. We hope that it will be useful to everyone who can do anything to improve nutrition and especially to medical assistants, medical students, nurses, midwives, agricultural assistants, community development and homecraft workers, and also to teachers in schools. All these people can teach other people. This, therefore, is mostly a book to teach you what and how to teach.

First you must learn how children grow (Chapter 1), then what happens when they fail to grow (Chapter 2). If children are going to grow, they must eat the right protein foods, so you must know what these foods are made of (Chapter 3). Energy foods and protective foods are also needed (Chapter 4). The right foods must be eaten together and some are especially important, so you must learn more about them (Chapter 5). You must also know how much food people of different ages need, and how much it costs (Chapter 6). When you know all this you can learn how to feed the normal child (Chapter 7), and how bad bottle-feeding can be (Chapter 8). If every child is going to be well fed, the bush has first to be cleared and fields planted and weeded. The food has then to be harvested, stored, cooked and eaten. Sometimes it has to be sent to market, sold and bought. It is as if food has to go along a path—a **food-path**—from the fields where it is grown to the body of the child who eats it. When this food-path gets blocked there is the danger of malnutrition,

so you must know about this path, and how it gets blocked (Chapter 9).

Some of the blocks in the food-path can be taken away by families themselves, if you teach them carefully (Chapter 10). Each family is important, so also are the many families who live and work in a district. People who live, work and meet together are called a **community.** A community of people working together can do many things that families cannot do by themselves. Last of all, therefore, you must learn how the families in a community can work together to remove the blocks in their food-path and fight malnutrition (Chapter 11). Near the end of the book there is an end-piece or Appendix. This tells you about grams and kilograms, if you do not know about these already. The Appendix also explains how this book can be used in class. We hope that you will teach families, but first of all you must learn what to teach, and how to teach it. At the end of the book there is a Vocabulary-Index, which tells you what words mean and where you can find out more about them.

You will see that this book has numbers on its pages and that it also has **sections.** Section 1.3 is the third section in Chapter One, and Section 4.12 is the twelfth section in Chapter Four. You will see that there is a dot (.) in the section number '1 *dot* 3'. The figures or pictures are also numbered in this way, but the numbers for figures have a dash in them. Thus, '1 *dash* 3', or 1–3, is the third *figure* in the first chapter. You will soon get used to this way of putting numbers on the figures and sections in a book; they make it easier to read and look up any part.

Food and language differ from one country to another. Because we have not been able to write a separate book for every country, we have written it for those where some English is spoken and where maize, millet and cassava are the main foods. This is mostly a book for Malawi, Tanzania, Zambia, Botswana, Rhodesia and Kenya, but it may be useful in other countries also. We have had to use examples of money from somewhere, so we have used Zambian money, the kwacha and the ngwee. There are 100 ngwee (n) in a kwacha (K). A kwacha is a bit more than an American dollar (K1 = $1.4).

Writing a book is a useful exercise. It makes us realize that not everything that we see in print is likely to be completely true *always*. We hope, therefore, that you who read this book will look carefully at what you read and ask yourselves, 'Is this true, and especially is this true for the place and the time where I work?' As you will read, nutrition varies greatly from time to time and from place to place, so keep asking yourself if what you read fits in with what happens in your district. This is part of what is meant by reading a book critically. Try, therefore, to criticize and comment on what you read—don't 'swallow' this, or any other book, whole!

Many people have helped us to write this book, but we would especially like to thank Derrick and Patrice Jelliffe, Tinika Boelens, Joe Kreysler, Francis Shattock, Ewan Thomson, Erica Wheeler,

Susan Cole-King, Pauline Whitby, Dorothea Lehmann, Jeta Norton, Kaye Turnbull, Susan Cousins, Jonathan Page, Gabrielle Ellison, Cherry Gardiner, Christine Sewell, Rik Canter, Joan Noak, Peter Cheese, Patrick Mwanza and Judith Mitchell. Celly Bacon's drawings were a cherished wedding present and John Biddulph gave us the idea of the 'slogans' which are to be found throughout the text. We hope that you will join with us in thanking War on Want who have helped to make the book as cheap as it is.

Much nutrition work was going on in Zambia when we wrote this book. We looked around and wrote down the best of what we saw. Once more we have but provided paper and ink for the ideas of others. This then, is not our book, but theirs, and yours, our readers.

MAURICE AND FELICITY KING
DAVID MORLEY
LESLIE AND ANN BURGESS

Please address all correspondence to:
   Maurice H. King
   c/o Oxford University Press
   P.O. Box 72532
   Nairobi, Kenya

Contents

Chapter One

GROWTH

1.1 Weight for age. Here is a picture of a child called John. He is one year old and is a happy, healthy child. You will see that he is being weighed by being hung from a weighing scale. If you look at the scale you will see that he weighs ten kilograms. **Kilogram** is a long word to write, so we will write 'kg' or sometimes 'kilo' instead. John weighs 10 kg. When he started life as one cell (see Section 3.2) in his mother's womb John weighed almost nothing. During the nine months that he lived there he grew so fast that he weighed $3\frac{1}{2}$ kg by the time he was born. During the first six months of his life outside the womb, while he was feeding at his mother's breast, John went on growing very fast. By the time he was six months old he had about doubled his birth-weight and weighed $7\frac{1}{2}$ kg. From then on he grew a little more slowly, so that by the end of his first year, when he weighed 10 kg, he weighed about three times as much as he did when he was born. We say he had tripled (multiplied three times) his birth-weight.

Next year, when John is two years old, he should weigh $12\frac{1}{2}$ kg. Because John is a healthy well-fed child and gets a little heavier and a little taller every month, we say he is *growing*.

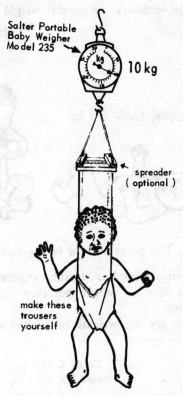

Salter Portable Baby Weigher Model 235

10 kg

spreader (optional)

make these trousers yourself

1-1, John being weighed

A CHILD DOUBLES HIS BIRTH-WEIGHT IN THE FIRST SIX MONTHS OF HIS LIFE

In the next figure you will see John again and some more children also. Luke was born this morning and weighs $3\frac{1}{2}$ kg, the same as John did when he was born. Matthew is six months old and weighs $7\frac{1}{2}$ kg, just as John did when he was that age. Mark is two years old and weighs $12\frac{1}{2}$ kg. Next year, when John is two, he should also weigh $12\frac{1}{2}$ kg. When they are all adults and their growing is finished, each of these children should weigh about 65 kg. Short men weigh less than this, and

some tall men weigh very much more, but 65 kg is the weight of an average or ordinary man. Women are usually a little smaller, and most women weigh about 55 kg. Short people weigh less than tall ones.

A CHILD TRIPLES HIS BIRTH-WEIGHT IN HIS FIRST YEAR

We see that young children grow very fast, and that there is a proper weight for all healthy growing children which depends upon how old they are. Children of the same age are not always exactly the same weight, but they are nearly. For example, some healthy one-year-old children are about 10½ kg, some about 10 kg and some about 9½ kg. So when we say that a healthy one-year-old child should weigh 10 kg, we mean that this is the average, ordinary, or normal weight of healthy

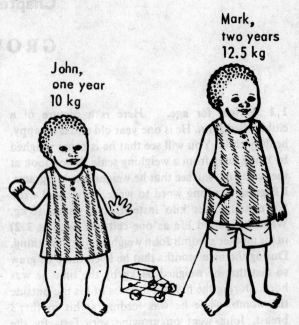

Mark, two years 12.5 kg

John, one year 10 kg

Matthew, 6 months 7.5 kg

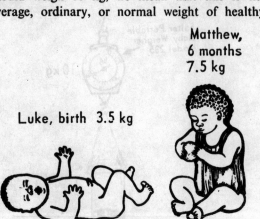

Luke, birth 3.5 kg

1-2, The older a child is the more he should weigh

one-year-old children. Healthy children are thus always near the weight that they should be for their age.

Here are the weights of healthy children of different ages:

TABLE 1
Weight For Age

| Child's age | | A healthy child's weight in kg | |
Months	Years	Fractions	Decimals
Birth		3½ kg	3.5 kg
4 months		6³⁄₁₀ kg	6.3 kg
6 months		7½ kg	7.5 kg
8 months		8⁴⁄₁₀ kg	8.4 kg
10 months		9³⁄₁₀ kg	9.3 kg
12 months	(1 year)	10 kg	10.0 kg
18 months	(1½ years)	11³⁄₁₀ kg	11.3 kg
24 months	(2 years)	12½ kg	12.5 kg
36 months	(3 years)	14½ kg	14.5 kg
48 months	(4 years)	16½ kg	16.5 kg
60 months	(5 years)	18½ kg	18.5 kg

The figures in the middle tell us that a child at birth weighs 3½ kg, a child of 4 months weighs six and three-tenths kilograms ($6\frac{3}{10}$ kg) and so on. Half ($\frac{1}{2}$) and three-tenths ($\frac{3}{10}$) are called **fractions,** so this is a list of children's weights in fractions of a kilogram. Fractions are not easy to use, so the figures on the right tell you the same thing but in an easier way using **decimals.**

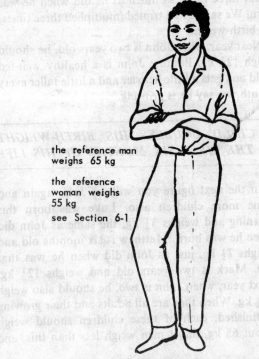

the reference man weighs 65 kg

the reference woman weighs 55 kg

see Section 6-1

1-3, John as a man weighs 65 kg

A HEALTHY ONE-YEAR-OLD CHILD WEIGHS ABOUT 10 KILOGRAMS

A child must be given enough of the right food if he is going to grow properly and reach the right weight for his age. A child who does not get enough of the right food is much lighter than he should be for his age. We say he is malnourished, and is suffering from malnutrition. Let us, for example, weigh Michael. He is one year old and we find he weighs 5 kg. But healthy one-year-old children weigh about 10 kg. Thus Michael only weighs half as much as he should do for his age, and is very malnourished indeed. Let us take another child, Gabriel. Gabriel is 18 months old and weighs $8\frac{1}{2}$ kg. But a healthy child of 18 months should weigh about $11\frac{1}{2}$ kg, so Gabriel only weighs about three-quarters as much as he should do, and is therefore malnourished, but not so badly malnourished as Michael. Both Michael and Gabriel are underweight for their ages. Michael is very underweight, and Gabriel is less underweight.

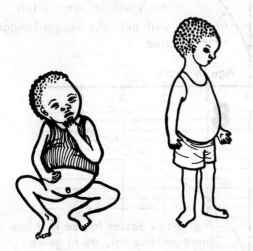

1-4, Michael and Gabriel

Later on you will read about how much of each kind of food a child must have each day if he is going to grow to the right weight for his age. You will also read about why malnutrition is so important, and how we can prevent it.

1.2 The weight-for-age graph. Most of the rest of this chapter is about a special kind of picture called a **graph**. By using a weight-for-age graph we can see if a child has reached the right weight for his age, and also if he is growing properly. The weights that you have just read are hard to remember, and it is sometimes difficult to find out how many months old a child is. The right kind of graph makes both these things much easier.

The best way to understand a graph is to think about how it is made. This is shown in Figure 1–5. Let us start by drawing a line (1). We divide it into five parts, one for each year of a child's age up to the time he is five. This is the age line (2). Now we can find where the ages of each of our healthy children come on this line (3). Luke has just been born, so his age is 0. Matthew is six months old. John is one year old, and Mark is two. We want some healthy older children, so let us take James who is three and weighs $14\frac{1}{2}$ kg, Philip who is four and weighs $16\frac{1}{2}$ kg, and Paul who is five and weighs $18\frac{1}{2}$ kg. Now let us draw weight lines for the weight of each child on top of the age line. We give each kilogram the same length and draw a line upwards for each child's weight (4). A heavy five-year-old child like Paul has a long line, and a small child like the newly-born Luke has a short line.

When you look at Picture 4 you will see that the short lines for the younger and lighter children are on the left and the longer lines **for** the older and heavier children are on the right. The tops of these weight lines can easily be joined together to give a smooth curved line (5). This is the weight-for-age line for healthy children. We will call it the **healthy-weight-for-age line.** (Sometimes, as we shall see, it is just called the 'top line'.) There is, however, no need to draw a separate line for the weight of each child, so instead we just mark the top of each line and join up the tops (6).

With a graph like this it is easy to find what weight a healthy child should be. All we have to do now is to look for his age on the age line at the bottom of the graph. We then follow a line *up* to the healthy-weight-for-age line and then straight *across* to the weight line. Picture 7 shows how we find the weight of a healthy one-year-old child. Because it is not easy to go straight up and straight across,

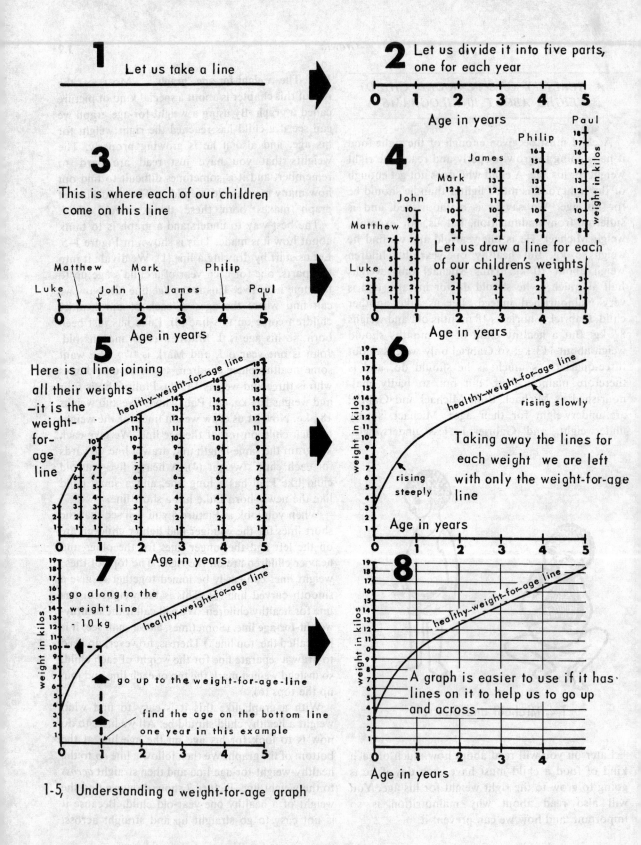

1 Let us take a line

2 Let us divide it into five parts, one for each year

0 1 2 3 4 5
Age in years

3 This is where each of our children come on this line

Matthew   Mark   Philip
Luke   John   James   Paul
0   1   2   3   4   5
Age in years

4 Let us draw a line for each of our children's weights

Matthew John Mark James Philip Paul
Luke
weight in kilos

5 Here is a line joining all their weights –it is the weight-for-age line

healthy-weight-for-age line
Age in years

6 Taking away the lines for each weight we are left with only the weight-for-age line

healthy-weight-for-age line
rising slowly
rising steeply
weight in kilos
Age in years

7 go along to the weight line – 10 kg

go up to the weight-for-age-line

find the age on the bottom line one year in this example

healthy-weight-for-age line
weight in kilos
Age in years

8 A graph is easier to use if it has lines on it to help us to go up and across

healthy-weight-for-age line
weight in kilos
Age in years

1-5, Understanding a weight-for-age graph

graphs are drawn with lines on them to make this easier (8). A graph like this is very useful, because we can easily find what the weight of a healthy child should be at any age between birth and five years.

You can see that from the time of birth until the age of one year the healthy-weight-for-age line climbs up the graph very steeply and that after one year it is flatter and climbs more slowly. This is because children grow very quickly in the first year of their life and more slowly after that. We can put this in another way—*the younger a child is, the faster he grows.*

So far our graph has been drawn in years from birth to five years. A year is a long time, and a child gets heavier each month, so it is better to divide it into months. The next graph in Figure 1–6 is drawn with a child's age in months. It goes from 0 (birth) to 60 months or five years (five years = 60 months). The graph stops at 60 months, so we cannot use it for children older than this.

By using a graph like this we can easily find if a child is the right weight for his age, or if he is underweight. We weigh him, ask his mother his age in months, and put a spot on the graph opposite the places for his age and his weight. The graph (1–6) shows you where our healthy well-nourished children, Matthew, Mark, Luke and John, come on this graph. They all come exactly on the healthy-weight-for-age line.

Let us see where our malnourished children come on our graph. Michael, who weighed 5 kg when he was one year old, comes well below the healthy-weight-for-age line and is very underweight indeed. Gabriel, who weighed $8\frac{1}{2}$ kg at the age of 18 months, comes below the healthy-weight-for-age line, but not so far below it as Michael. It is easy to see that Gabriel is a little malnourished but that he is not so malnourished as Michael.

Weight-for-age graphs are even more useful in another way. We can use them to see if a child is *growing* as he should do. Let us weigh John every two months and each time put a dot for his weight on the graph. Let us join this row of dots together to make a line. You can see from Figure 1–7 that John's row of dots climbs up the graph and that it stays close to the healthy-weight-for-age line. His

row of dots is not exactly on the line, but this does not matter. Just as the weights of healthy children are close to the line, but not always exactly on it, so also the rows of dots showing their growth are usually close to it, but may not always be exactly on it. We see that John is not only the right weight for his age, but that he is also growing well.

When Michael first came to the clinic he was very malnourished indeed. His mother would not let him come into hospital, but she did bring him to the clinic to be weighed. A nurse tried to teach her how she could feed him, but the teaching was bad, and she could not do what she was taught. Michael did not get enough to eat, and although his age increased, his weight stayed nearly the same. The row of dots for his weight did not climb up the card. He failed to grow, and he became more and more malnourished. After a few months he died from malnutrition.

Gabriel's mother did much better. She grew plenty of food in her garden and fed him as the nurse in the clinic taught her. Each time she brought Gabriel to the clinic he weighed more than the month before. He grew well. The row of dots for his weight climbed up the card and soon reached the healthy-weight-for-age line.

You can see, therefore, that a weight-for-age graph is useful for seeing if a child is well or badly nourished, and also for seeing if he is gaining weight and growing. If you are teaching a mother, and you see that her child is growing, you know that you are teaching her in the right way. So, by using a weight-for-age graph to see if a child is growing, we can see if our teaching is right. Best of all, a weight-for-age graph lets us see a child's weight and growth immediately, without any working out or arithmetic.

As children grow older, they grow in other ways besides growing in weight. They grow taller or grow in height. Their heads and their chests and their arms get larger. All these things and many others can be measured, but growth in weight is the easiest thing to measure in a busy clinic. Children must be healthy before they will grow, and *by measuring growth we come as nearly as we can to measuring health.* This is why so much of this book is about growth in weight, and how we can measure it.

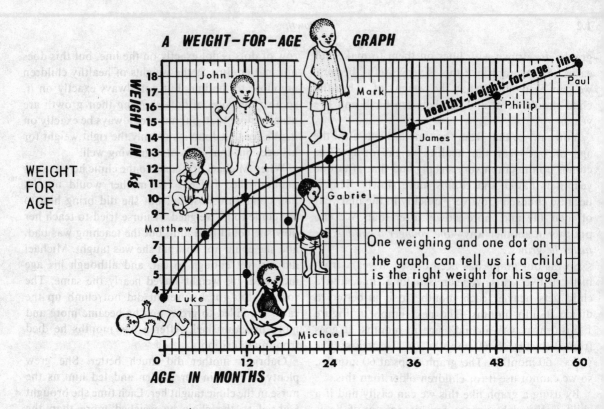

A WEIGHT—FOR—AGE GRAPH

WEIGHT IN kg

WEIGHT FOR AGE

John

Mark

healthy—weight—for—age line

Paul

Philip

James

Matthew

Gabriel

Luke

Michael

One weighing and one dot on the graph can tell us if a child is the right weight for his age

AGE IN MONTHS

1-6, A weight-for-age graph

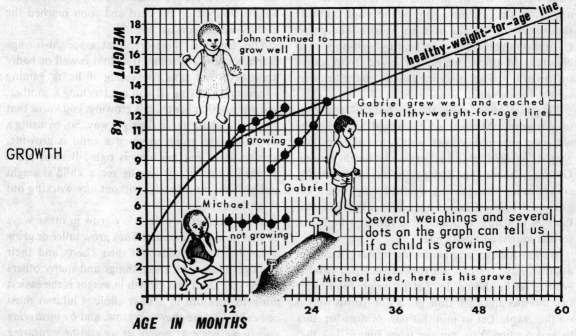

WEIGHT IN kg

GROWTH

John continued to grow well

healthy—weight—for—age line

growing

Gabriel grew well and reached the healthy-weight-for-age line

Michael

Gabriel

not growing

Several weighings and several dots on the graph can tell us if a child is growing

Michael died, here is his grave

AGE IN MONTHS

1-7, A weight-for-age graph showing growth

BY MEASURING GROWTH
WE MEASURE HEALTH

Two of the most important things about a healthy child are that he should be growing and that he should be about the right weight for his age. But these are not the only things that matter. A child should also be walking and talking as well as other children of the same age. He should be active and lively, and interested in the world around him. He should have a dark shiny skin, strong black hair and be without any of the symptoms, like cough or diarrhoea, which spoil health. One of the best ways a mother can keep her child healthy is to take him to an under-fives clinic every month.

1.3 The 'under-fives clinic' and the 'road-to-health' chart.   An under-fives clinic is a special kind of clinic for children from the time they are born until they are five years old. Children who are brought to these clinics are given special medicines called **vaccines.** These vaccines stop them getting measles, poliomyelitis (polio), smallpox, tuberculosis (TB), diphtheria, whooping cough (pertussis) and tetanus. The vaccine which prevents **D**iphtheria, **P**ertussis and **T**etanus is called **DPT**, or **triple vaccine**. Children who have been given these vaccines in the right way are said to be **immunized** against the

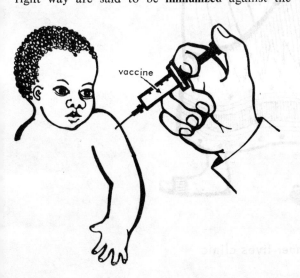

1-8, Immunization

diseases they prevent. *DPT and polio vaccines must be given THREE times if they are to protect the child,* but the other vaccines need only be given once. At under-fives clinics mothers are also taught how to feed and look after their families, and if children are sick they can often be cured without going to hospital.

One of the most important jobs for these clinics is to try to make sure that children are well nourished and are growing steadily. Each child is given his own weight-for-age graph printed on strong card and kept for him by his mother in a strong plastic bag. The mother in Figure 1–9 is bringing both her children and their cards to an under-fives clinic.

The card for the under-fives clinic has an inside and an outside, and the weight-for-age graph is broken up into several parts. On the inside of the card the part for the first year of a child's life is on the left, the part for his second year is in the middle, and the part for his third year is on the right. The graph for a child's fourth and fifth years is printed on the outside of the card. The weight in kilos is written up the left hand side of each part of the graph. The cards used in different countries are not always exactly the same. The cards shown in this book are those used in Zambia.

EXPLAIN TO MOTHERS WHAT AN
UNDER-FIVES CLINIC TRIES TO DO

It is easy to weigh a child, but it is sometimes not so easy to find out how many months old he is, because few mothers know this exactly, and it is not easy to work out, even if you know his birthday. If you want to see how difficult this is, ask several people how many months old a child will be in, say, July next year, if he was born in, say, February last year. Many people will get the answer wrong, and it will take them a minute or so to work it out. An easier way to find out a child's age in months is to write the months of his life along the bottom of a weight-for-age graph in a special way. This is how it is done.

Along the bottom of the inside of the card you will

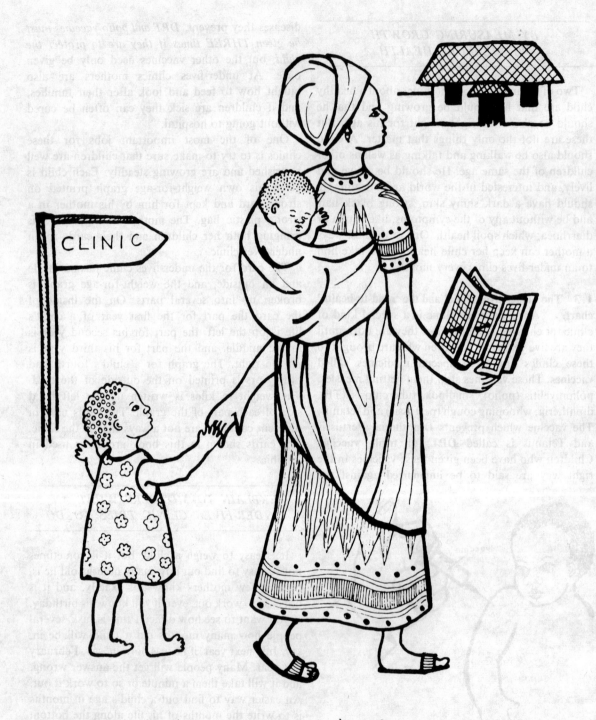

1-9, A mother and her children going to an under-fives clinic

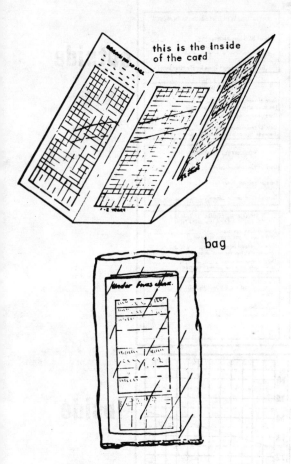

this is the inside of the card

bag

1-10, An under–fives clinic card and its plastic bag

see three rows of twelve boxes or spaces. There are twelve months in a year, and one of these rows of twelve boxes is for each of the first three years of a child's life. Each box is for a different month. The left-hand box in each row has a very thick line around it. This thick-lined left-hand box in each row is for the month in which the child was born. Peter, for example, was born in March, so March is written in all five of the thick-lined boxes on the card in Figure 1-11.

Let us take another example. Raphael was born in August, so August must be written in all the thick-lined boxes. The other boxes in each part of the card are for the months of the rest of the year. For Peter, who was born in March, for example,

the next months are April, May, June, July, August, September, October, November, December, January and February. For Raphael, who was born in August, the next months are September, October, November, December, January, February, March, April, May, June and July. The twelve months of the rest of the year are always filled in like this. *Each row of boxes always starts with the month in which a child was born in the special thick-lined box on the left.*

We have now to put in the years on the card. Opposite the first of the thick-lined boxes we put the year the child was born, and opposite the other thick-lined boxes we put the years after that. If a child was born in April 1967 we put '67 opposite the first thick-lined box and '68, '69, '70 and '71 opposite the other boxes. Whenever you come to January put the number of the new year beside it. In Figure 1-11 '68, '69, '70, '71 and '72 have been put underneath the five Januarys on Peter's card.

PUT THE CHILD'S BIRTH MONTH IN EVERY THICK-LINED BOX

Mothers can sometimes tell you their child's birthday, even if they cannot work out his age right. But what can we do if she does not know the month or the year of his birth? Ask her carefully to see if she can time it by some special happening, such as an election, or a harvest, or a drought, or something else. In Tanzania good happenings to use are Christmas, Saba Saba, Independence Day, and the dry and rainy seasons. Mothers can usually remember if their child was born before or after a happening of this kind. If, for example, a child was born just before Christmas two years ago, he was probably born in November or December of that year. It is often useful to ask a mother if her child was born before or after the child of one of her friends who knows the age of her child.

This way of using local happenings or events is called a **local-events calendar**, and is very useful in finding a child's age. Because local events vary from one place to another, a local-events calendar must be made for each district. There is an example from Malawi at the end of this chapter.

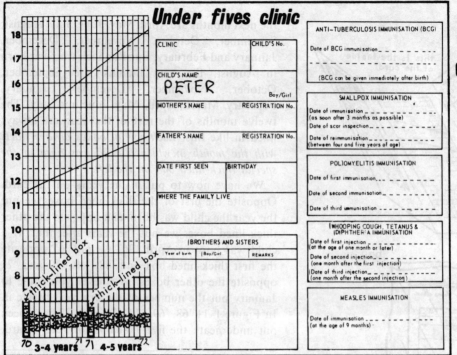

outside

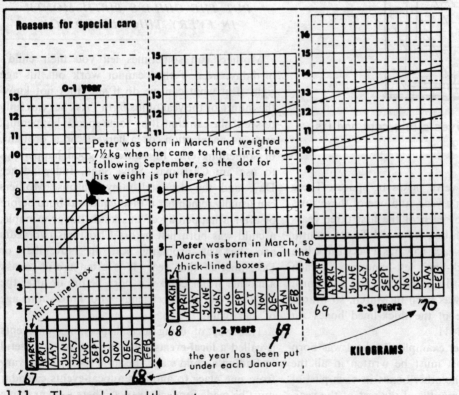

inside

1-11,   The road-to-health chart

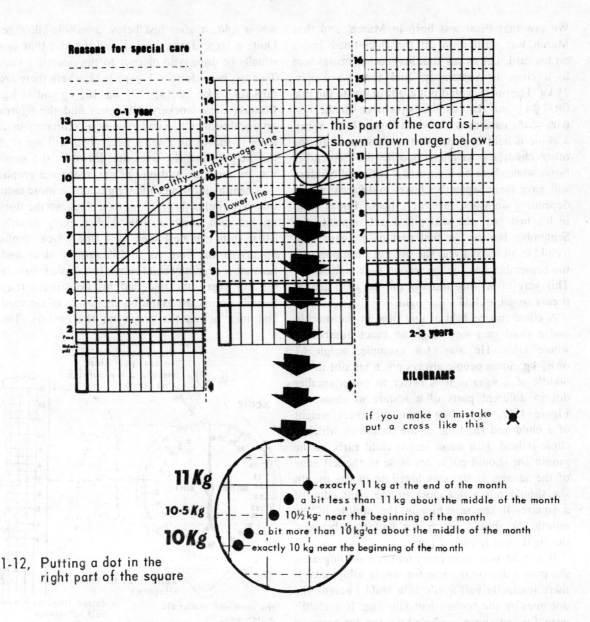

Reasons for special care

0-1 year

healthy-weight-for-age line

lower line

this part of the card is shown drawn larger below

2-3 years

KILOGRAMS

if you make a mistake put a cross like this ✖

11 Kg ——— exactly 11 kg at the end of the month
— a bit less than 11 kg about the middle of the month
10·5 Kg — 10½ kg near the beginning of the month
— a bit more than 10 kg at about the middle of the month
10 Kg —— exactly 10 kg near the beginning of the month

1-12, Putting a dot in the right part of the square

If we cannot be sure about the month of a child's birth, we have to make a guess. Provided that we guess the month nearly right, it will usually be good enough. Every child should be weighed and given a weight chart by the midwife who delivers him. When this is done it is easy to find a child's age.

EVERY CHILD SHOULD BE GIVEN A ROAD-TO-HEALTH CHART AT BIRTH

Whenever a child comes to a clinic, a nurse weighs him and puts a dot for his weight opposite the box of the month in which the clinic is held.

We saw that Peter was born in **March**, and that March was written in all the thick-lined boxes on his card. Let us say that his mother brings him to a clinic in September, and that he weighs $7\frac{1}{2}$ kg. The nurse would put a dot opposite the line for $7\frac{1}{2}$ kg and the box for September on the first part of the card as is shown in Figure 1-11. When a clinic is held in September a nurse puts all the other children's weights opposite the September boxes somewhere on their cards. Different children will have their September boxes in different places depending on when they were born. For a child in his first year she will put a dot opposite the September box on the first part of the card. For a child in his second year she will put a dot opposite the September box for the second year, and so on. This way of writing months on the card makes it easy to get a child's age right.

A clinic can be held at any time in the month, and a child may not weigh an exact number of whole kilos. He may, for example, weigh $6\frac{1}{2}$ or $8\frac{3}{4}$ kg. Some people always put a big dot in the middle of a square. It is better to put a smaller dot in different parts of a square as shown in Figure 1-12, depending upon the exact weight of a child and the time of the month in which a clinic is held. If a nurse sees a child early in the month she should put a dot close to the left edge of the square. If she sees him late in the month she should put a dot close to the right edge of a square. If she sees him in the middle of the month she should put a dot half way between the right- and left-hand lines.

If a child weighs an exact number of kilograms, she puts a dot on the line for whole kilograms. If there is exactly half a kilo in a child's weight, the dot goes on the broken half-kilo line. If a child's weight is just above a·whole kilo, the dot goes just above a whole-kilo line, and if it is just below a

whole kilo, it goes just below a whole-kilo line. Quite a large dot is needed, and the best that can usually be done is to place it to the nearest $\frac{1}{4}$ kilo. This has been done in Figure 1-12, where there are dots for 10 kg, $10\frac{1}{4}$ kg, $10\frac{1}{2}$ kg, $10\frac{3}{4}$ kg and 11 kg. Because clinic workers sometimes find the figures on a scale difficult to understand, a commonly used scale is shown in Figure 1-13. You will see that the weights and the lines are drawn in the same way on the scale and on the weight-for-age graph.

A healthy growing child weighs a little more each time his mother brings him to a clinic, so the dots on his card climb a little higher every month. These dots can be joined by a line which climbs up across the card as a chi'd grows older and heavier. If a healthy child comes to a clinic regularly for five years, the line that his dots make rises steadily across the graph on the inside of the card and then across the graph on the outside. The

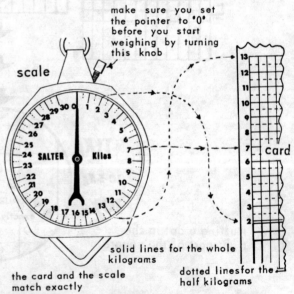

make sure you set the pointer to '0' before you start weighing by turning this knob

scale

SALTER   Kilos

card

solid lines for the whole kilograms

the card and the scale match exactly

dotted lines for the half kilograms

1-13,   A scale for the under-fives clinic

*Note: The scale shown in Figure 1-13 is made by Messrs. George Salter of West Bromwich, Birmingham, England, specially for under-fives clinics. The divisions on the scale match those on the road-to-health chart, and there is a wide range zero adjustment, so that the pointer can be brought to zero even when there is a heavy pan or seat on which to weigh the child. It is most important that this adjustment be made before a child is weighed, or there may be a large error. Intending purchasers should ask for the 'Portable Baby Weigher Model 235', costing about $ 12. This scale is best used with pairs of hanging trousers which hang from a hook on the scale. These can be used either with or without the frame shown in Figure 1-1. A basket can also be hung from the scale. If trousers are being used, provide several, so that mothers waiting their turn in the queue can put their children into them, so enabling weighing to be done very quickly. Trousers can be used satisfactorily, even with very young children, and can conveniently be made locally.

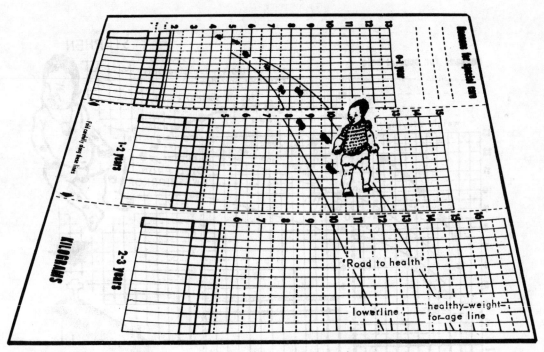

1-14, A child on the road to health

line of dots that a child's weight makes on the card is called his **growth curve.**

So far we have only thought about one line on the graph. This is the top line, and we have called it the healthy-weight-for-age line. This is the average line that healthy well-fed children follow in most parts of the world. It was drawn by finding the average weights-for-age of very many healthy children with rich parents who could feed them well. The dot for the weight of a healthy child is usually close to this line. The more malnourished he becomes the further the dot for his weight falls below this line. If the dot for his weight is only just below the healthy-weight-for-age line we need not worry, but if it is far below we know he is malnourished and must try hard to see that he is properly fed. We therefore need a second line on the graph to tell us when to worry about a child's weight. We will call this second line the **lower line.**

The place between the two lines is called the 'road to health', and the card for the under-fives clinic is often called the **road-to-health chart** or card. A chart is a kind of map. It is called the road-to-health chart because this is an idea that mothers can easily understand. They like to think of their children walking along a path on the chart which leads to health. The path on the chart is like a path through the bush, and the dots on the graph are like a child's footsteps. If a child walks off the road to health towards the bottom of the card he becomes thin and malnourished. Workers in under-fives clinics, therefore, try to make sure that all children are on the road to health and are above the lower line.

If there are no children below the lower line, there are no children who are much underweight for their age. The only children who might be malnourished would be the very few children like Stephen in Figure 1–15. If this is so, the clinic workers can be very happy. If some children are heavier than they should be for their age and are above the top line, this seldom matters. There are usually a few fat over-nourished children, and we do not need to worry about them in the countries for which this book was mainly written.

Road-to-health graphs are useful in two main ways. They can tell us if a child is the right weight

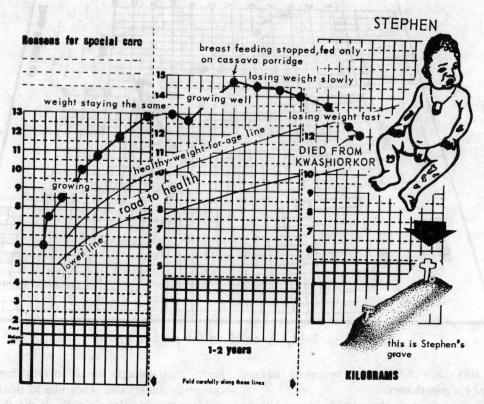

Reasons for special care

weight staying the same

healthy-weight-for-age line

growing

road to health

lower line

Food
Industry
grid

growing

STEPHEN

breast feeding stopped, fed only
on cassava porridge

losing weight slowly

growing well

losing weight fast

DIED FROM
KWASHIORKOR

this is Stephen's
grave

1-2 years

Fold carefully along these lines

KILOGRAMS

1-15, The story of Stephen

for his age, or if he is underweight. Even one weighing and one dot on the graph can tell us this. But, if a child has been weighed each month for several months and there are several dots on his graph, we can also tell if he is growing or not. A child whose line of dots is climbing up the card is growing, but a child whose line of dots is staying level is not growing. Even if a child is below the road to health but is growing well, he will probably soon climb back onto it again and become the right weight for his age. *Even though his weight is below the lower line, if he is growing well and his growth curve (his line of dots) is rising up the chart, he is doing well.*

Sometimes a child may be on the road to health or even above the upper line because he may have eaten well in the earlier months of his life. But even though he is above the upper line, his line of dots may become level or start falling. This

is important, because it means that he has now stopped growing and is malnourished. However, because he started so far above the lower line, it may be several months before his line of dots falls below it. Occasionally, children like this can even die from malnutrition before their weight has fallen below the lower line.

This is what happened to Stephen, who grew so well until he was about 18 months old that the line of dots on his road-to-health chart was well above the upper line. Then his mother became pregnant again, so she stopped breast-feeding him and sent him away to stay with his grandmother. His grandmother was very poor and fed him only on cassava porridge. He lost weight, stopped growing and became so malnourished that he got kwashiorkor when he was a little over two years old (see Section 2.5). He was so fat to start with that this happened *while he was still on the road to health.*

Three days after he went to hospital Stephen died.

We cannot find children like Stephen by weighing them once. They have to be weighed for several months before we can see that they are not growing. *Whether a child is growing or not is more important than what weight he is.* A line of dots from several weighings is thus more useful than one dot from one weighing, because it is the only way that we can tell if a child is growing or not.

GROWTH IS MORE IMPORTANT THAN POSITION ON THE WEIGHT CHART

1.4 Using the road-to-health chart for a nutrition survey. Road-to-health charts can be used in another way. The weights of many children can be put on one chart. This has been done in Figure 1–16. Chart A is from the Woodlands area of Lusaka where top civil servants live. These people are well paid and have plenty of money with which to buy food for their families. Two medical students (Messrs Patel and Saasa) weighed 158 children in Woodlands under the age of five. Of these children 122 were Zambians, and the rest came from other countries. A dot has been put on the chart for the weight of each of them. Only the inside of the road-to-health chart is shown here. You will see that Chart A has dots for the weights of 103 children under the age of three years and that all but one are on the road to health and many are above it. Almost all the children living in Woodlands are thus very well nourished.

Chart B is from the 'shanty-town' called Kapwepwe on the edge of Lusaka. A shanty-town is a community of people living close together in mud-brick houses without mains water, or proper drains, or roads, and usually also without clinics or schools. Most of the people who live in them are poor, and many have no jobs. (In Zambia shanty-towns are also called 'illegal townships' or 'squatter compounds'.) The weights of 106 children from Kapwepwe are shown on Chart B. You will see that 32, or nearly one-third of them (30 per cent), are below the road to health. These are the underweight children whom you will read

about in the next chapter.

In counting these children we have counted all children whose dot touches the line as being on the road to health. We have also started counting children where the road to health begins, which is at about five months.

More than half the children in Lusaka live in the shanty-towns like Kapwepwe, and very few of them are fortunate enough to live in rich, well-nourished areas like Woodlands. Perhaps you will begin to see what a big problem malnutrition is in countries like Zambia.

By using a road-to-health chart in this way and putting the weights of many children on it, we are measuring the nutrition of a community. Measuring the nutrition of a community like this is one way of doing what is called a **community nutrition survey.** A survey is only another name for a way of looking carefully at a group of people or things. In the 'things to do' section at the end of this chapter, you will learn how to do your own community nutrition survey.

Before we leave road-to-health graphs, there is one more very important thing to say about them. It is this. We use them to find out if children are well nourished and are growing. If children are underweight and are not growing, our job is to show their mothers how to feed them better. *Weighing a child does nothing by itself.* It is teaching his mother how to feed him that really matters, *not* charting his weight! However, weighing a child regularly and charting his weight will tell you if your teaching is succeeding.

TEACHING IS MORE IMPORTANT THAN CHARTING

If mothers are going to keep their weight charts, they must be taught about them. Tell mothers to bring their weight charts *whenever they take their children to a hospital or clinic.*

In the next chapter you will learn *why* it is so important that children should be the right weight for their age and be growing. But, before telling you about this, here is another way to tell if a child is well or badly nourished.

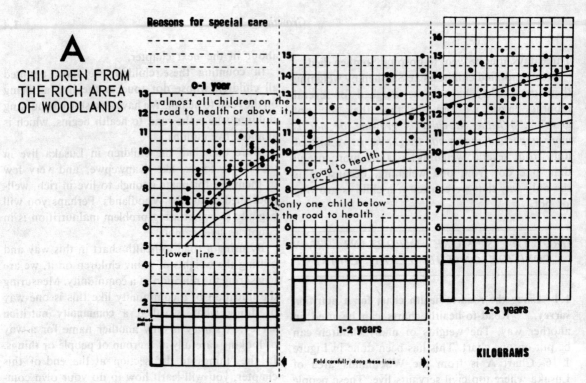

A

CHILDREN FROM THE RICH AREA OF WOODLANDS

Reasons for special care

0-1 year

almost all children on the road to health or above it

road to health

only one child below the road to health

lower line

Feed
Relax
pill

1-2 years

KILOGRAMS

Fold carefully along these lines

2-3 years

1-16, Using the road-to-health chart to do a community nutrition survey

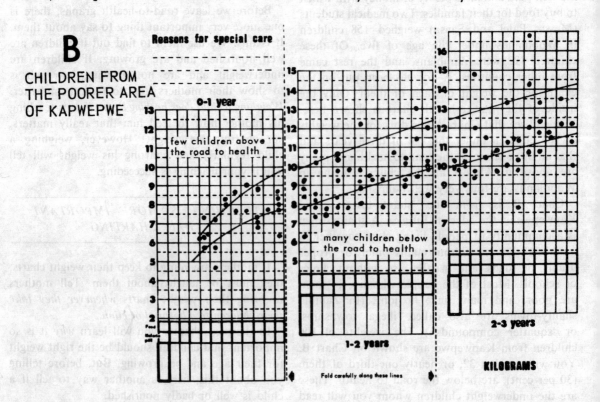

B

CHILDREN FROM THE POORER AREA OF KAPWEPWE

Reasons for special care

0-1 year

few children above the road to health

many children below the road to health

Feed
Relax
pill

1-2 years

KILOGRAMS

Fold carefully along these lines

2-3 years

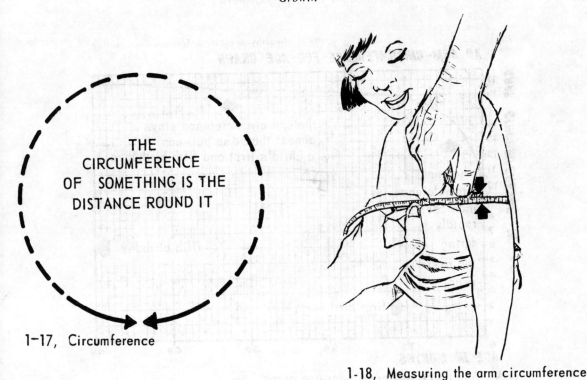

THE CIRCUMFERENCE OF SOMETHING IS THE DISTANCE ROUND IT

1-17, Circumference

1-18, Measuring the arm circumference

1.5 Using arm circumference to measure a child's nutrition. If you have understood the idea of a weight-for-age graph, you will easily understand the idea of an arm-circumference-for-age graph. In the next chapter you will see how a healthy child has thick arms, how an underweight child has thin arms, and how a marasmic child has very thin arms indeed. We can thus measure a child's nutrition by measuring the thickness of his arms. This is easily done. All that we have to do is to put a tape measure round a child's upper arm and measure how many centimetres round it is. (Instead of centimetres we usually write cm.) When we measure round something, we say that we are measuring its circumference. A healthy child will have thick arms and a big arm circumference. A thin malnourished child will have thin arms and a small arm circumference. Even if the lower arm of a malnourished child with kwashiorkor is swollen with fluid, the muscles of his upper arm will be thin and he will have a small arm circumference.

Here is a graph (Figure 1–19) to show the arm-circumference-for-age of healthy children. You will see that, just as in the weight-for-age graph, there is a line along the bottom for a child's age from 0 to 60 months. But, instead of there being weight in kg up the line at the left, there is arm circumference in cm from 0 to 17 cm. You will see that the top line has been called the 'healthy-arm-circumference-for-age line'. It starts at 10.5 cm, which is the arm circumference of a healthy child at birth. The line rises steeply from birth, and by the time a child is one year old his arm circumference is nearly 16 cm.

A child's arm, therefore, gets much thicker during his first year. *But, during the next four years of a child's life, that is from the time he is one until the time he is five, the line on the graph is nearly flat.* You will see from this line that his arm circumference only rises from a little under 16 cm to a little over 17 cm during these four years. *A healthy child's arm circumference, therefore, only grows by a little over one centimetre from*

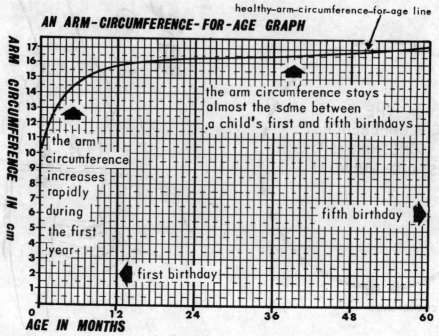

healthy-arm-circumference-for-age line

AN ARM-CIRCUMFERENCE-FOR-AGE GRAPH

the arm circumference stays almost the same between a child's first and fifth birthdays

the arm circumference increases rapidly during the first year

fifth birthday

first birthday

ARM CIRCUMFERENCE IN cm

AGE IN MONTHS

1-19, An arm-circumference-for-age graph

the time he is one until the time he is five. This is very useful, because, whatever exact age a child is between one and five, his arm circumference should be between 16 and 17 cm. If a child's arm circumference is much less than this, his arm is thinner than it should be and he is malnourished. Not needing to know a child's age is very useful, because, as we have already seen, this is often difficult to find out.

Look back to the weight-for-age graph. You will see that the healthy-weight-for-age line also climbs very steeply from birth to the age of one year *but that it goes on climbing quite steeply after that*. It is unlike the healthy-arm-circumference-for-age line which is quite flat from the age of one year, onwards. This is only another way of saying that a healthy child goes on getting heavier between the age of one and five years, whereas the circumference or thickness of his arm stays about the same. Another way of saying this is to say that between the ages of one and five a child's arm circumference is largely independent of his age. This is useful because it is also the time that a child is usually

in the greatest danger from malnutrition. It is also often easier to measure a child's arm circumference than it is to weigh him. This is because a tape measure is cheaper and lighter to carry than a scale. A measure can even be made from a piece of cardboard. So you see that the arm circumference can be a very useful measure of nutrition.

When we thought about weight for age, we saw that not all one-year-old children were exactly 10 kg. Some weigh a little more and some a little less. In the same way not all healthy children have an arm circumference which is exactly 16.5 cm. Thus they are not all exactly on the healthy-arm-circumference-for-age line, but they are always quite close to it. When we thought about weight for age, we found that we could think of children as being malnourished if they were below the lower line on the road-to-health chart. In the same way we can think of children as being malnourished if their arm circumference is below the lower line on the graph. This line is the 14-cm line, and we will call it the **lower line**. *It is useful to remember that*

ARM-CIRCUMFERENCE-FOR-AGE GRAPHS

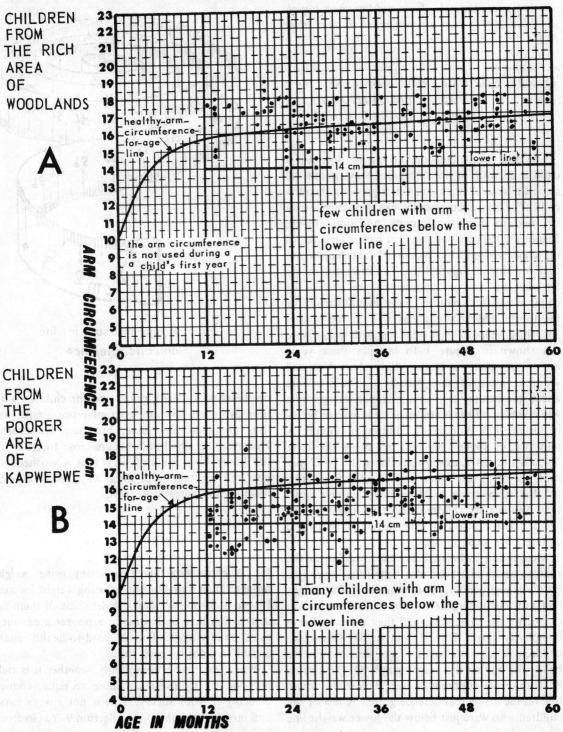

CHILDREN FROM THE RICH AREA OF WOODLANDS

A

healthy-arm-circumference-for-age line

14 cm

lower line

few children with arm circumferences below the lower line

the arm circumference is not used during a a child's first year

ARM CIRCUMFERENCE IN cm

CHILDREN FROM THE POORER AREA OF KAPWEPWE

B

healthy-arm-circumference-for-age line

14 cm

lower line

many children with arm circumferences below the lower line

AGE IN MONTHS

1-20. A community nutrition survey using arm circumference

a child between the ages of one and five years is malnourished if his arm circumference is less than
14 cm.

AN ARM CIRCUMFERENCE OF LESS THAN 14 CM SHOWS MALNUTRITION IN A ONE- TO FIVE-YEAR-OLD CHILD

The arm circumference is no use for seeing if a
child is growing or not because it stays about the
same for several years, even in a growing, healthy
child. The arm circumference can, however, easily
be used to do a community nutrition survey.
Figure 1–20 shows you the arm circumferences of
the same children from Woodlands and Kapwepwe
that you saw in Figure 1–16. The only differences
are that no arm circumferences are shown for
children under 12 months, but they are shown for
the fourth and fifth years as well as the second
and third years. The fourth and fifth years were
not shown in Figure 1–16 because these years
are on the other side of the weight chart. You will
see that most of the Woodlands children are
above the healthy-arm-circumference-for-age line,
while almost all the Kapwepwe children are below
it. Of the 116 Woodlands children in Picture A
only two, or about 2 per cent, are below the *lower
line*. Of the 124 Kapwepwe children 26, or 21 per
cent, are below the *lower line*. These graphs show
us that Kapwepwe children have thinner arms
than Woodlands children and that about a fifth
(21 per cent) are so thin that they show that these
children are malnourished.

Most children who are below the lower line on the
road-to-health chart are also below the lower line
on the arm-circumference-for-age chart. But weight
and arm circumference do not measure nutrition
in exactly the same way, and they do not always
completely agree. Thus 27 out of 81 Kapwepwe
children *between the ages of one and three* were
below the line on the weight graph. Of these same
81 Kapwepwe children 24 were below the lower
line on the arm-circumference graph. A few of the
children who were just below the lower weight line
were just above the lower arm-circumference line,
and the other way round. The underweight children

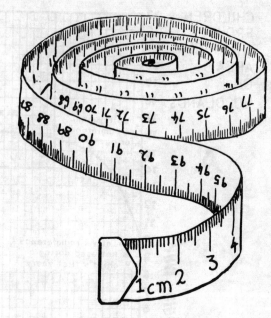

1-21, A tape measure for the arm circumference

on the road-to-health graph and the children with
thin arms on the arm-circumference graph are
thus not quite the same, but they are nearly.
However, the children who are close to either of
the lower lines are not very well nourished, so
you will see that both these ways of measuring
malnutrition agree quite well.

1.6   THINGS TO DO

**(a) A community nutrition survey using weight
for age.** Do a nutrition survey using weight for age.
If several people are doing it, let some of them do
it in a rich area and some in a poorer area, such
as a shanty-town. Use a road-to-health chart
and fill in a dot for each child.

When you visit a community, whether it is rich
or poor, try to give each house an equal chance
of being in your survey. This is not always easy,
and more is said about it in Section 9.26. Go from
house to house and weigh as many children as
you can. Try to get at least a hundred. If the children

in your area are well nourished most of your dots will be above the lower line on the weight chart, and most children will be on the road to health or above it. If the children in your area are malnourished many of them will be below the lower line on the chart and off the road to health. You may be able to get road-to-health charts and the loan of a scale from an under-fives clinic.

This is a simple community nutrition survey, and it will be useful in making the community diagnosis of malnutrition in Section 9.25.

Before you visit a village or shanty-town, be sure you ask the chief or headman first!

(b) A community nutrition survey using arm circumference. Do your survey exactly as described above, but use arm circumference instead of weight. If several people want to do a survey and they have not got enough scales, they can easily measure the arm circumference. This can be done with tape measures, or even with a narrow piece of thin cardboard marked off in centimetres. One of these has been shown in Figure 1–22 and has been called a 'child nutrition indicator'. An indicator is something which shows you things.

14 cm marks the difference between healthy and malnourished children

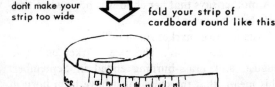

use thin card and don't make your strip too wide

fold your strip of cardboard round like this

use a strip of thin cardboard and mark it out in centimetres like this

1-22, A 'child nutrition indicator'

Remember these things when you measure the arm circumference, and look at Figure 1–18:
Use a cloth, or better still a fibreglass tape measure which does not stretch (see Section 12.3).

Put your tape *gently but firmly* round the arm, and don't pull so tight that wrinkles come in the skin.

Always measure the *left* arm *half way between the point of the shoulder and the tip of the elbow* (olecranon).

Let the left arm hang freely by the child's side. The arm must be *straight* and *not* bent at the elbow.

You can record your answer in various ways. One of them is to copy the graph in Figure 1–20 and put a dot for each child. But for this you will want to know a child's age, and the usefulness of the arm circumference is that this is not necessary—provided that he is between one and five years old. Another way is to measure children's arm circumferences and group them as has been done in Figure 1–23. Put a stroke for each child, and count in fives. Do this by putting each fifth stroke across the other four. This kind of count is called a **tally** and makes counting easier.

arm circumference in centimetres		numbers of children
18 - 19	ll	**2**
17 - 18	ll	**2**
16 - 17	ℍℍ ℍℍ ℍℍ Oℍ	**19**
15 - 16	ℍℍ ℍℍ ℍℍ ℍℍ ℍℍ ℍℍ ll	**32**
14 - 15	ℍℍ ℍℍ ℍℍ ℍℍ l	**21**
13 - 14	ℍℍ ℍℍ ℍℍ	**15**
12 - 13	ℍℍ lll	**8**
11 - 12	l	**1**
		100

well nourished — badly nourished

– – – – – – – – – 14 cm – – – – – –

24% (15 plus 8 plus 1) of these children are malnourished because their arm circumference is less than 14 cm

1-23, A tally for the arm circumference

In a well-nourished area there will be few, if any, children with an arm circumference below 14 cm. The worse the nutrition of the area the more children will there be below 14 cm, and the fewer children will there be with fatter arms. The tally in Figure 1–23 was made from the arm circumferences of the youngest 100 children in Kapwepwe in Figure 1–20. You will see that 24 per cent (15+8+1) of the children had an arm circumference of less than 14 cm.

(c) Weighing children in an under-fives clinic. See if you can visit an under-fives clinic and help to weigh the children and fill in their road-to-health graphs.

(d) Making a height-for-age graph for some bean plants. Some people find it difficult to really understand a weight-for-age graph. It may ,help them to make another kind of graph. This is height-for-age instead of weight-for-age. Plant some beans in a tin of earth. Keep them watered. Take one bean plant and measure its height in centimetres each week. Take a piece of paper. Put the weeks 1, 2, 3, 4 . . . in a line along the bottom and centimetres in a line up the side. Your graph will start at 0, and the line for the height of your bean plant will slowly climb up the paper. We start to weigh children at birth when they weigh about $3\frac{1}{2}$ kg. If we wanted to start right at the beginning, when a child weighed nothing at all, we should have to start when he was inside his mother's womb, and this is not easy to do! Just as some children are heavier and grow faster than others, so some of your bean plants will grow faster and be taller than others.

(e) Making a local-events calendar. In this chapter we have said much about a child's weight for his age, but to find this out we must know a child's age. A good way to do this is to use a local-events calendar, as explained in Section 1.3. Here are some rules for making a local-events calendar that were given us by Mr. Biswick and Mr. Matambo of Malawi.

Make a separate calendar for each place, as the people in different places remember different things.

Make it with the help of people in the village, the clinic, or the local government offices.

Get the times of planting, weeding, harvesting and selling; the seasons; and the holidays and feasts. Find out when important things happened in that place, such as a visit from the president, a census, a flood or a famine, the opening of a new school, or a change of headman. In one village everyone remembered the time that someone was eaten by a crocodile. If you can, put the exact date of each event on your calendar.

When you are using your calendar, cross-check what a mother tells you. For example, if a mother says her child was born at the beginning of the rainy season, ask her if he was born before or after Christmas, or how big he was when they planted maize. Do not believe any birthdate a mother gives you unless she shows you a certificate, or you have checked that she has got the date right with your calendar. Mothers may know the month their child was born, but make a mistake with the year. Check a child's birthdate with those of his brothers and sisters or friends whose birthdates you know.

EVERY UNDER-FIVES CLINIC MUST HAVE A LOCAL-EVENTS CALENDAR

Here is an example of how the local-events calendar in Figure 1–24 might be used.

A mother says that her child was born when they were burning grass.

'Was the rice market running?'

Mother says, 'No'. The rice market ended in August, and grass-burning ended in September. This means that the child must have been born in September.

'Was the child born when the President opened the lakeshore road?'

Mother says, 'No, but he was born a few weeks afterwards'. This again shows that the child was born in September, because the President opened the road in August.

Make quite sure by asking the mother if the child was born when the mangoes had started. Mother says, 'No, they started a few weeks later'.

SEASON	ANNUAL EVENT	MONTH	EVENTS IN 1968
Dzinja (rains)	Begin cassava planting Late rice planting End of mangoes	January	Eid Daha
	Begin rice weeding Cassava planting Abundance nchila fish	February	President opens new rest house; Kampungu mill closes
	Rice weeding Cassava planting	March	Easter
Mwera (cold, windy)	End weeding of rice Sanjika season Cassava planting	April	
	Begin rice harvest Begin maize harvest Begin digging groundnuts Begin Ntchisi tobacco market	May	
	Cassava weeding End maize harvest Continue rice harvest	June	Ascension
	Begin rice market Cutting grass for thatching Initiation of children—Jando	July	
Mwavu (hot)	Continuation of Jando End rice market	August	President opens new road, speaks at airfield
	Building houses End of burning grass	September	
	End of building houses Preparation of fields Mangoes start	October	Shabani
Yosuula (breaking ground)	Early maize and groundnut planting Continuation of preparing fields	November	Ramazan
	Early rice planting Rains start Continue planting maize and groundnuts	December	Christmas Eid Fitar

1 - 24, A local-events calendar from Malawi

Now we know for sure that the child was born in September 1968.

Once you have made a local-events calendar, and used it for a little while, you will know it by heart, and be able to use it very easily. The calendar in Figure 1–24 is for one year only. A calendar is, however, needed for at least five years and needs to be very carefully made month by month for the last three years. Many clinics will find it useful to have a calendar recording the most important events each year going back much further than this.

A local-events calendar may seem a lot of trouble to make, but perhaps this chapter will have shown you that one of the most important things that we can know about a child is his true age.

Chapter Two

WHEN GROWTH FAILS

2.1 The underweight child. The first chapter was about how children grow. We saw how a healthy child is always about the right weight for his age, and how a child who is growing gets heavier each time he is weighed. This chapter is about what happens if a child does not grow as he should.

NORMAL   UNDERWEIGHT
                    shorter

2-1, The underweight child

If a child does not get enough to eat he does not grow. He does not weigh as much as he should do for his age. We say that he is 'underweight for his age'. In some parts of Africa 40 children in every 100 (40%) are much underweight for their ages, and there are districts where even more children are underweight. By this we mean that the dots for their weights come below the lower line on the road-to-health chart. We want a name for a child who does not weigh as much as he should do for his age, so we will call him the **underweight child**.

Why do underweight children matter? They matter for three reasons.

THE THREE REASONS

2.2a The first reason: underweight children grow up less clever than they should be. If a child does not eat enough food, and especially enough of the body-building food called protein, his body and his brain do not grow as well as they should. Although malnutrition is harmful all through a child's life, we can think about it harming a child around the time of birth, before he goes to school, and while he is at school.

Around the time of birth. A child's brain grows fastest just before he is born, while he is still in his mother's womb, and during the first few months of life afterwards. His brain is thus especially likely to be harmed if his mother does not eat enough food to give him what he needs while he is in her womb, and also if he lacks food soon after he is born.

Malaria can also cause a child to be malnourished in the womb. This is how it happens. A child in his mother's womb is nourished through the cord (the umbilical cord) that joins him to the afterbirth, or placenta. During pregnancy the placenta sticks close to the wall of the womb, and nutrients (see Section 3.1) from the mother go through it on their way to the child. If a mother has malaria, it can harm the placenta, and so stop nutrients getting to the child. He does not grow so well and is often lighter when he is born than a child with a healthy placenta. Malaria is thus an important cause of malnutrition inside the womb. This is why pregnant mothers, in places where malaria is common, should always be given tablets to cure their malaria. This is an important kind of malnutrition, and it is easy to prevent.

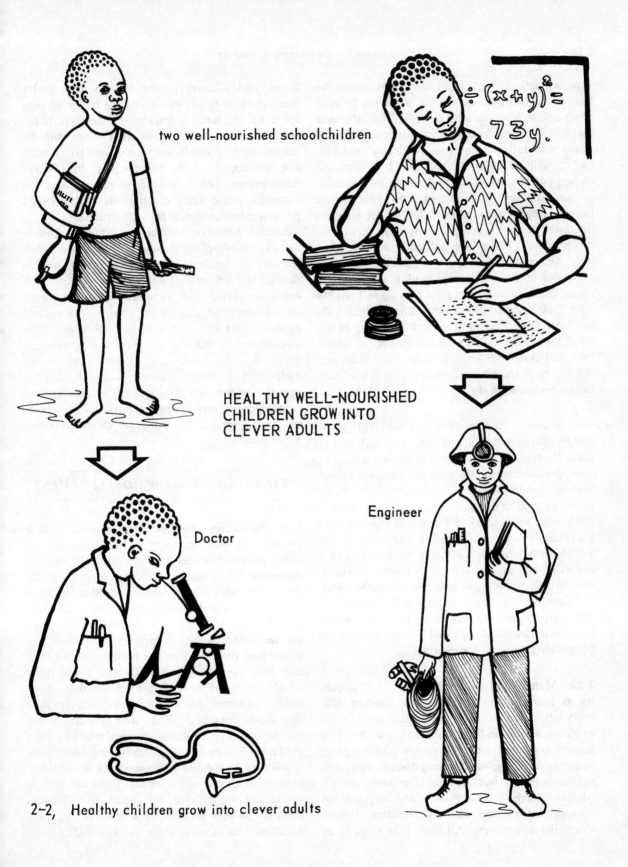

two well-nourished schoolchildren

$$\div (x+y)^2 = 73y.$$

HEALTHY WELL-NOURISHED
CHILDREN GROW INTO
CLEVER ADULTS

Engineer

Doctor

2-2, Healthy children grow into clever adults

Before school. A child has many things to learn in the first five years of his life before he goes to school, such as learning to walk, and talk, and play. If he lacks food at this time, he becomes sleepy and dull and does not run about and talk like a well-fed child of his age. Malnourished children often start walking later than they should, or stop walking, if they started to walk before becoming malnourished. Such children are also less interested in what is going on around them, and do not play well. If they are dull and sleepy because they are malnourished, their families are less interested in them, and do not play with them so much. Children learn a lot from playing and talking with their families. So malnourished children do not learn from their families and their play in the way they should. When such children get to school they find that other children, who have been well fed in the years before they came to school, are better in class than they are.

At school. If a child is not well fed, he is hungry, sleepy and dull, and does not think well in class. He does not learn so well as he would do if he were well nourished. He does not pass the exams that he should pass, and when he gets a job, he is not so good at doing it as he might have been.

Thus we are coming to think that children who are malnourished, either while they are in the womb, or before they go to school, or while they are at school, do not grow up to be as clever as they should be. We can say this in another way. Children who are malnourished and underweight are likely to grow up less clever than they would have been if they had been well fed, and had always been the right weight for their age.

2.2b Malnutrition and development. If a country is going to go forward and develop fast, every adult, and therefore every child, needs to be as clever, as able and as skilful as he can be. This matters not only for the few people who are going to do the difficult jobs, like being doctors, engineers or businessmen, but also for the many people who are going to do the more ordinary jobs. A country needs good farmers, builders, typists, mechanics and drivers. All these jobs have to be

learnt, and a clever person can do them better than one who is not so clever. The better all jobs are done, the faster a country will develop. If the workers of a country have been made dull by malnutrition in childhood, it will not go forward and develop so fast. Malnutrition thus slows development. This is one of the reasons why the countries where many children are malnourished go forward more slowly than they need.

So far we have only talked about malnutrition in children slowing development. But when adult workers are malnourished, development is also slowed. In Sections 7.21 and 9.2 you will read how many workers, and especially many farmers, are malnourished, and are not able to work as hard as they would do if they were well nourished. They lack especially the energy food that they need to be able to work hard. When workers are malnourished, they cannot work hard, the country cannot go forward as it should, and development slows. Thus malnutrition in adults, as well as malnutrition in children, slows development.

MALNUTRITION SLOWS DEVELOPMENT

2.2c Measuring what malnutrition does. It is not easy to measure what malnutrition does to make people less clever. This is partly because cleverness is itself not easy to measure, and partly because it takes a long time for children to grow into adult men and women. We can weigh children now, but we will have to wait 20 years before we can see if underweight children grow up to be less clever than those who are the right weight for their age. But, even though it is difficult to be quite certain, more and more people feel sure that underweight children do grow up less clever than they might have been. If we wait 20 years before we do anything, millions of children will have grown up less clever than they should have been. It will then be too late to do anything about them. If there were only a few underweight children, it would not matter quite so much. But, because there are so very many of these children, we must do all we can to make their nutrition better now.

This is why many people are so worried about malnutrition and so keen to prevent it. It is also why this book has been written.

UNDERWEIGHT CHILDREN MATTER BECAUSE THERE ARE SO MANY OF THEM

2.3 The second reason: underweight children become ill and die more easily. Nobody has any doubt about this. When underweight children become ill with a disease such as measles they are more likely to die than are big, strong, well-nourished children. Underweight children cannot fight diseases so well. Some people like to think of an underweight child as being like a house in which the ants have eaten all the poles (sticks). The house looks quite well and stands up during the dry season, but, when the rains come, the roof falls in and it is washed away. A strong house in which the poles have not been eaten by the ants is not harmed by rain. In the same way an underweight child seems fairly well, until he gets measles,

or some other disease which kills him. A strong well-nourished child is much less hurt by diseases and nearly always gets well again. This idea of a house in the rains is a good one to teach mothers. It was given us by Mr. Chikakuda of Malawi.

In countries where children are well nourished they hardly ever die from measles. A good saying to remember is that *a community is malnourished so long as children die from measles.*

Measles is an example of an **infection.** By this we mean that it is caused by a very small living thing or organism getting into a child's body and living there. Micro means small, so we call these very small living things **micro-organisms.** Another name for them is germs. A person with a micro-organism living inside him is said to be infected by that micro-organism. Not all diseases are caused by infections. Marasmus, for example, is caused by lack of food. However, many important diseases of children are infections, such as most kinds of diarrhoea, tuberculosis (TB), and whooping cough. Each of these diseases is caused by infection with a different micro-organism.

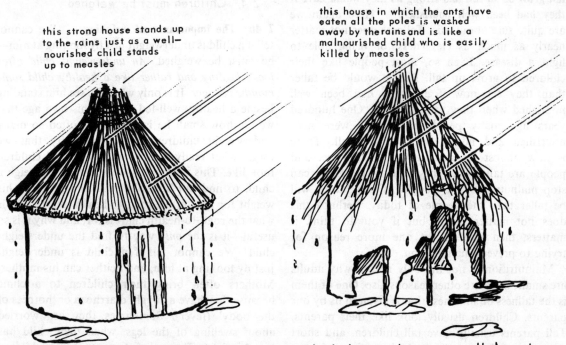

this strong house stands up to the rains just as a well-nourished child stands up to measles

this house in which the ants have eaten all the poles is washed away by the rains and is like a malnourished child who is easily killed by measles

2-3, A malnourished child is like a house in which the ants have eaten all the poles

Malnourished children also get other infections, besides measles, more severely than they would do if they were well nourished. They get diarrhoea and tuberculosis more often and die from them more easily. In one district underweight children were found to get diarrhoea four times as often as well-nourished children. As you will read in Section 7.20, one of the best ways of preventing diarrhoea is to make sure that all children are well nourished and are on the road to health.

UNDERWEIGHT CHILDREN DIE FROM INFECTIONS MORE EASILY

Underweight children are also in danger of getting even more malnourished. If their nutrition gets a little worse, or if they get diarrhoea, or some other infection, they may become so malnourished that they get the very bad kinds of malnutrition called kwashiorkor or marasmus. They may die because of this. *The underweight child is thus always in danger.*

2.4a The third reason: underweight children do not grow up so tall and strong as they would have if they had been well nourished. Here again we are quite sure about this. Tallness does not matter nearly as much as cleverness, or being able to fight a disease. Even so, most people like their children to grow up tall. People would be taller than they are now if everyone had been well nourished when they were children. One hundred years ago many people in Europe were mal-nourished and adults were quite small. There is now almost no malnutrition in Europe, and people are taller than they used to be. If we can stop malnutrition, the people of the future will be taller than the people of today. Perhaps this does not matter much, but if you do think it matters, then here is just one more reason for trying to prevent malnutrition.

Malnutrition is not the only reason why adults are small; there are other reasons also. One of them is the tallness or shortness that is given to us by our parents. Children usually look like their parents. Tall parents usually have tall children, and short parents usually have short children. Our height is

UNDERWEIGHT CHILDREN CAN ONLY BE FOUND BY WEIGHING THEM

thus partly due to the tallness or shortness that was given to us by our parents, and partly due to the food that we had while we were growing. A child who is not given enough food while he is growing is not able to make use of the tallness given to him by his parents. He does not grow as tall as he would do if he were well fed. Do not worry if you are short. Your shortness may have been given to you by your parents!

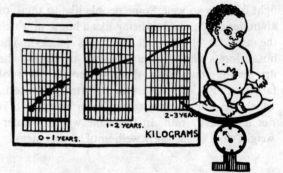

2-4, Children must be weighed

2.4b The importance of weighing. We cannot tell if a child is underweight just by looking at him—he must be weighed. *An underweight child often looks healthy and rather like a healthy child some months younger.* It is only when we see him standing beside a healthy well-fed child of his own age that we see how small he is. There are often so many underweight children in a community that we forget what really healthy well-nourished children look like. This is why it is so important to weigh a child, to find out how old he is and to check his weight for age on the road-to-health chart. This is what the road-to-health chart is for, and why it is so useful—it is the *only* way to find the underweight child! We cannot tell if a child is underweight just by looking at him, and neither can his mother. Mothers often bring their children to a clinic because they have a cough, diarrhoea or 'hotness of the body' (fever). Sometimes they are worried about swelling of the legs, when their child has kwashiorkor. They almost never bring children to a clinic because they are thin and underweight. There may be so many thin, underweight children in a village that mothers think it is right for their children to be like this.

Just as mothers cannot tell if their children are underweight, nor can doctors, medical assistants or nurses either. *This means that every child coming to a clinic or hospital must be weighed and given a road-to-health chart.* Their mothers should also be asked to bring them to the under-fives clinic. This is especially important if they are underweight, but all children should come.

EVERY CHILD COMING TO A HEALTH CENTRE OR HOSPITAL MUST HAVE A WEIGHT CHART

2.4c How many malnourished children are there? Some lucky children get all the food they need. These are the healthy well-nourished children who are on the road to health. Many children get less food than they need to grow and keep healthy, and are below the road to health. These are the underweight children that you have just read about, and who are important because there are so many of them.

Some children eat enough food, but it is the *wrong kind of food.* They get a disease called **kwashiorkor.** Other children eat *so little food of any kind* that they get a disease called **marasmus.** In a community where there is much malnutrition perhaps 40 children in every hundred will be underweight (40%), perhaps two (2%) may have marasmus, and perhaps only one (1%) or less will have kwashiorkor. Because the nutrition of children differs greatly from one community to another, these numbers will be different in different districts. In a district where the nutrition is not quite so bad, perhaps only 20 per cent of the children will be underweight, 1 per cent will have marasmus, and there will perhaps be only one child in 500 with kwashiorkor. As we shall see in Section 9.25, the nutrition of children also varies greatly from season to season and from year to year.

In Malawi and Zambia, and in many other countries, only about seven out of ten children

who are born live to reach their fifth birthday. Three children in every ten die. Some die soon after birth. Many die because they are malnourished, or because diseases like measles can kill them when they are underweight. Of the seven children who live, perhaps three will have had malnutrition at some time before they were five years old, and may not grow up so clever as they might have been.

THE NUTRITION OF CHILDREN VARIES GREATLY FROM PLACE TO PLACE AND FROM TIME TO TIME

2.5 Kwashiorkor. This is an African word which comes from Ghana. It means the 'illness of the displaced child'. By displaced we mean that a child has been taken away from his mother's breast because she has become pregnant again. Many tribes recognize kwashiorkor. The Bemba call it *ulunse* and the Soli *buwise*. The Nyanja name for the disease is *unjise*.

A child with kwashiorkor does not usually look thin. He may have plenty of fat underneath his skin which makes his body look round and his cheeks look fat. His legs and hands may look too fat because they are swollen with water (**oedema**), and if you press on the leg of a child with kwashiorkor your finger may leave a hole or dent behind it. A child may look fat, but underneath he is thin, because his muscles have got thin and weak. His stomach may also look big and fat, but this is because the muscles of his stomach are also weak and loose. If you look at his shoulders and the tops of his upper arms you can see that they are thin.

The skin of a child with kwashiorkor often becomes pale, or a bit red, and not as black as it should be. It becomes thin and weak, and may start coming off like old paint from a door. His hair gets pale and thin and may become straight and easy to pull out. He is sad and sits still in his mother's arms and does not want to run about and play. Sometimes he stops walking altogether.

Children get kwashiorkor because they do not

Of every ten children who are born _ _ _ _

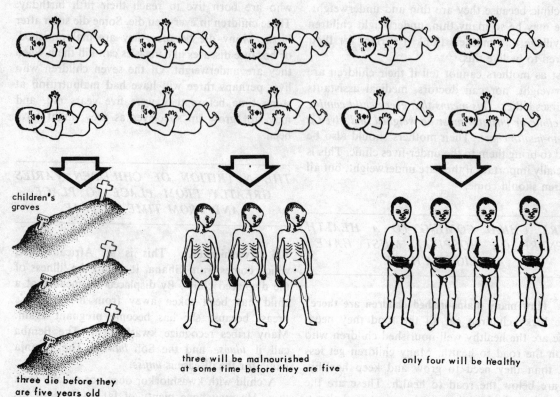

children's
graves

three die before they
are five years old

three will be malnourished
at some time before they are five

only four will be healthy

2-5, Of every ten children who are born

eat enough of the body-building food called
protein that is needed to make strong muscles,
skin and blood. But some children may have
eaten enough energy foods before they got ill
to make them quite fat. A child with kwashiorkor
usually weighs less than the right weight for his
age. But, because he may still be quite fat, and
because of the water that makes his legs swollen,
he may not be very underweight. Sometimes
children like Stephen in Section 1.3 may even get
kwashiorkor while they are on the road to health.
Children with kwashiorkor always stop growing.

Mothers sometimes think that any child who is
fat must be well nourished. When you are teaching
mothers you may have to show them that fat
children with kwashiorkor are malnourished
because they are eating *the wrong kind of food.*
They may be getting nearly enough energy food,
but they are not getting enough body-building
protein.

CHILDREN GET KWASHIORKOR BECAUSE THEY EAT TOO LITTLE PROTEIN

The commonest age for a child to get
kwashiorkor is when he is about 18 months, but it
can happen at other times, especially when he
stops breast-feeding.

2.6 Marasmus. Marasmus is really only
another word for starvation, or not having enough
food of any kind to eat. Children with marasmus
are always very underweight, and sometimes only
weigh half as much as they should do for their
age. Look how very thin the child in Figure 2–6 is.
His arms and legs are like sticks, and you can see
his ribs. His muscles are very thin, and his arm
circumference (Section 1.5) is very small indeed.
His face is thin, like the face of an old man, and
his head looks big, because his body is small.

MARASMUS

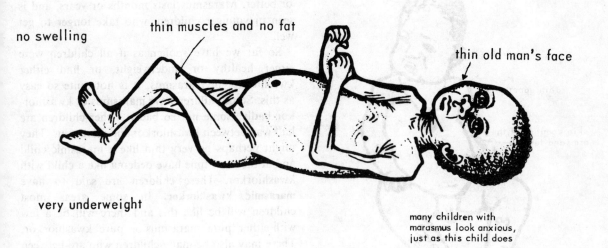

no swelling

thin muscles and no fat

thin old man's face

very underweight

many children with marasmus look anxious, just as this child does

KWASHIORKOR

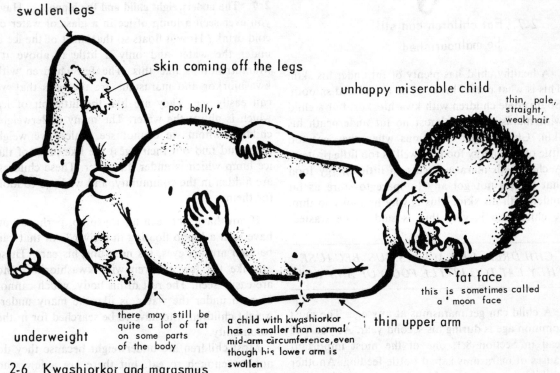

swollen legs

skin coming off the legs

'pot belly'

unhappy miserable child

thin, pale, straight, weak hair

fat face
this is sometimes called a 'moon face'

thin upper arm

a child with kwashiorkor has a smaller than normal mid-arm circumference, even though his lower arm is swollen

there may still be quite a lot of fat on some parts of the body

underweight

2-6, Kwashiorkor and marasmus

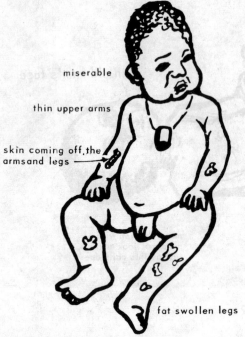

miserable

thin upper arms

skin coming off the
arms and legs

fat swollen legs

2-7, Fat children can still be malnourished

A healthy child has plenty of fat under his skin. This is what makes his body so round and smooth. So do some children with kwashiorkor, but a child with marasmus has almost no fat underneath his skin. Children get marasmus when they eat too little of the energy foods as well as too little protein. A child with marasmus eats so little energy food that he has not got any to spare to store as fat underneath his skin. This is why he looks so thin. A child who is very thin is said to be wasted.

CHILDREN GET MARASMUS BECAUSE THEY EAT TOO LITTLE FOOD OF ANY KIND

A child can get marasmus at any age. The most common age is during his second year. As you will read in Section 8.1, one of the most important causes of marasmus is bad bottle-feeding. Another is children not being given enough porridge with added protein from the age of four months onwards.

Marasmus and kwashiorkor differ in other important ways. Children get kwashiorkor quite quickly over a few weeks, and are soon either dead or better. Marasmus lasts months or years, and is seen in younger children, who take longer to get well.

So far we have spoken as if all children were either healthy or underweight, or had either kwashiorkor or marasmus. It is not quite so easy as this. Some children have marasmus or kwashiorkor badly, some not so badly. Other children are half way between kwashiorkor and marasmus. They might perhaps be very thin like a marasmic child and at the same time have oedema like a child with kwashiorkor. These children are said to have **marasmic kwashiorkor.** In some areas most children will be like this and there will be a few with either 'pure' marasmus or 'pure' kwashiorkor. There may also be many children who are between the underweight child and the child with either marasmus or kwashiorkor.

2.7   **The underweight child and the hippo.** Have you ever seen a lump of ice in a glass of water or cold drink? How it floats so that most of the ice is under the water and only a little is above it? Malnutrition is like this. The few children with kwashiorkor and marasmus are the ones that we can easily see. They are like the little bit of ice which is above the water. The many underweight children whom we cannot see (unless we weigh them and find out their ages) are like most of the ice lump which is under the water. These children are hidden in the community, and we have to look for them.

If you have not seen an ice lump, perhaps you have seen a hippo floating in a river? All that can be seen are his eyes, his nose and his ears. These are like the few children with kwashiorkor who are easily seen. The rest of his body, which cannot be seen under the water, is like the many underweight children who have to be searched for in the community.

Most children are underweight because they do not get enough to eat, but there are a few who are underweight because they have some other disease. Because this is a book about nutrition we will not say anything more about these children here.

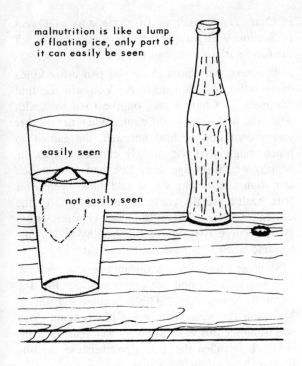

malnutrition is like a lump of floating ice, only part of it can easily be seen

easily seen

not easily seen

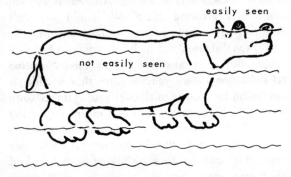

malnutrition is like a hippo, most of him cannot be seen

easily seen

not easily seen

2 - 8, The underweight child, the ice lump, and the hippo

2.8 Protein Joule Malnutrition or PEM. In the next chapter we shall learn that the part of the food that is used for building and repairing the body is called protein. The following chapter tells us about the foods that give us the energy to run about and work, and which we store as fat underneath our skin. We shall also see that this energy is measured

in **joules.** To be healthy and well nourished a child must eat enough protein and enough joules of energy food. A child whose food does not contain enough protein and energy becomes malnourished. We say he is suffering from **Protein Energy Malnutrition** or **PEM.** This is a new word which is now used instead of PCM, or protein calorie malnutrition. Underweight children eat some protein and energy food, but they do not eat enough, so they suffer from mild PEM. A child with marasmus is starving and gets much too little protein and too few joules of energy food. He suffers from severe PEM. A child with kwashiorkor also suffers from severe PEM. He also lacks protein, but he may be getting nearly enough energy.

PEM is a useful word for all kinds of malnutrition due to lack of protein and energy food. It includes the underweight child suffering from mild PEM, and also children with severe PEM, who may have marasmus or kwashiorkor, or something in between.

Of every ten children who are born in many countries at least three die before they are five years old. Sometimes as many as half of all the children who are born die before they are five years old. Many of them die because they are malnourished and suffer from PEM. They often die from marasmus or kwashiorkor, or because some other disease such as measles is able to kill them when they are weak, underweight and malnourished. Almost no children need die, and it is our job to work very hard to keep them alive and healthy. In the next two chapters we shall read about the foods that children need to make them grow and keep them healthy. Before we do so, it is useful to learn more about the weight chart in malnutrition.

2.9 The weight chart in malnutrition. In the first chapter we learnt how a healthy child is always about the right weight for his age, and how growth is more important than position on the road-to-health chart. Now that we know about

PEM, kwashiorkor and marasmus, we can compare the growth curves of some malnourished children with the growth curve of a healthy child.

The growth curves of this section are from Uganda, and are the work of Michael Church and Paget Stanfield. You will see that each chart is for five years, and that we have left out the months and only put in a few of the weights.

Chart 1 shows the growth curve of a well-nourished child, whom we will call Anne. You will see that her growth curve stays close to the healthy-weight-for-age line. Although she lost weight when she had infections, such as coughs or diarrhoea, she soon caught up again, *because she was well fed*. When children lose weight for a short time and then catch up again, we say their weight falters. To **falter** is to wait or hesitate.

Chart 2 is the growth curve of a child called Andrew. Unfortunately, Andrew was not given enough protein foods with his porridge from the age of four months onwards. Like Anne, he also had infections, and his weight faltered, but he could not catch up properly afterwards because he was not well fed. Because he did not have enough food to make him grow, and to let his weight catch up after infections, his growth curve became flat. When he was 19 months old he weighed only $7\frac{1}{2}$ kg and got kwashiorkor.

Many children who get kwashiorkor have a growth curve like that of Andrew. It is as if they were going along **the road to PEM** that is shown in Chart 3. You will see that children start on the road to health for the first six months while they are breast-fed. But, from the age of four months onwards they are not given enough porridge with protein foods. They stop growing, their weight curve flattens, and they go along the road to PEM.

The road to PEM is not printed on the road-to-health chart, but mothers can understand it if you make a big teaching chart and explain it to them. As we saw with Stephen in Section 1.3, children can get kwashiorkor at other places on the chart, but the end of the road to PJM is the place where they usually get it.

Children can become malnourished at any age, but the most common time is during their second year, which is the time that Andrew got kwashiorkor

in Chart 2. We shall see from the story of David in Section 9.23 just how many things can block the food-path of a child at this age.

The next two charts show you two other kinds of growth curve you may see. You will see that Elizabeth in Chart 4 was on the road to health when she first came to the clinic. When her mother was shown how to feed her well, she gained so much weight that she quickly climbed above the healthy-weight-for-age line. She had been much less than the weight she should have been. Her true healthy-weight curve is that shown by the dotted line. She is one of the many children whose growth curve rises above the healthy-weight-for-age line when they have enough to eat.

Sarah in Chart 5 had kwashiorkor with oedema. She was well fed and got better quickly. But she began by losing weight. This is because she started by losing the water that made her oedema. You will often see this as children get well from kwashiorkor. It is called the 'tick sign', because the line on the chart looks like a tick.

2.10 Measuring rehabilitation with the weight chart. Chart 7 shows what happens when a child with kwashiorkor, such as Andrew, is well fed and starts growing again. We could say that Andrew was cured, but we usually say that he was 'rehabilitated', which means made well again. But it means more than this. **Nutrition rehabilitation** means making sure that a child is not going to become malnourished again as soon as he goes home to his family. It means improving a child's nutrition, *and teaching his mother how to look after him so that he does not get PEM once more*. This can be done by taking both him and his mother into hospital, so that he can be cured with good food and she can be taught how to feed him. Children can be rehabilitated in hospital, but it is cheaper to rehabilitate them in a special rehabilitation unit, like that described in Section 11.4b. Chart 7 shows Andrew's rehabilitation growth curve when he and his mother went to stay in a rehabilitation unit.

If we are going to be able to measure how good we are at rehabilitating a child and his mother, we must think more carefully about weight and

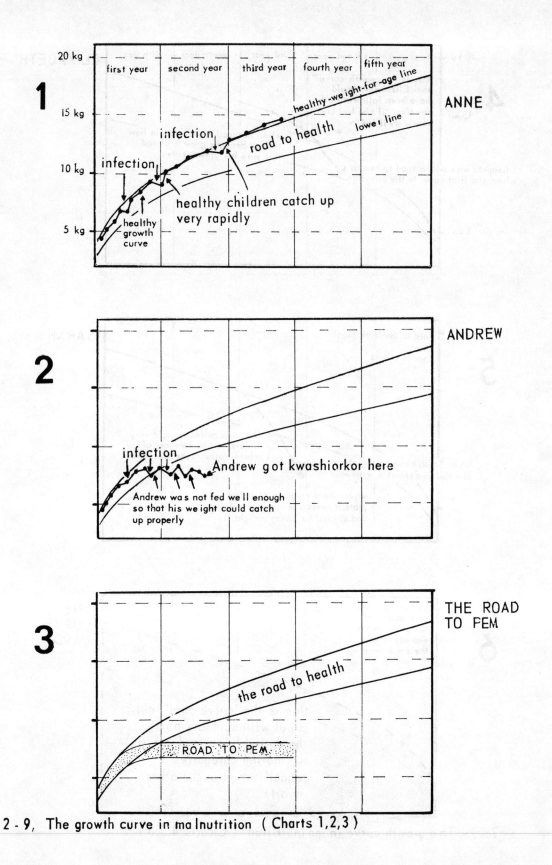

1 ANNE

20 kg
15 kg
10 kg
5 kg

first year · second year · third year · fourth year · fifth year

healthy-weight-for-age line

road to health

lower line

infection

infection

healthy growth curve

healthy children catch up very rapidly

2 ANDREW

infection

Andrew got kwashiorkor here

Andrew was not fed well enough so that his weight could catch up properly

3 THE ROAD TO PEM

the road to health

ROAD TO PEM

2-9, The growth curve in malnutrition (Charts 1,2,3)

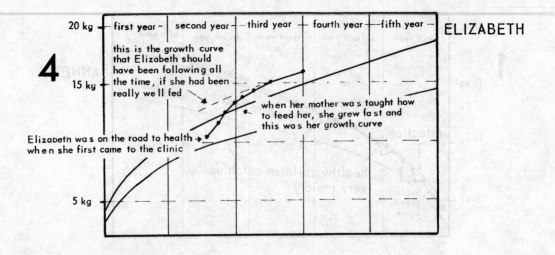

4

20 kg — first year – | second year – | third year – | fourth year – | fifth year – **ELIZABETH**

this is the growth curve that Elizabeth should have been following all the time, if she had been really well fed

15 kg

when her mother was taught how to feed her, she grew fast and this was her growth curve

Elizabeth was on the road to health when she first came to the clinic

5 kg

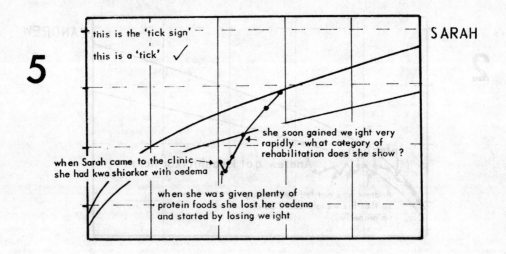

5

this is the 'tick sign'

this is a 'tick' ✓

SARAH

she soon gained weight very rapidly – what category of rehabilitation does she show ?

when Sarah came to the clinic she had kwashiorkor with oedema

when she was given plenty of protein foods she lost her oedema and started by losing weight

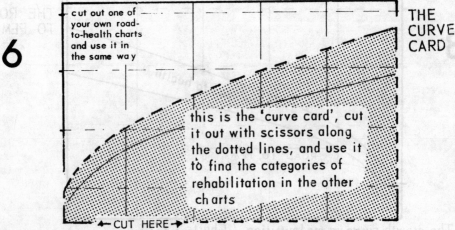

6

cut out one of your own road-to-health charts and use it in the same way

THE CURVE CARD

this is the 'curve card', cut it out with scissors along the dotted lines, and use it to find the categories of rehabilitation in the other charts

← CUT HERE →

2 - 9. The growth curve in malnutrition (Charts 4,5,6)

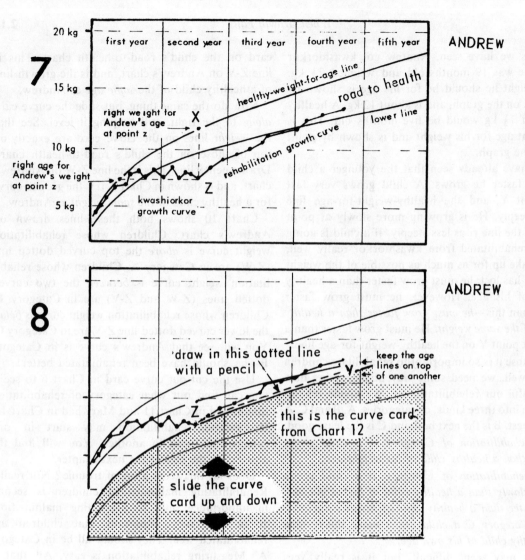

7

20 kg

first year | second year | third year | fourth year | fifth year   ANDREW

15 kg

healthy-weight-for-age line   road to health

right weight for
Andrew's age
at point z   X   lower line

10 kg

right age for
Andrew's weight
at point z   rehabilitation growth curve

kwashiorkor
growth curve   Z

5 kg

8

ANDREW

'draw in this dotted line
with a pencil   Y   keep the age
                                                lines on top
                                                of one another

                              Z

this is the curve card
from Chart 12

slide the curve
card up and down

2 - 9, The growth curve in malnutrition (Charts 7,8)

age. As we have seen, Andrew got kwashiorkor when he was 19 months old and weighed $7\frac{1}{2}$ kg. The weight he should be for his age is shown by point X on the graph, and is about 12 kg. A healthy child of $7\frac{1}{2}$ kg would be five months old. This is the right age for his weight and is shown by point Y on the graph.

We have already seen that the younger a child is, the faster he grows. A child grows very fast at point Y, and the healthy-weight-for-age line rises steeply. He is growing more slowly at point X, and the line rises less steeply. If a child is going to be rehabilitated from kwashiorkor really well, and make up for as much as possible of the weight that he has lost, he must grow faster than a healthy child of his age. However, he must grow faster even than this—*he must grow faster than a healthy child of the same weight.* He must grow faster than a child at point Y on the healthy-weight-for-age line.

Because it is so important to rehabilitate children really well, we need some way of measuring how successful our rehabilitation is. We divide rehabilitation into three kinds, or categories, A, B and C. A is the best, B is the next best and C is the least good.

In rehabilitation of Category A a child grows faster than a healthy child of his weight-age.

In rehabilitation of Category B a child grows more slowly than a healthy child of his weight-age, but faster than a healthy child of his own age.

In Category C a child grows more slowly than a healthy child of his own age.

This may seem difficult, but it is really very easy. All we have to do is to cut one of our own road-to-health charts along the healthy-weight-for age line, as in Chart 6. This is given you as an example, so cut it out. Let us call the road-to-health card we have cut out the **curve card,** and see how well Andrew was rehabilitated.

Put the curve card on top of the child's road-to-health chart showing his rehabilitation curve. Keep the curve card level (horizontal) with its *age* lines exactly on top of those of the child's chart. Slide it *up and down* until you find the place where the child's weight at the start of rehabilitation touches the edge of the curve card. This is point Z on Andrew's chart and is shown in Chart 8. Draw a pencil line along the edge of the curve card on the child's road-to-health chart. This is line Z-V on Andrew's chart, and is the growth line of a healthy child of the *same age* as Andrew.

Now do the same thing, but slide the curve card *along* to the right, still keeping it level. See that the *weight* lines on the curve card are exactly on top of those on the child's road-to-health chart. Draw a pencil line. This is the line Z-W on Andrew's chart, and is shown in Chart 9. It is the growth curve for a healthy child of the *same weight* as Andrew.

Chart 10 shows both these lines drawn on Andrew's chart. Children whose rehabilitation weight curve is *above* the top curved dotted line (Z-W) are in Category A. Children whose rehabilitation weight curve is *between* the two curved dotted lines (Z-W and Z-V) are in Category B. Children whose rehabilitation weight curve is *below* the lower curved dotted line Z-V are in Category C. You will see that Andrew's curve is in Category B—he should have been rehabilitated better!

Use the cut-out curve card in Chart 6 to see if you can find out what category of rehabilitation Simon had in Chart 11 and Mary had in Chart 12. Be careful—rehabilitation may start in one category and end in another! You will find the answers at the end of the next chapter.

Does all this seem a lot of trouble? Not really. Rehabilitating malnourished children is second in importance only to preventing malnutrition. It is also very important that children are rehabilitated well. They should all be in Category A. Measuring rehabilitation is easy. All that is necessary is to cut out a curve card and draw two lines with a pencil! A better curve card can be made out of plastic sheet, such as an old x-ray film with the 'picture' washed off. Weight charts, like that in Figure 1–11, which are divided into pieces or panels for each year, can be used in the same way as Chart 6 in this section. You will, however, find it necessary to slide your curve card along when you come to the step between the panel for one year and that for the next.

2.11 THINGS TO DO

(a) Visiting a children's ward. See if you can visit the children's ward in a hospital, and ask

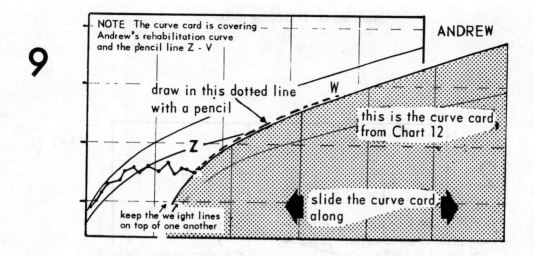

9

NOTE The curve card is covering Andrew's rehabilitation curve and the pencil line Z - V

draw in this dotted line with a pencil

this is the curve card from Chart 12

ANDREW

W

Z

slide the curve card along

keep the weight lines on top of one another

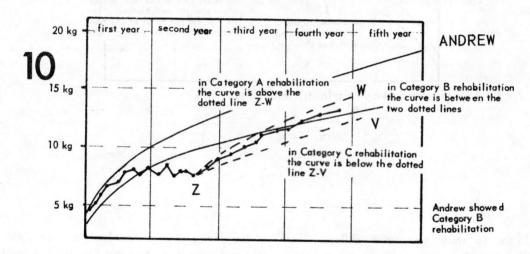

10

20 kg

first year — second year — third year — fourth year — fifth year

ANDREW

15 kg

in Category A rehabilitation the curve is above the dotted line Z-W

W

in Category B rehabilitation the curve is between the two dotted lines

V

10 kg

in Category C rehabilitation the curve is below the dotted line Z-V

Z

5 kg

Andrew showed Category B rehabilitation

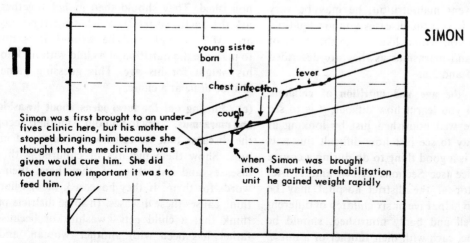

11

SIMON

young sister born

fever

chest infection

cough

Simon was first brought to an under-fives clinic here, but his mother stopped bringing him because she thought that the medicine he was given would cure him. She did not learn how important it was to feed him.

when Simon was brought into the nutrition rehabilitation unit he gained weight rapidly

2 - 9, The growth curve in malnutrition (Charts 9,10,11,)

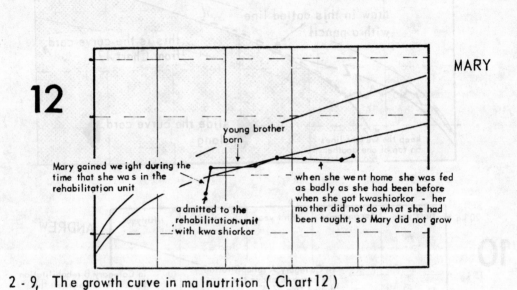

MARY

young brother
born

Mary gained weight during the
time that she was in the
rehabilitation unit

when she went home she was fed
as badly as she had been before
when she got kwashiorkor - her
mother did not do what she had
been taught, so Mary did not grow

admitted to the
rehabilitation unit
with kwashiorkor

2 - 9, The growth curve in malnutrition (Chart 12)

the doctor to show you some children with kwashiorkor and marasmus. If you are members of a nutrition club or nutrition group who are trying to prevent malnutrition, he may be very pleased to show you the diseases you are fighting. Tell him that you would like to see the signs of kwashiorkor and marasmus as they are described in Sections 2.5 and 2.6.

(b) Guessing the age and nutrition of children. In Section 2.4 you learnt how difficult it is to see if children are well nourished just by looking at them. One way to see just how difficult this is is to try it. This is a good thing to do during a course or a conference (see Sections 11.24b and 11.24c) and the doctor at the district hospital may be very pleased to help. Five or six children of different ages, both well and badly nourished, should be seated in a line, each with their mother or a nurse. Each child should be given a number. Members

of the course should then look at each child in turn and write down how old they think a child is and whether they think he is well or badly nourished. They should then gather together and ask the doctor to tell them what the right answers are. Many people will be wrong! It is difficult to measure the nutrition of a child without knowing his weight for his age. This guessing game can also be done at a clinic.

(c) Finding out the local ideas about kwashiorkor and marasmus.   Try to find out if mothers recognize the diseases that we call kwashiorkor and marasmus. Show them pictures of children with these diseases and ask them if they have their own words for them. If they have, ask them what they think causes these diseases. In some districts people think that a child gets kwashiorkor because his father has been with another woman, and not because he has not been eating the right food.

Chapter Three

PROTEINS

3.1 Nutrients.   In the last chapter we saw what happens when children do not get the food they need. In this one and the next we shall see what foods are made of.

All foods are made of nutrients. There are six kinds of nutrients.

PROTEIN — for body-building and repair

CARBOHYDRATES
FATS AND OILS } for energy and warmth

VITAMINS
MINERALS } for protection from some diseases

WATER

If adults are to stay healthy and children are to grow, they must have enough of each of these nutrients which come from the food they eat. The first nutrient to think about is protein, and what it is for.

3.2 Protein for growing or body-building.   Our bodies are built of very many small pieces called cells in the same way that a village is made of houses. Cells are mostly made from protein just as some houses are mostly made from bricks. A child starts off as one cell inside his mother's womb and is far too small to see. This cell takes in protein and builds another cell. Each of these cells takes in more protein and builds two more cells. This goes on until there are millions of cells, which take on different shapes to make the different parts of a child's body, such as his muscles, his eyes, his heart, and his brain. We saw in Section 1.1 that while a child is in his mother's womb he grows from one cell weighing almost nothing to a birth weight of $3\frac{1}{2}$ kg. Because a child is growing very fast at this time, he needs lots of protein. This comes to him through the cord (the

umbilical cord) that joins him to the inside of his mother's womb. A pregnant mother must thus eat plenty of protein if she is to have enough for herself as well as enough for the child that is growing inside her.

When a child is born, his body, and especially his brain, go on growing. We saw in the first section of this book that he grows so fast that he doubles his birth-weight in the first six months of his life and triples it during his first year. If a child is to be able to grow as fast as this, he needs plenty of protein food. In the first months of his life this comes to him in his mother's milk, but, from the age of four months onwards, he must have plenty of protein foods added to his porridge. After a child is one year old he grows more slowly, *but he is still growing* and so he still needs plenty of protein food.

3.3 Protein for repair.   When a child becomes an adult, he stops growing—that is he stops getting taller and only gets heavier if he gets very fat. An adult, therefore, no longer needs protein for growing. But the different parts of his body are wearing out all the time. Each cell lives for a while and then dies, and a new cell has to be made. One of the red cells of the blood, for example, only lives for about 120 days, after which it wears out and a new red cell has to be made. Protein is needed to make these new cells, so an adult has to eat protein to repair his body. The cells of a child's body are also wearing out, so a child needs protein for repair as well as protein for growth.

If you wear a pair of shoes for long enough the soles will wear out, but if you wear no shoes the soles of your feet do not wear out. This is because new skin cells are being made all the time underneath the old skin. The hard skin that touches the ground is being worn away, but the new skin

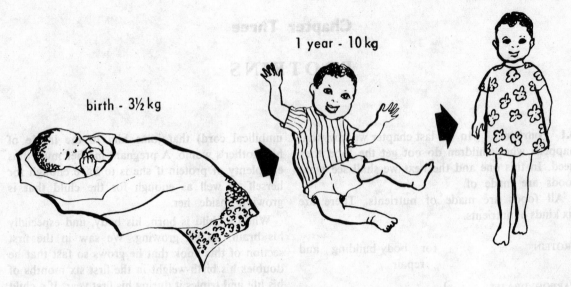

2 years - 12½ kg

1 year - 10 kg

birth - 3½ kg

PROTEIN IS NEEDED FOR GROWTH

adult woman - 55 kg

15 years - 50 kg

5 years - 18 kg

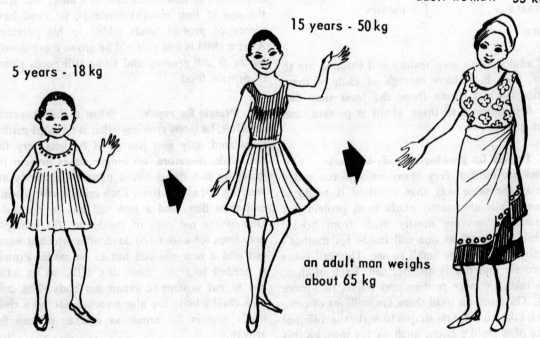

an adult man weighs
about 65 kg

3-1, Protein is needed for growth

shoes wear out and
need repairing

feet never wear out because
they are being repaired all
the time with protein in
the food

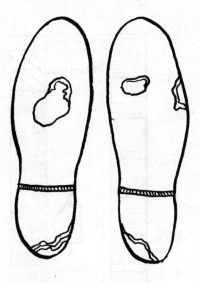

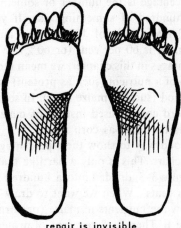

repair is invisible,
we cannot see it,
but it is happening
all the time

3-2, Protein is needed for repair

underneath is growing all the time to repair it. After you have cut your hair it is also 'repaired' again, and new hair is made out of protein. When you cut yourself, the hole in your skin is repaired in the same way by new skin cells made out of protein. We can understand repair most easily by thinking about the skin and the hair, but the same thing is happening to all parts of the body all the time.

When the body is harmed by a cut or a burn, some of the skin is cut or burnt off, and the harm must be repaired with protein. In much the same way, when the body is harmed by an illness, such as measles, or malaria or tuberculosis (TB), some of the cells inside the body are harmed and wear out faster than usual. This is easy to see in children, who often get thin and stop growing when they are ill. Sick people, especially sick children, therefore, need extra protein to repair the harm caused by an illness.

We can now make a list of the people who need protein, and what they need it for.

People who need protein.
Healthy adults need protein to repair their bodies.

Pregnant women need protein for repair and for building the baby who is growing inside them.
Nursing mothers need protein for repair and also to make milk to feed their growing child.
Children need protein for repair and for growth.
Sick adults need extra protein to repair the harm caused by their illness.
Sick children need extra protein for repair as well as protein for growth.

3.4 Some foods contain more protein than others, and some proteins are better for body-building than others. Now that we know why we need protein, the next thing to think about is the kind of foods that contain it and how good it is for body-building. There are two very important ideas here.

Firstly, nearly all foods are mixtures of nutrients, and some of them contain more protein than others. Few foods are made of one nutrient only. Most foods are mixtures of nutrients and contain some water, even though they look dry. Some foods, such as green plants like cabbage, are nearly all water.

A good way to think about how much of each kind of nutrient there is in a food is to use 'per cent'. 'Cent' is only another name for a hundred. A percentage is the number of something there is in a hundred of something else. If you have to get 60 marks out of 100 to pass an exam, the pass mark is 60 per cent (or 60%). When we use percentages in this chapter, we mean the number of grams of a nutrient (such as protein) in 100 grams of a food (such as maize meal). In some countries the word corn is used instead of maize. So maize meal is the same as corn meal.

A good way to show these percentages is to use a bar chart. This is only a bar like that in Picture A, Figure 3–3, divided into a hundred equal parts or 'per cents'. When we want to draw a bar chart to show the nutrients in maize (or corn), we draw Picture B. There is 8 per cent of protein in maize, which is only another way of saying that there are 8 grams of protein in 100 grams of maize. We are going to show protein in black on our bar charts, so we draw the length of 8 'per cents' on our bar in black. We are going to show fat or oil with dots. There is only 1 per cent of oil in maize, so we draw the length of 1 'per cent' as dots. Carbohydrate is drawn with thin lines crossing. Maize is mostly carbohydrate—it is 78 per cent carbohydrate—so we draw the length of 78 'per cents' with thin lines crossing. Water is shown with thick lines sloping. Maize meal has about 10 per cent of water, so we draw the length of 10 'per cents' with sloping lines.

The percentages of the nutrients in a food do not always add up to a hundred. Our percentages for maize meal only add up to 97 per cent (8+1+78 +10). There is 3 per cent missing to make up to 100 per cent. In the bar charts for the other foods there are also a few per cent missing. This is because it is not always easy to measure the nutrients in foods exactly, and because there are other things in food, like fibre, which are not nutrients, and which are not shown in the bar charts. Fibre is the string-like part of some foods which the body cannot use. Because fibre, and other things which are not nutrients, cannot be used by the body, they pass out of the body in the stools (the waste from the bowel).

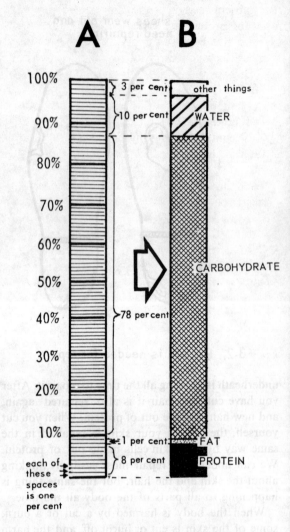

3-3, The nutrients in maize meal as an example of a bar chart

Vitamins have been left out of all bar charts, and minerals out of most of them, even though they are important. This is because there is too little of them to draw—much less than 1 per cent.

MOST FOODS ARE MIXTURES OF NUTRIENTS

Although most foods are mixtures, many of them contain a lot of one nutrient and a little of the other nutrients. Foods are often called after the nutrient there is most of. Foods which contain a lot of protein are called **protein foods** because protein is the most important nutrient in them. Foods which contain a lot of fat or carbohydrate and perhaps only a little protein are called **energy foods** (see Section 4.2). Foods in which the most important nutrients are vitamins or minerals are called **protective foods** (see Section 4.14). Some 'foods' contain hardly any nutrients at all, except water, so they are called **'non-foods'** (see Section 4.15).

Even though there is only a little protein in some foods, such as dark green leaves, it is important and must not be forgotten. Some foods are not mixtures. Cooking oil is all oil, and sugar is all carbohydrate. These foods contain no protein at all.

Secondly, some kinds of protein are better than others for body-building. Our bodies are made from cells which are partly made from protein; so also are the bodies of animals and plants. Our bodies are very like those of cows and goats. Their proteins are very like our proteins. Our bodies are very unlike those of maize or beans. Their proteins are very unlike our proteins. Because it is usually easier to make something out of something else which is very like it, animal proteins are usually better for body-building than plant proteins. *Thus proteins differ as to how good they are for body-building.* Some are better than others. Later on we shall describe a measure of how good they are for body-building. We shall also see that, even though plant proteins are usually less good for body-building than animal proteins, they can be made better by mixing them. We shall also see that they are very important, because they are cheaper and much easier to grow.

So we see that one food might contain a lot of

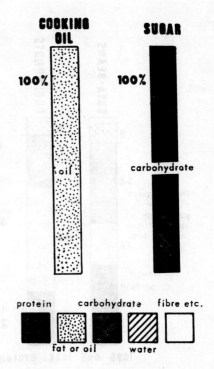

3-4, Some foods are one nutrient only

protein, but it might not be very good for body-building, and that another food might have only a little protein in it, but that this protein might be very good for body-building. *How much protein there is in a food, and how good that protein is for body-building, are thus two quite different things.*

When you have understood these two very important ideas you can read more about them. The first thing to think about is how much protein there is in various plant and animal foods.

3.5 The plant foods that give us protein. Here is a table of some plant foods and the protein they

TABLE 2
The Percentage of Protein in Some Plant Foods

Soya beans	} Legumes	34%	} Enough protein to be called protein foods
Groundnuts		23%	
Dry beans and peas		20%	
Maize (corn), wheat, Irish potatoes and the millets	called 'good' staples	8–10%	} Protein very useful, but not enough to be protein foods
Dark green leaves		3–7%	
Cassava, sweet potatoes, *matoke*	called 'poor' staples	1%	} Too little protein to be useful
Cabbage		1%	

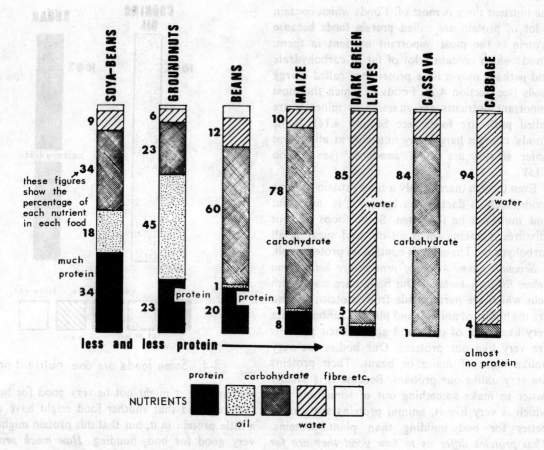

these figures show the percentage of each nutrient in each food

less and less protein →

NUTRIENTS

protein · carbohydrate · fibre etc.

oil · water

3-5, The plant foods that give us protein

contain. Those that contain the most protein are at the top of the table.

As we shall see in Section 3.10, the family of plants called legumes contain the most protein. Of these the soya bean contains much the largest amount; about 34 per cent. Groundnuts contain 23 per cent, which is why they are such a good food for young children. Dry beans of other kinds contain 20 per cent of protein and are nearly as good. Next on the list are the good **staples**, such as maize, corn, wheat, and the millets like finger millet and sorghum. The staple is the main food of a country. All the good staples have 8–10 per cent of protein. Then come the dark green leaves, such as cassava leaves, which contain 3–7 per cent of protein. Older leaves contain more protein than younger ones, but this is not so easily

digested. At the bottom of the list come the poor staples, like cassava flour and the kind of plantain (a sort of banana) that the Baganda tribe of Uganda call *matoke*. These poor staples have only 1 per cent of protein, and so also have the pale green plants like cabbage, which are almost all water.

Grains like wheat, millet, maize and rice are sometimes called **cereals**. They all have 8–10 per cent of protein and differ from the roots like cassava, sweet potatoes and *matoke* which only only have 1–2 per cent of protein.

You will see that maize has 8 per cent of protein while cassava has only 1 per cent. This is a very important difference. It shows why people who live in villages where cassava is the main food are usually more malnourished than people in villages where maize is the staple food.

You will also see from the figure that groundnuts contain 45 per cent of oil and 23 per cent of carbohydrate. This carbohydrate and oil gives us much energy. Groundnuts are thus especially useful because they give us a lot of energy food, as well as much protein.

Don't worry to learn all these figures by heart— it is more important to be able to compare one food with another. It is useful to know, for example, that maize has about eight times as much protein as cassava, and that there is more protein in soya bean than in ordinary beans.

3.6   The animal foods that give us protein.   Here is a list of the animal foods that give us protein. The list is an easy one to remember because all the foods from animals give us protein, except for butter, which is the fat from milk, and lard, which is the fat from animals. You may be surprised

to see mother's milk among the animal proteins. Man is, however, only a special kind of animal, and mother's milk is the most important animal-protein food for a young child.

TABLE 3
Animal-Protein Foods

Milk, especially mother's milk and dried skim milk
Cheese
Fish of all kinds, whether fresh or dried
Eggs
Meat of all kinds, including game animals, monkeys,
   rats and mice
Blood, liver and all the inside parts of an animal
Chicken
Snails
Insects, including grasshoppers, locusts, lake flies,
   caterpillars and flying ants

Some animal foods contain more protein than others. Here is a figure to show how much protein they contain.

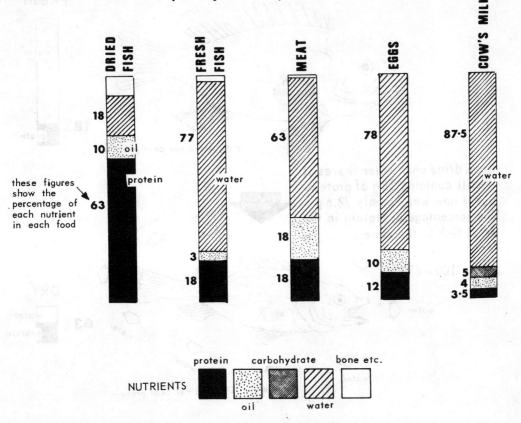

3-6, The animal foods that give us protein

Why is there only 18 per cent of protein in fresh fish while there is 63 per cent in dried fish? Some people find this difficult to understand, so let us catch some fishes each weighing 100 g. As we have seen, 'per cent' means the number of something that there is in a hundred of something else. One of our fishes contains 18 g of protein, so it is 18 per cent protein, which means that there is 18 g of protein in 100 g of fish. Let us forget about the bones and the oil in the fish and say that all the rest of it is water. There will therefore be 100−18=82 g of water in one of our fishes. Now let us dry some of our fishes and get rid of most of the water in them. When a fish is dry we find that it weighs only 28.6 g, but there will still be exactly the same weight of protein in it as there

was when it was wet, i.e. 18 g. However, there will now be only 28.6−18=10.6 g of water and not 82 g, as there was when the fish was fresh. All the rest of the water will have gone into the air. The percentage of protein in our dried fish will now be:

$$\frac{18}{28.6} \times 100 = 63\%.$$

Here is another way of looking at it. *There is the same weight of protein (18g) in each of our fishes.* A fresh fish weighs 100 g and because it contains 18 g of protein, it is 18 per cent protein. However, one of our dried fishes only weighs 28.6 g. Thus we need $3\frac{1}{2}$ dried fish to weigh 100g ($3\frac{1}{2} \times 28.6=$ 100). So, in $3\frac{1}{2}$ dried fishes there is $3\frac{1}{2} \times 18=63$ g of protein. 100 g of dried fish, therefore, contain

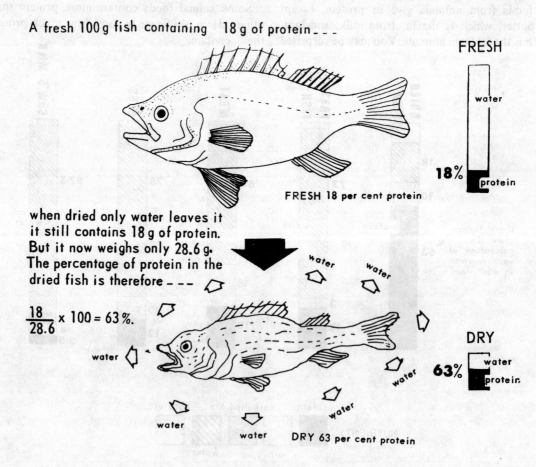

A fresh 100 g fish containing 18 g of protein _ _ _

FRESH

water

18% protein

FRESH 18 per cent protein

when dried only water leaves it it still contains 18 g of protein. But it now weighs only 28.6 g. The percentage of protein in the dried fish is therefore _ _ _

$$\frac{18}{28.6} \times 100 = 63\%.$$

water

DRY

water
protein

63%

DRY 63 per cent protein

3_7, Why there is a greater percentage of protein in dried fish

63 g of protein. In other words there is 63 per cent of protein in dried fish.

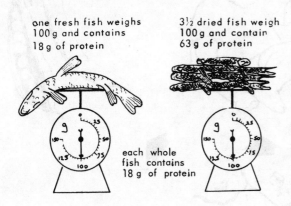

one fresh fish weighs
100 g and contains
18 g of protein

3½ dried fish weigh
100 g and contain
63 g of protein

each whole
fish contains
18 g of protein

3-8, A hundred grams of fresh fish and a hundred grams of dried fish

If you still find it difficult to see why there should be more protein in dried fish than in fresh fish, the example of the shirt may help you. A wet shirt is heavy because it contains much water. It might perhaps be 20 per cent shirt and 80 per cent water. When it is dry it will be much lighter. It might perhaps be 90 per cent shirt and only 10 per cent water. *There will, however, be the same weight of shirt, whether it is dry or wet*, just as there is the same weight of protein in a fish, whether it is dry or wet.

Just as dried fish contains a higher percentage of protein than fresh fish, so also many other foods contain a higher percentage of protein when they are dry. Dried meat contains a higher percentage of protein than fresh meat. Fresh beans and peas, for example, contain 3 per cent of protein. But, when most of the water has gone out of them and they are light and dry, they contain about 20 per cent of protein.

3.7 What proteins are made of.   So far in this chapter we have seen that foods are mixtures of nutrients, and that one of the most important of these is protein. We have seen that protein is needed for building and repairing the body. We have also seen that some foods contain much protein and some only a little. We have seen, for example, that there is very little protein in cassava (1%), more in maize (8%) and even more in dried fish (63%). *We have now got to think about how good that protein is for body-building, which is quite different from how much protein there is in a food.* For example, there is only 3.5 per cent of protein in fresh milk, but milk protein is very good for body-building. There is 34 per cent of protein in soya beans, but soya bean protein is not so good as milk protein for body-building. Most of the rest of this section is about how some proteins can be better than others for body-building.

This is a very important idea to understand, so before we go on, let us look at it in another way, with another example—good and bad cement in blocks. Some cement is good and makes strong blocks. Other cement is bad, especially if it has got damp, and makes weak blocks. When we use cement to make blocks, the strength of our blocks depends on how much cement we use (whether we use a lot or a little) and how good our cement is (whether it is strong or weak). It is the same with protein foods. *The usefulness of a food for body-building depends on how much protein it contains (whether it contains a lot or a little) and how good or 'strong' that protein is for body-building.*

How can one protein be better than another for body-building? You will have first to learn what proteins are made of. We shall use three ideas to explain this. We have already used part of the first one.

FIRST IDEA

The idea of amino acids as the clay which makes bricks. In Section 3.2 we thought of our bodies being made of cells in the same way that a village is made of houses. The cells of the body are made of proteins in the same way that a house is made of bricks. These proteins are made of smaller things called **amino acids,** in the same sort of way that bricks are made of clay. Everything in the world, including the clay that makes bricks and the amino acids that make proteins, is made of very much smaller things still. These very small things are called **atoms.**

Let us start right at the beginning with the smallest things. These are the atoms which are

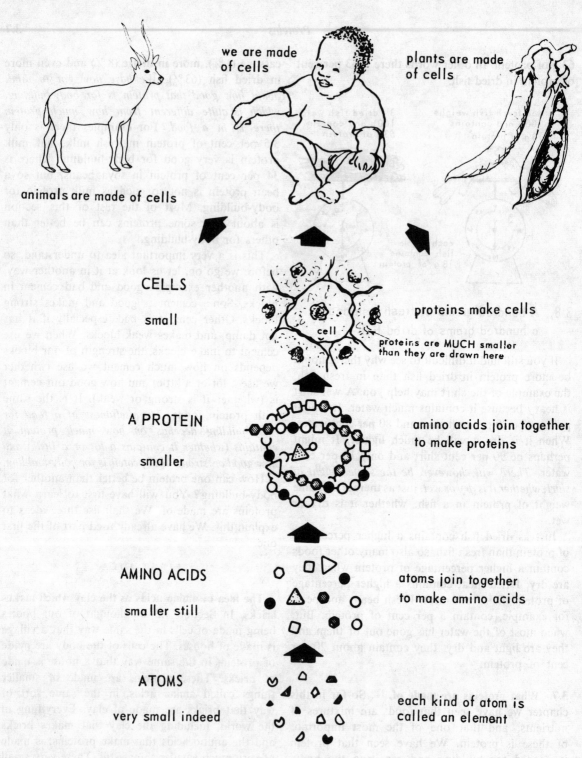

we are made
of cells

plants are made
of cells

animals are made of cells

CELLS

small

proteins make cells

cell

proteins are MUCH smaller
than they are drawn here

A PROTEIN

smaller

amino acids join together
to make proteins

AMINO ACIDS

smaller still

atoms join together
to make amino acids

ATOMS

very small indeed

each kind of atom is
called an element

3-9, Atoms build amino acids which build proteins which build ourselves.
and animals and plants

very very small indeed and from which, as we have said, everything in the world is made. There are about a hundred different kinds of atom, and each kind of atom is called an **element.** Amino acids are made of the elements called **carbon, hydrogen, oxygen, nitrogen** and sometimes **sulphur.** About ten of these atoms join together to make an amino acid. When atoms are joined together in this way they make a **molecule.** There are about twenty different kinds of amino acid molecule. The names of two of them are **methionine** and **lysine.** About a hundred amino acids of various kinds join together to make a protein molecule, which is thus very much larger than an amino acid molecule. As we shall soon see, there are millions of different kinds of protein molecule.

Cells are best thought of as very small bags filled with a kind of watery jelly called **protoplasm.** The bag and the protoplasm are made of millions of protein molecules of many different kinds. Protoplasm also contains much water, some carbohydrate and fat, a few minerals, and many other molecules, most of them small ones. There are hundreds of different kinds of cell, and our bodies are made of millions of them; so also are the bodies of all the larger plants and animals. Cells are too small to see, except with a microscope; so is everything smaller than a cell. There have to be very many cells together before we can see them with our eyes alone.

We have just seen that amino acids, and therefore proteins, are made of atoms of the elements carbon, hydrogen, oxygen, nitrogen and sometimes sulphur. It is the nitrogen in them that makes them different from the energy foods, the carbohydrates and the fats, which are made only of the elements carbon hydrogen and oxygen. This is one of the reasons why protein foods can be burnt to give energy, but energy foods cannot be used for body-building.

When plants make proteins they have to build the amino acids they want from atoms. They take carbon atoms from a gas called **carbon dioxide** in the air. They get hydrogen and oxygen atoms from water. They get the energy they need to grow from the sun. The nitrogen (and the sulphur) they get from the ground. Some of the most important plant foods or **fertilizers** are those which

contain nitrogen that plants can use to make their amino acids and thus their proteins.

Animals cannot make amino acids in this way. They have to eat the amino acids in the proteins of plants or other animals. We too are animals and have to get the amino acids we need from the plant and animal proteins we eat.

The idea of a village (our bodies), houses (cells), bricks (proteins) and clay (amino acids) teaches us that our bodies are made of very many very small pieces. These are made of even smaller pieces still, and so on downwards until we get to atoms, which are very small indeed.

SECOND IDEA

The idea of amino acids as beads in a necklace. A better way to think of amino acids is to think of them as beads. When beads are joined together they make a necklace or chain of beads. When amino acids are joined together they make an **amino acid chain.** When a necklace is rolled together it makes a ball. When a long amino acid chain is rolled together it makes a protein. Several different coloured beads can be threaded together in lots of different ways to make many different necklaces. In the same way several different amino acids can be joined together in many different ways to make many different proteins. *The way in which the amino acids in their proteins are joined together is what makes a man different from a maize plant, a chicken or any other living thing.* It is as if the protein 'necklaces' of every living thing were different.

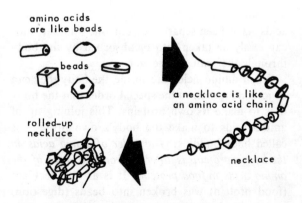

amino acids are like beads

beads

a necklace is like an amino acid chain

rolled-up necklace

necklace

3-10, A protein is like a rolled-up necklace

When a man eats a protein food, say a fish, it is broken down or digested inside his gut (stomach and intestines). First the cells in the food are broken down so that the proteins come out of them. Then these protein chains are broken down into separate amino acids. It is as if lots of different necklaces were broken into separate beads. This breaking down or digesting is done by special things called **enzymes** in the gut. Proteins are quite

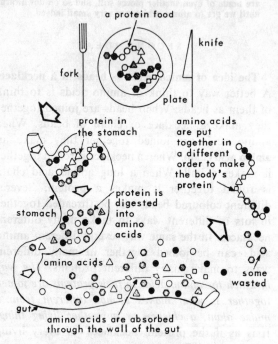

3-11 Digestion and absorption

big, but amino acids are very small. Once amino acids have been separated from one another, they can easily be taken into or absorbed by the body through the wall of the gut.

When amino acids are inside the body they can be joined together in the special order that the body uses to make its own proteins. This joining up of amino acids to make the body's own proteins is called body-building. *The order of amino acids in the body's proteins is different from the order of the amino acids in food proteins.* It is as if a necklace (food protein) was broken into beads (digestion) and the beads were put together in a different order to make a *different* necklace (the body's proteins).

Don't confuse digestion with absorption. Digestion is the breaking down of food in the gut into small pieces. The small pieces of protein are the separate amino acids. Absorption is the taking into the body, *through the wall of the gut*, of these small pieces from the food. It may seem strange to think that food is outside the body even though it is inside the stomach or intestine. What we mean by inside the body is inside the cells and the blood. The small pieces from the food, such as amino acids, have got to be absorbed through the wall of the gut into the blood. They can then be carried by the blood to all the cells of the body which need them. When amino acids in the blood are taken into the cells of the body, they can be used to make new proteins and thus new cells. This is why we say that protein foods and the amino acids that they are made of are body-building. Anything which is not absorbed passes out of the body in the stool (waste from the bowel).

This idea of beads (amino acids) making a chain or necklace (an amino acid chain) which rolls up into a ball (a protein) teaches us that amino acids join into a chain when they make a protein. It also teaches us that the necklaces or protein chains of every kind of living thing are different. When food proteins are eaten their amino acid chains are broken down by digestion into separate amino acids. During body-building we join up these separate amino acids in a different order to make our own kinds of protein.

THIRD IDEA

The idea of amino acids as letters in a sentence. *Another and much better way of thinking* about amino acids and proteins is to think of amino acids as the letters which a printer uses to make a sentence. A sentence is like an amino acid chain. The protein is the sentence rolled into a ball. If you can think of a protein in this way it will be a very good example and tell you many things about proteins. We will use part of the second sentence of this paragraph as an example: 'ANOTHER AND MUCH BETTER WAY OF THINKING . . . '. You will see that it has some vowels and some consonants. Vowels are the letters A, E, I, O and U. All the other letters are consonants.

There are 26 letters in the alphabet from which a sentence can be made. In the same way there are

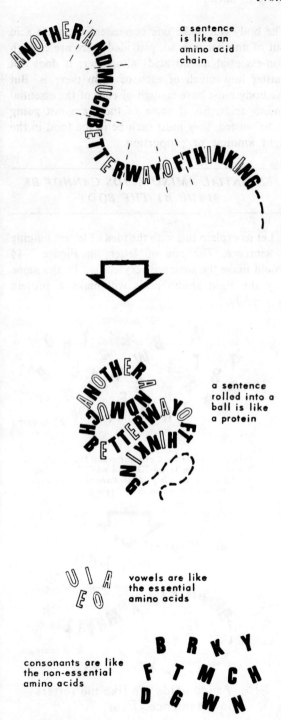

a sentence is like an amino acid chain

a sentence rolled into a ball is like a protein

vowels are like the essential amino acids

consonants are like the non-essential amino acids

3-12, Amino acids are like the letters in a sentence - One

20 different amino acids from which the amino acid chain of a protein can be made. Just as a long sentence can contain many letters, so a protein contains many amino acids, usually several hundred. In order to make a sentence you have to have the right number of each kind of letter, and they have to be put into the right order. If the order of the letters in a sentence is changed, the meaning of the sentence may be different. If the order of the amino acids in a protein is changed, the protein is different. If one letter in a sentence is exchanged for another one, the meaning of that sentence may be different. In the same way, if one of the amino acids in a protein is exchanged, that protein is different. Just as it is possible to make millions of different sentences using the 26 letters of the alphabet, so it is also possible for there to be millions of different proteins using only 20 amino acids. All living things contain many different proteins. This is only possible because there are so many millions of different proteins.

20 AMINO ACIDS CAN MAKE MILLIONS OF DIFFERENT PROTEINS

Let us take an example. Medical readers may be interested to know that normal haemoglobin, which is the red protein in blood, differs from the haemoglobin in sickle cell patients by just one amino acid in several hundred. An amino acid called valine is changed for one called glutamic acid. Haemoglobin is a protein, and changing one amino acid in its long chain makes it into quite a different kind of haemoglobin. Because there is just one amino acid changed in their haemoglobin, these patients suffer from sickle cell disease.

The body can make some amino acids out of other ones, but there are about eight of them it cannot make. The amino acids that the body *can* make are called the **non-essential amino acids.** The eight amino acids that the body *cannot* make are called the **essential amino acids.** Essential means necessary, or something that somebody must have. These essential amino acids have to be eaten in the food proteins. Lysine and methionine are both essential

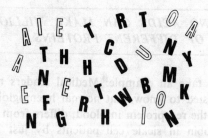

R ➤ P

just as a printer might make an R into a P by
cutting off one of its legs, so the body can make
one non-essential amino acid out of another

3-13, Amino acids are like the letters
in a sentence - Two

amino acids. It is as if our printer was able to
make some non-essential letters out of other ones,
but there were some essential letters he could not
make from others and would have to be given.
For example, it would be as if he could make one
consonant out of another, such as a P out of an R
by cutting off one of its legs, but that he had to
be given the essential vowels A, E, I, O and U,
because he could not make them.

*The proteins in our bodies are made of special
amounts of each kind of amino acid. These amounts
are quite different from those in most protein foods.*

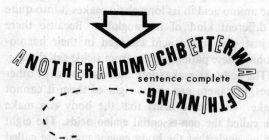

this pile of letters will make the sentence
perfectly in the same way that the right
amino acids can make a protein

sentence complete

3-14, Amino acids are like the letters
in a sentence-Three

The body can make one non-essential amino acid
out of another one, so, provided there are enough
non-essential amino acids altogether, it does not
matter how much of each of them there is. But
the body must have enough of *each* of the essential
amino acids. So, if some of them are not going
to be wasted, they must each be in the food in the
right amount or proportion.

ESSENTIAL AMINO ACIDS CANNOT BE
MADE BY THE BODY

Let us explain this with the idea of letters making
a sentence. The pile of letters in Figure 3–14
would make the sentence very easily. In the same
way the right amino acids will make a protein
very easily.

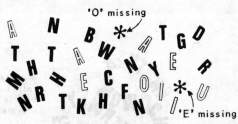

'O' missing

'E' missing

this pile of letters cannot make the sentence
because there is an 'O' and an 'E' missing,
in the same way a protein cannot be made
if there are amino acids missing

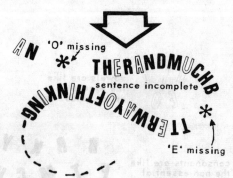

'O' missing

sentence incomplete

'E' missing

3-15, Amino acids are like the letters
in a sentence - Four

But this pile of letters (3–15) could not make
the sentence because there is an O and an E
missing.

In the same way the body cannot make a protein if some essential amino acid, such as lysine or methionine, is missing.

However, our printer could still make *one* sentence if he took *two* piles of letters. There would, however, be a lot of letters wasted. In the same way some protein can be made from a mixture of amino acids that are not in quite the right proportion, but more are needed and some are wasted.

The scarcest letter in a pile (the one of which there are fewest compared with the number needed) will decide how useful that pile of letters is for making a sentence. In the same way the scarcest amino acid in a protein will decide how useful that protein is for body-building. It is often said

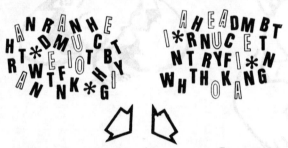

these are the same piles of letters as in Figure 3–15, two of them could make the sentence but there would be many wasted, in the same way protein can be made from imperfect mixtures of amino acids, but many are wasted

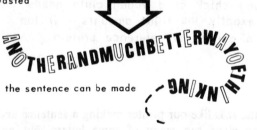

the sentence can be made

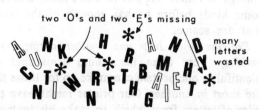

two 'O's and two 'E's missing

many letters wasted

3-16, Amino acids are like the letters in a sentence - Five

that 'a chain is as strong as its weakest link (part)'. In the same way a protein is as useful for body-building as its scarcest essential amino acid.

When the proteins of either egg or mother's milk are digested they give us just the right proportions of amino acids that we need for making our own body proteins. There are no amino acids which are especially scarce, and there are none of which there are too many. It is as if our printer were making his sentence out of just the right pile of letters, as shown in Figure 3–14. The proteins of egg and mother's milk are thus perfectly used for body-building and are thus the best body-building foods there are. They are 100 per cent used for body-building.

All other proteins when they are digested give us a less perfect mixture of amino acids for body-building. When they are digested they give us a less useful mixture of amino acids, like the pile of letters in Figures 3–15 and 3–16. We have to eat more of these other proteins to get the amino acids we need. In eating these proteins we get many amino acids that we do not need (like the pile of letters at the bottom of Figure 3–16) and which we have to burn for energy (see Section 4.1). If we don't get the amino acids we need, we cannot make the protein our body needs and we become malnourished.

This idea of letters (amino acids) making a sentence (a protein) teaches us three things:
1. That the order of the amino acids in a protein is important, and that the order is different in different proteins.
2. That there has to be the right number of each kind of amino acid to make a protein, and that different proteins contain different amounts of each amino acid.
3. That our bodies can make some amino acids out of other ones, but that there are some (the essential amino acids) that it cannot make.

This idea of letters in a sentence is a good one, and we shall use it later on.

Reference proteins. We have just seen that some proteins such as egg and mother's milk contain amino acids in exactly the same amounts as the body wants them. The order of the amino acids in egg protein is different from that in our protein, but this does not matter because digestion breaks them down anyway, and body-building builds them up in the order our bodies want.

Because the proteins of egg and mother's milk are so perfect for body-building, they are sometimes

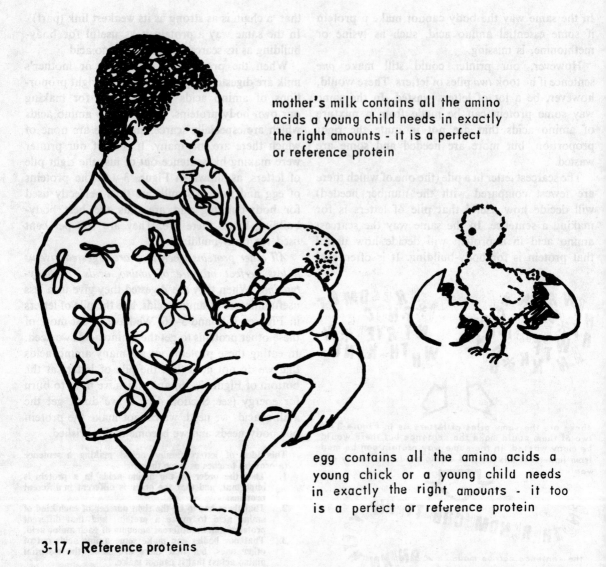

mother's milk contains all the amino acids a young child needs in exactly the right amounts - it is a perfect or reference protein

egg contains all the amino acids a young chick or a young child needs in exactly the right amounts - it too is a perfect or reference protein

3-17, Reference proteins

called **reference proteins.** A reference protein is a protein which is so good for body-building that the usefulness of other proteins can be compared with it or referred to it. Other proteins, especially those in plants, such as maize or groundnuts, are made of amino acids in different amounts from those in the body. They have too many of some amino acids and not enough of others. Maize contains too little of the amino acid lysine, but enough of the amino acid methionine. Peas contain too little methionine but enough lysine. They can be used for body-building, but there is much

waste. It is like our printer making a sentence and being given too many of some letters, but not enough of others. He has to waste many letters of some kinds before he has enough of the letters that are scarce.

Proteins often help one another during body-building. Very often the amino acids that are plentiful in one protein can make up for those that are short in another. Our printer might have two piles of letters from which to make his sentence, one pile with two E's short and an O too many, and the other with two E's too many and an O short. He could make the sentence if he used more than one pile of each kind. He would, however, waste many letters in searching for the one that he wanted, and he would only be able to make one sentence. If, however, he were to take one left-hand pile and one right-hand pile he could make *two* sentences with no waste at all.

In the same way it is possible to get many of the amino acids that we need by eating a very large amount of maize, or a very large amount of peas. But if maize *and* peas are mixed we can get the amino acids from much less food. This is because the lysine in pea protein can make up for the lysine that is lacking in maize protein, and the methionine in maize protein can make up for the methionine that is lacking in pea protein. Thus a mixture of maize meal and pea flour contains the essential amino acids in a better

proportion for body-building than either maize or pea flour alone.

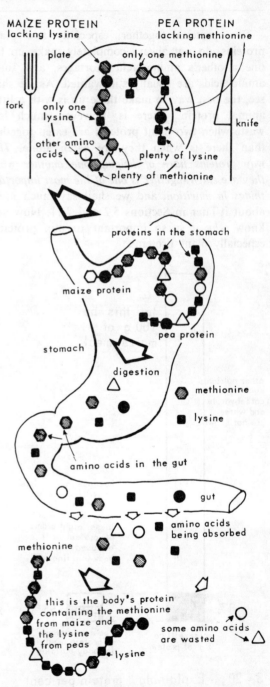

two 'Es' missing and an 'O' too many

two 'Es' too many and an 'O' missing

even though both these piles of letters are not complete, when mixed together they make two sentences very nicely

ANOTHERANDMUCHBETTERWAYOFTHINKING

ANOTHERANDMUCHBETTERWAYOFTHINKING

3-18, Amino acids are like the letters in a sentence - Six

3-19, Proteins often help one another when they are eaten together

PLANT PROTEINS ARE BETTER FOR BODY-BUILDING WHEN THEY ARE MIXED

Two proteins together, especially two plant proteins, do not always completely make up for one another's amino acid shortages, and some amino acids are usually still wanted. As we shall see, the best way to make these up is with a little animal protein. There is, however, much less waste when two plant proteins are eaten together than there is when they are eaten alone. *This way proteins have of helping one another when they are eaten together is one of the most important things in nutrition*, and we shall say much more about it later in Sections 5.2 and 7.11. Now you know *why* it is so important to mix proteins, especially plant proteins.

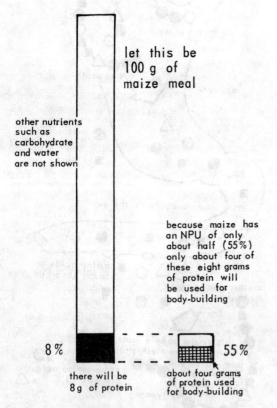

let this be
100 g of
maize meal

other nutrients
such as
carbohydrate
and water
are not shown

because maize has
an NPU of only
about half (55%)
only about four of
these eight grams
of protein will
be used for
body-building

8%   55%

there will be   about four grams
8g of protein   of protein used
                        for body-building

3 - 20,   Explaining protein per cent
          and the NPU using maize
          meal as an example

3.8 Some proteins are better than others for body-building: the NPU.   In the last section we saw that the proteins of egg and mother's milk contain all the amino acids that are needed for body-building in exactly the right amounts. They are thus called reference proteins and can be used for body-building with no waste. In other words they are used for body-building 100 per cent. A special way of saying this is to say that the proteins of egg and mother's milk have a **Net Protein Utilization,** or **NPU,** of 100 per cent. Utilization means 'use'. Net means what is left when what is wasted has been taken away. The 'net utilization' thus means the amount to which proteins are used for body-building, when the amino acids that cannot be used have been burnt for energy by the body (see Section 4.2). Proteins that are only partly used for body-building have NPU's of less than 100 per cent. Maize protein, for example, can only be 55 per cent used for body-building, which means that it can only be about half used. Maize protein thus has an NPU of 55 per cent.

THE NPU MEASURES HOW GOOD A PROTEIN IS FOR BODY-BUILDING

You will see that we have used 'per cent' (%) in two quite different ways. For example, we have said that maize has 8 per cent of protein, and that the usefulness of this protein for body-building (its NPU) is 55 per cent. If you find this difficult to understand, Figure 3–20 may help. Let the bar chart on the left be 100 g of maize meal. Because maize is 8 per cent protein, it will contain 8 g of protein, which is drawn black at the bottom of the bar. This 8 g is shown again in the small bar chart on the right. Because the NPU is only about half (55 per cent), only about half of the 8 g, that is only about 4 g, are used for body-building. The 4 g that can be used for body-building are shown with small squares.

Another way to explain this is to say that 'a part of a part of a food is used for body-building' or that 'a percentage (NPU per cent) of a percentage (protein per cent) of a food is used for body-building'. It may also help to say that the percentage of protein in a food is a measure of the *quantity* of protein in it, and that the NPU measures its *quality*.

From this we see that the percentage of protein in a food is one thing. How good that protein is for body-building (its NPU) is quite another.

Here is a table of proteins and their NPUs.

TABLE 4
The NPU's of Some Proteins

Food	NPU(%)	
Egg protein	100 ⎱	reference
Mother's milk protein	100 ⎰	proteins
Fish protein	83	
Meat protein	80	animal
Cow's milk protein	75	proteins
Sweet potato protein	72	towards
Irish potato protein	71	the top
Liver (beef) protein	65	
Rice protein	57	
Soya bean protein	56	
Millet protein	56	
Maize protein	55	
Wheat (white flour) protein	52	plant
Groundnut protein	48	proteins
Bean protein	47	towards
Pea protein	44	the bottom

(Data from FAO's *Protein Requirements*, 1965)

If you look at Table 4, you will see that the animal proteins come towards the top of the table, and the plant proteins towards the bottom with the lowest NPUs. *On the whole, animal proteins have higher NPUs and are better used for body-building than plant proteins.*

Among the plant proteins, those that have higher NPUs, and are thus better used for body-building, are the proteins of the sweet potato (NPU 72%) and the Irish potato (NPU 71%). It is a pity that the sweet potato has so little protein in it, even if it is so good for body-building. Among the other plant proteins, those of maize, rice, soya bean and millet come next with NPUs of about 55 per cent. These foods contain much more protein. Rice, maize, millet and Irish potatoes contain about 8 per cent, and soya beans as much as 34 per cent. Thus, not only is the protein in these plant foods quite good for body-building, but they contain a lot of it, especially the soya bean.

In Figure 3–19 we saw that proteins often help one another, if they are eaten together. This is also shown by their NPUs. If maize is eaten alone it has an NPU of 55 per cent. The NPU of beans alone is 47 per cent. But, if the right mixture of maize and

beans is eaten *together*, the NPU of the mixture may be 70 per cent. As we have seen, this is because maize helps to supply the methionine that beans lack, and beans help to supply the lysine that maize lacks. The NPU of most mixed foods is likely to be higher and better for body-building. This is why we teach families that 'A good food is a mixed food'.

This has been a difficult chapter, and it may help if we list some of the things that we have learnt so far.

> There are about 20 amino acids.
> By putting these amino acids together in different ways, many different proteins can be made.
> Eight of these amino acids are said to be essential, because the body cannot make them.
> A perfect or reference protein has the amino acids in exactly the amounts the body wants.
> If one or more amino acids are missing from a food protein, it cannot be used for body-building.
> Lack of some amino acids in one food protein can often be made up by mixing two, or more, food proteins together.

3.9 The differences between plant and animal proteins.

Amino acids are made by plants such as maize and beans, and by green plants of all kinds. When, for example, cows eat grass, they use the amino acids in the grass, especially the essential ones, to make their own proteins. When we eat beef (cow's meat) we eat the amino acids that have been made by the grass, eaten by the cow, and made into beef. Cows make a little beef from a lot of grass, and a kilogram of beef protein contains more essential amino acids than a kilogram of grass protein. Our stomachs are different from the stomachs of cows, and we cannot eat grass. We can get some of the protein we need from other green leaves, but we cannot get it all. If we try to live on leaves alone our stomachs feel full, and we get pains. We have, therefore, to get the proteins we need from plants like maize, beans and groundnuts, which contain more protein than green leaves. If we are fortunate, we can get at least some of our proteins from eating animals, or the things that animals make, such as milk and eggs.

In Section 3.8 we saw that animal proteins, like those in eggs, meat, milk and fish, have more essential amino acids. They are very like those in our bodies, they have high NPUs, and they are very good for body-building, even if they are eaten alone.

The plant proteins, like those in maize, beans and groundnuts, have fewer essential amino acids. They are less like the proteins in our own bodies. They nearly all have lower NPUs, and they are good for body-building, but *only if they are eaten together*. Plant proteins are also much cheaper than animal protein, and it is usually easier for people to grow plants than to keep animals. Here is a list of the differences between these two kinds of protein.

TABLE 5
The Differences Between Animal and Plant Proteins

Animal proteins	Plant proteins
Contain more essential amino acids	Contain fewer essential amino acids
Higher NPU's	Lower NPU's
Very like the proteins in our own bodies	Not very like the proteins in our own bodies
Very good for body-building, even if eaten alone	Very good for body-building, only if eaten together
Expensive	Cheaper
It is often difficult to keep animals	It is usually easy to grow protein-containing plants, such as legumes

Plant proteins are important because they can be grown almost anywhere and are cheap. They do not need rivers like fish, and are not harmed by tsetse flies like cows. Although the animal proteins, like meat, milk, eggs and fish, can help, they are expensive, and there will never be enough of them at a cheap enough price to give everyone the protein they need. Most families will have to get most of the proteins they need from plants, especially the good staple foods (see Section 4.3) and legumes.

3.10 Legumes and dark green leaves. Beans and peas and groundnuts are examples of plants called **legumes**. There are many hundreds of different kinds of legumes, and they contain more protein than most other plants. Legumes are also useful because they take nitrogen out of the air and leave it in the soil so that other plants can use it. A crop of legumes, therefore, leaves the soil richer in nitrogen than it was before. One of the most important ways of helping families to eat enough protein is to grow plenty of legumes, especially the soya bean.

THERE IS A LOT OF PROTEIN IN LEGUMES

The soya bean is a famous legume because it contains 34 per cent of protein. It comes from China, and although it is not yet widely grown in Africa some farmers are growing it. The Chinese get much of their protein from soya beans and are well nourished. However, these beans have one particular difficulty. They must be cooked in special ways, or they will not be digested. A good way to eat them is to leave them to sprout (grow a little) in the dark before they are cooked and eaten.

Many new ways are now being found to process (change) soya bean protein, and make it into different kinds of food. Soya bean protein can even be made into something that looks and tastes very like meat, and is nearly as good as meat for body-building, but is much cheaper. We shall soon see many more new foods made from soya beans. This is another reason why more soya beans must be grown.

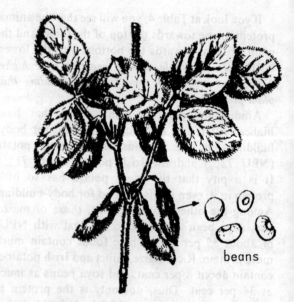

3 - 21, The soya bean

Some plants, such as the soya bean, require micro-organisms (very small living things, or germs) in the soil to help them to grow. If you plant soya beans in a new place where they have not grown before, you may have to sow the bean seeds and the micro-organisms that these beans need to grow. These micro-organisms can most easily be got by taking a little soil from a place where soya beans have been growing successfully before, and planting it with the bean seeds.

Dark green leaves. Although eating legumes is the best way of eating vegetable protein, dark green leaves are also very important. They are found everywhere in the bush, and some of them, such as cassava leaves, are even found at the end of the dry season. They are especially important, therefore, as an always-ready way of getting a little plant protein, and of getting a different kind of plant protein to make a mixture. If mothers have no protein, or only very little, ask them to gather lots of leaves. It is difficult for an adult to get all the protein he needs from eating leaves, and a child certainly cannot; so, in hungry times, we should ask mothers to give children the best protein foods they have, such as beans, and let adults eat leaves.

It is often thought that the light green leaves of cabbages are a better and more 'prestigious' food than the dark green leaves. However, cabbage contains almost no protein, and the dark green leaves of the bush contain five times as much. We should *not* teach mothers either to grow or to eat cabbage.

3.11 What makes a protein food good for children.

Chapter 6 is about feeding children, but this is the best place to think about the things which make a protein food good for feeding children. If a food contains a lot of protein—that is it contains a high percentage of protein—it is good for feeding children. If the protein in it has a high NPU and is thus good for body-building, this also makes the food a good one. If there is a lot of protein in a small space or bulk, this is also good (Section 7.8). If the protein food is cheap and tastes nice, this too is good.

If the food also has plenty of joules of energy, this makes it even better. Mother's milk is the best food for young children. It may not seem to contain very much protein, but this is because it has all the other nutrients a child needs, including all the water. Also, the protein it has is so good that it is 100 per cent used for body-building, and none is wasted.

TABLE 6
Things that Make Protein Food Good for Children

A high percentage of protein
The usefulness of the protein for body-building, or a high NPU
Small bulk
Cheapness
A good taste
Easy to prepare, so a mother will make it often

3.12 THINGS TO DO

(a) The protein game. Here is a 'protein game' that can be played in class. Let the teacher write on the board a sentence which shall be the perfect or reference protein and which is 100% Used for body-building. Let him take this sentence as an example: 'A YOUNG CHILD NEEDS PLENTY OF PROTEIN'. Let the vowels be the essential amino acids that the body cannot make, and let the other letters be the non-essential amino acids that the body can make. Then let all the members of the class take a 'protein' and see how good it is for body-building. Let these proteins be the first words of one of the sections of this book. Let the class count how many letters (amino acids) they need to get all the vowels (essential amino acids) in the 'young child' sentence. The member of the class who gets these vowels in the smallest number of letters has the best protein for body-building and so wins the game.

The young child sentence contains one A, four E's, two I's, three O's and one U. If we try the game on the 'protein' of this section and start with 'Things to . . .', we find that we get the A, the E's, I's and O's very easily but that we have to wait until we get to the U in Used before we get a U, and so get all the vowels (essential amino acids) that we need. Starting with 'Things to . . .' we have to go through 152 letters, or amino acids, until we get this U and so get all the essential amino acids we need. The 'protein' of this section is not therefore, a very good one. The protein of Section 3.11 is much better, and we get all our essential amino acids in only 52 letters.

How good is the 'protein' of your section?

(b) Teaching about proteins. One of the best ways of teaching about proteins is to use a necklace or string of beads. The easiest beads to use are the plastic ones that children play with, and which fit into one another without the need for a string to hold them together. By using beads like this you can teach about the way amino acids make a chain, about the way the chain rolls up to make a protein, about the importance of the order of the amino acids in a protein, about the different proportions (amounts) of different amino acids in different proteins, about reference proteins, and about how two proteins can help one another in body-building. If you have not got beads, use bottle tops with a hole in them, small rolls of coloured paper, buttons, or corks. Perhaps the best way of all is to use the members of the class as amino acids, and to get them to make an amino acid chain by holding onto each other's hands to make a line. They can then make a protein by all coming together into a pile! Their protein can be 'digested' by leaving go of their hands, and they can 'body-build' a new protein by joining up again in a different order. The class will not forget this lesson in a hurry! This, by the way, is an idea for teaching students in a class, not mothers in a clinic!

The 'letters' part of this chapter is sometimes thought to be difficult. It can be made easier by writing each of the letters of the sentence 'Another and much better way of thinking . . .' on a piece of paper and cutting them out. Can the sentence be made from the pile of letters so made, if there is an O and an E missing? Can one sentence be made from two such piles?

(c) Answers from Section 2.10 on categories of rehabilitation. If you used the curve card in the right way you will have found that Simon showed Category A rehabilitation all the time. Mary started in Category A, continued in Category B and ended in Category C.

Chapter Four

ENERGY FOODS,
VITAMINS AND MINERALS,
NON-FOODS AND WATER

ENERGY FOODS

4.1a Energy. A tractor needs diezel if it is going to plough the ground and do work. When the tractor is running this diezel is burnt and used up. Diezel is an energy food for the tractor. In the same way our bodies need energy foods if we are going to move and work. But we are different from tractors. When a tractor's engine is turned off it does not use any more diezel. But our bodies use energy from our food all the time until we are dead. While we are asleep our heart keeps pumping, and we have to breathe and keep warm. This uses up some energy. When we move and walk around we use up more energy. If we run fast or do heavy work, like digging or carrying a heavy load, we use up still more energy; *so we need plenty of energy for heavy work*.

Just as tractors need diezel to give them the energy to plough, so our bodies need energy foods. There are two kinds of energy food—carbohydrates and fats or oils. Most carbohydrates are the white powdery foods like sugar or flour. For example, a man digging can use the energy of the carbohydrate in maize to give him the energy that he needs to dig. It may surprise you to think that the body can 'burn' food to make heat and energy. It really is burning, but it goes on so slowly that there is no smoke or flame, and our bodies become only slightly warm. A tractor burning diezel gets hot as well as doing work, and in the same way we keep warm by burning energy foods. Our bodies are cooler at night when we are asleep and get hotter when we are awake and work hard.

The gas called carbon dioxide is made when food is burnt in the body, and when diezel is burnt in a tractor. Carbon dioxide goes out of a man in his breath and out of a tractor in its exhaust. We have already seen that plants take carbon dioxide from the air and energy from the sun to make the energy foods and proteins that they contain. Carbon dioxide thus goes round in a circle from plants to man and animals and then back again. By burning up energy food man uses energy that plants have taken from the sun.

In an earlier section we saw that cells make our bodies, as houses make a village, and that proteins make cells, as bricks make a house. Just as it is hard work and uses energy to lift bricks and make a house, so our bodies use energy to make cells out of protein. *Children therefore need energy for growing.* Protein foods give us the proteins from which our cells are built, while energy foods give us the energy to do the building. Thus a pregnant mother needs energy to give to her child who is growing in her womb. A nursing mother needs energy to put into the milk to give the child at her breast. Children of all ages need the energy with which to grow, to run and play, and to walk to school.

4.1b Joules. Sometimes we want to measure energy. We want to measure how much energy a man needs to do a certain amount of work or to run a mile. We also want to measure how much energy there is in each of the foods that he eats. We use joules to measure energy in the same way that we use grams to measure weight and metres to measure length. The joule is said to be the **unit** of energy in the same way that the kilogram is the unit of weight and the metre the unit of length.

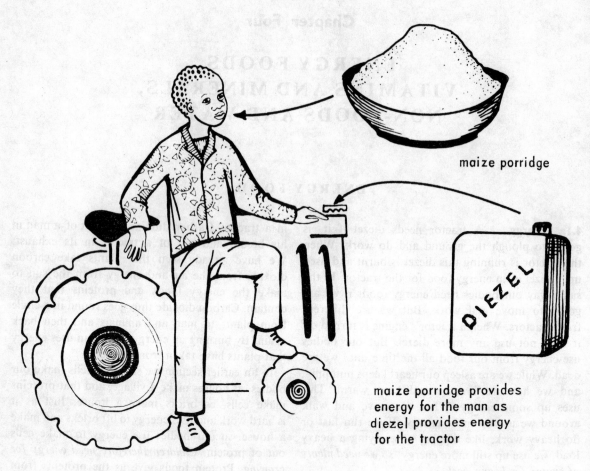

maize porridge

maize porridge provides
energy for the man as
diezel provides energy
for the tractor

4-1, Energy foods for a man and his tractor

Until a little time ago people working in nutrition used another unit for measuring energy—the calorie.* The calorie was used in some sciences but not in others. This was very inconvenient, so all scientists are now going to use the same system of units. A system is something made of parts that work together. All scientists are now going to use the **SI system,** or International System of units. Joules are part of the SI system of units, so are grams, metres and seconds, but not calories, feet or pounds. This book is written in SI units, so you will read here about millimetres (a thousandth part of a metre), kilograms (a thousand grams) and joules, but not about calories or inches, because they are not SI units. There are many other SI units besides those you have just read, such as the volt and the ohm. These are used in other sciences but not in nutrition.

If you are starting to learn nutrition, it will be easy for you to think about measuring energy in joules. If you have already started to learn nutrition using calories, you will have to change to joules.

*Note: The calorie previously used in nutrition was the 'big Calorie', kilocalorie, kcal, kal, or Cal. It was thus equal to about four kilojoules. The exact figure is 1 kcal = 4.184 kJ. Thus when 2,500 Calories was specified as a man's daily energy need this is equal to about 4 × 2,500 kilojoules, which is 10,000 kilojoules or 10 megajoules. More exactly it is 4.18 × 2,500 Calories, which is 10.45 megajoules.

We had not used joules before we came to write this book, but as we used them we came to like them more and more. If you are used to calories and try to work in joules, you will find that they grow on you!

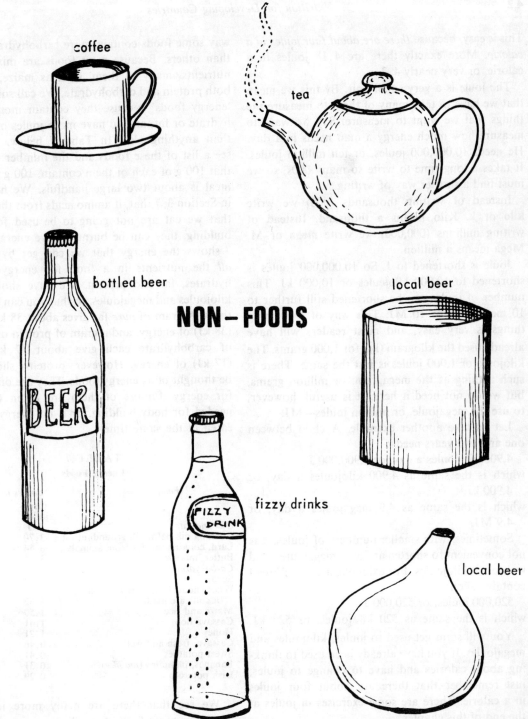

coffee

tea

bottled beer

NON – FOODS

local beer

BEER

fizzy drinks

FIZZY DRINK

local beer

4-2, Non - foods

This is easy, because *there are about four joules in a calorie.* More exactly there are 4.18 joules in a calorie, or very nearly 4.2.

The joule is a very small unit. By this we mean that we have to take many of them to measure the things that we want to measure. Say we want to measure how much energy a man needs in a day. He needs 10,000,000 joules, or ten million joules. It takes a long time to write so many 000s, so we must find a shorter way of writing.

Instead of writing thousands (000) we write **kilo** or k. Kilo means a thousand. Instead of writing millions (000,000) we write **mega** or M. Mega means a million.

Joule is shortened to J. So 10,000,000 joules is shortened to 10,000 **kilojoules** or 10,000 kJ. This number of joules can be shortened still further to 10 **megajoules** or 10 MJ. This way of shortening things is very easy, and most readers will have already used the kilogram (kg) for 1,000 grams. The kilojoule or 1,000 joules is just the same. There is such a thing as the megagram, or million grams, but we do not need it here. It is useful, however, to use the megajoule, or million joules—MJ.

Let us take another example. A child between one and two years needs:

4,900,000 joules a day, or 4,900,000 J

which is the same as 4,900 kilojoules a day, or 4,900 kJ

which is the same as 4.9 megajoules a day, or 4.9 MJ.

Sometimes, with smaller numbers of joules, it is not convenient to shorten as far as megajoules, and we stop at kilojoules. For example, a slice of bread contains about:

520,000 joules, or 520,000 J

which is the same as 520 kilojoules, or 520 kJ.

You will soon get used to joules, kilojoules and megajoules. If you have already been used to thinking about calories and have to change to joules, just remember that there are about four joules in a calorie. There are some exercises in joules at the end of this chapter.

4.2   Energy foods.   We have already seen that most foods are mixtures of nutrients and that some foods contain more protein than others. In the same

way some foods contain more carbohydrate or fat than others. Because most foods are mixtures of nutrients, many of them, such as maize, contain both protein and carbohydrate. We call some foods 'energy foods' because they contain more carbohydrate or fat, and so have more joules of energy, than anything else. In Table 7 below, you will see a list of these foods and the number of joules that 100 g of each of them contain. 100 g of maize meal is about two large handfuls. We have seen in Section 3.7 that, if amino acids from the protein that we eat are not going to be used for body-building, they can be burnt to give energy. Table 7 shows the energy that we can get by burning *all* the nutrients in a food for energy—carbohydrates, fat and protein. We have shown both kilojoules and megajoules, so that you can compare them. A gram of *pure* fat gives about 38 kilojoules (38 kJ) of energy, and a gram of protein or a gram of carbohydrate each give about 17 kilojoules (17 kJ) of energy. However, proteins should not be thought of as energy foods. They are only burnt for energy if more of them are eaten than are needed for body-building, or if no energy food is eaten at the same time.

TABLE 7
Energy Foods

Food	Joules in 100 g	
	mega-joules MJ	kilo-joules kJ
Oils and fats		
Cooking oil, palm oil, groundnut oil	3.70	3,700
Lard, cooking fat, fat from animals	3.54	3,540
Butter, margarine	3.01	3,010
Carbohydrates		
Sugar	1.62	1,620
Wheat flour, from which bread and biscuits are made	1.52	1,520
Maize and rice	1.50	1,500
Cassava flour	1.41	1,410
Honey	1.21	1,210
Cassava, fresh and wet	0.46	460
Sweet potatoes	0.41	410
Bananas, plantains (*matoke*)	0.31	310
Irish potatoes	0.29	290

We see that there are many more joules of energy in some foods than there are in others. In some foods, such as cabbage, there is so little energy that they are not in the list. 100 g of cabbage only contain about 71 kilojoules (71 kJ). There are 1,500 kJ in 100 g of maize meal. A man can easily get the energy he needs from a plate of maize *nshima*, but he will get very little from a plate of cabbage.

Oils and fats are the best energy foods there are, but they are also expensive, and few families have enough money to get many of the joules they need from oils and fats, nor do many people want to eat so much fat. Oils and fats are useful for cooking and for adding more joules of energy to foods. In Section 7.8 you will read how useful it is to add some joule-giving margarine to a child's maize porridge.

Carbohydrates and fats only provide energy. They cannot be used for body-building because they contain no amino acids. For example, if a child is fed only on an almost pure carbohydrate food like cassava, he will not grow. This is because the cassava will only give him the energy to run about and play. Because it contains so little protein and thus so few amino acids, it cannot build and repair his body.

4.3 Staple foods. You will often hear the important carbohydrate food of a place called the **staple.** Many people get both their energy food and most of the protein they need from their staple. In many parts of Africa maize or cassava are staple foods. In other countries rice (India) or potatoes (Ireland) or bread (Europe) are the staple foods. Some Ugandans eat a kind of green banana called a plantain. The Ugandan name for these plantains and the staple food they make from it is *matoke*.

As we saw in Section 3.4 good staple foods, such as wheat, maize, rice and millet, contain about 8 per cent of protein and are thus much better than staples like bananas and cassava, which only contain about 1 per cent of protein. People who have these high-protein staples are thus usually better nourished than those who have low-protein staples. In the old days, several kinds of millet, such as finger millet, bulrush millet, or sorghum were the staple foods of Africa. Maize, cassava and bananas were brought to Africa from other countries. It is good that maize has come, but it is not so good that Africa now has both cassava and bananas. Cassava was often brought

to a village as a famine or starvation food that would only be eaten if the millet failed. But what has happened is that cassava, which is so easy to grow, has been grown more, and millet, which is more difficult to grow, has been grown less and less. Children are now, therefore, being fed, not on millet porridge as they used to be, but on cassava porridge, which contains only an eighth as much protein.

No wonder, therefore, that malnutrition is getting worse in cassava districts. This is a pity, and we should encourage people to grow either millet or maize instead of some of their cassava. Cassava does, however, have several advantages. You can eat its leaves, whereas you cannot eat the leaves of maize, and it is easy to store. It can stay in the ground for two years before it is eaten. Cassava also lives through a year when there is so little rain that maize will not grow. This is why cassava is a useful famine food. In places where the rains sometimes fail it is wise for families to grow *some* cassava, but to eat it only when there is not enough maize. The sweet potato is another food whose leaves and roots can both be eaten.

A GOOD STAPLE GIVES A FAMILY MUCH OF THE PROTEIN IT NEEDS

Maize and other grains can be made into meal in several ways. The whole grain can be made into meal and nothing thrown away. This is ordinary maize meal which contains 8 per cent protein and costs 7 ngwee a kilo in Zambia. Maize can also be made into meal in such a way that the outer part of the grain and the **germ** are thrown away. The germ is the part of the grain where the plant is going to start growing from. This kind of maize meal is whiter than ordinary maize meal and is called refined maize meal. The outer part of the grain and the germ contain much of the protein of maize; so refined maize meal contains less protein than ordinary maize meal, which is made from the whole of the grain. In Zambia refined maize meal is often called 'breakfast' meal. It costs 10 ngwee a kilo and only contains 7 per cent of protein. It is thus not such a good buy as ordinary maize meal.

OUTSIDE

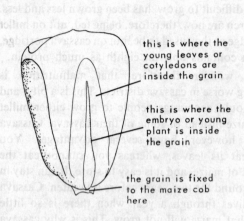

this is where the young leaves or cotyledons are inside the grain

this is where the embryo or young plant is inside the grain

the grain is fixed to the maize cob here

4-3, A maize grain

CUT IN HALF

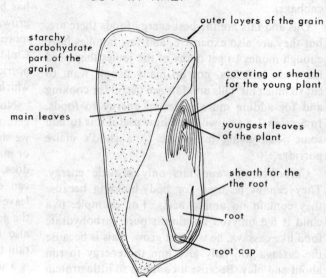

starchy carbohydrate part of the grain

outer layers of the grain

covering or sheath for the young plant

main leaves

youngest leaves of the plant

sheath for the the root

root

root cap

MAIZE IS A BETTER FOOD FOR CHILDREN THAN CASSAVA

VITAMINS AND MINERALS

4.4 What vitamins and minerals are. We have said that a house is made of bricks, and that our bodies are made out of cells, which are mostly made from proteins. When we build a house we need a few other things besides bricks, and the energy to do the building. We need nails and a lock to fasten the door. A lock may not seem an important part of the house, but it is necessary to keep the house safe. In the same way the body needs a few special things if it is to work properly and stay healthy. These are the **vitamins** and **minerals.** The body can make most of the things it needs from energy foods and the amino acids in protein, but it cannot make vitamins or minerals. Only very small amounts of these (only a few milligrams or even less) need to be eaten each day to keep the body healthy.

The vitamins are special molecules made mostly by plants. They are often given the letters A, B, C, D, etc. Minerals are elements which are found in the ground and which the body can get

from food or water. **Iron** that helps to make the blood red, and **calcium** that helps to make bones hard, are both minerals. The foods which contain plenty of vitamins or minerals are often called **protective foods.** If people eat too little of any of them, they get certain diseases. There are particular diseases caused by a lack of each vitamin or mineral. People are therefore protected from that illness by eating enough of the vitamin or mineral. Protection means guarding or keeping away. When you talk to mothers, talk about protective foods rather than about vitamins and minerals, because they will find this easier to understand.

VITAMINS ARE ONLY NEEDED IN VERY SMALL AMOUNTS

As we have already seen, most foods are mixtures of nutrients. Many of them contain vitamins and minerals as well as protein and energy food. Thus, when a child lacks protein, he usually lacks vitamins and joules as well. *So, if he can be given the protein and joules he needs, he will usually get the vitamins and minerals he wants at the same time.* This is why the section on vitamins is shorter here than it is in some other books.

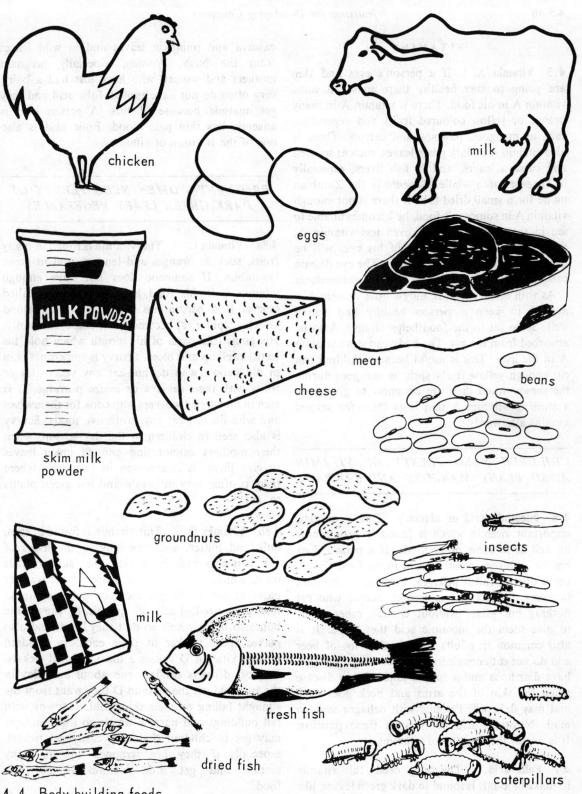

chicken

eggs

milk

meat

MILK POWDER

cheese

beans

skim milk powder

groundnuts

insects

milk

fresh fish

dried fish

caterpillars

4-4, Body-building foods

VITAMINS

4.5 Vitamin A.   If a person's eyes and skin are going to stay healthy there must be some vitamin A in his food. There is vitamin A in many orange or yellow coloured fruits and vegetables, such as mangoes, pawpaw and carrots. There is also vitamin A in dark green leaves, such as spinach and cassava leaves, and in fish livers, especially in *kapenta* eaten whole. *Kapenta* is the Zambian name for a small dried fish. If there is not enough vitamin A in someone's food, he becomes unable to see in the dark. If he has even less vitamin A, the clear front part (cornea) of his eyes will be harmed and he may become blind. The eye disease caused by lack of vitamin A is called **keratomalacia.**

As with other vitamins, only a little vitamin A is needed to keep a person healthy and seeing well. Some fat in the food helps vitamin A to be absorbed from the gut. The body can store vitamin A in the liver. This is useful because children can eat enough yellow fruits such as mangoes during the season when they are common to give them a store of vitamin A that lasts them for several months afterwards.

CHILDREN NEED PLENTY OF VITAMIN A, SO PLANT MANGOES AND PAWPAWS

4.6 Nicotinic acid or niacin.   This is another important vitamin which is found in groundnuts as well as in some other foods. If a person does not have enough nicotinic acid in his food he will get a disease called **pellagra.** Pellagra is common in many districts and is seen in people who eat nothing but maize without enough other foods to give them the nicotinic acid they need. It is also common in adults who drink a lot of beer and do not eat enough food. Patients with pellagra have diarrhoea and a special kind of skin disease when the skin of the arms and neck goes dark and may flake off. Patients with pellagra may go mad. Nicotinic acid soon cures these patients. It is one of the B group of vitamins.

4.7 Folic acid.   The body needs this vitamin to make blood. It is found in dark green leaves, like cassava and pumpkin leaves and in wild leaves from the bush. Women, especially pregnant mothers and women who have just had a baby, very often do not have enough folic acid and may get **anaemic** because of this. A person who is anaemic has thin pale blood. Folic acid is also one of the B group of vitamins.

PREGNANT WOMEN NEED PLENTY OF DARK GREEN LEAFY VEGETABLES

4.8a Vitamin C.   This vitamin is found in many fruits, such as oranges and lemons, and in green vegetables. If someone does not have enough vitamin C in his food he gets a disease called **scurvy.** If a person has scurvy his small blood vessels (capillaries) become weak and break easily. His gums (the parts of his mouth which hold his teeth) swell up and bleed. Scurvy is sometimes seen in old people who do not eat any vegetables or fruits with their cassava or maize porridge. It is seen in unmarried workers who cook for themselves and who do not eat any protective foods. Scurvy is also seen in children in the dry season, when their mothers cannot find enough green leaves to give them. It is common in Botswana where there is often very little rain and few green plants to eat.

4.8b Vitamin D.   This vitamin is found in eggs, milk and butter, and especially in the livers of fish. It is also made in the skin when sunlight falls on it, which is the way that people in the warmer parts of the world get most of the Vitamin D that they need. Lack of vitamin D causes the bones to become soft so that they bend, and also makes them thicker at their ends. In children lack of vitamin D causes a disease called **rickets.** In most districts children run about and play in the sun, and get the vitamin D they want from the sunlight falling on their skins. But in towns with tall buildings and narrow streets so little sunlight may get to children that they easily get rickets, especially if they are wrapped up in many clothes and get little vitamin D in their food.

MINERALS

4.9 Salt.   Salt is a mineral made of the elements sodium and chlorine. Even the poorest villagers try to buy some salt. Salt makes food taste better, but there is usually enough in most foods to give the body all it needs. There is thus seldom any need to add extra salt to food. The ash from burnt plants or trees is sometimes mixed with water, and the liquid part of the mixture is added to food. The Bemba call this *ifishikisa*. It contains salt and smaller amounts of other minerals.

Soda is sometimes bought and added to green vegetables to make them greener when they are cooked. Soda is another mineral and is rather like salt.

4.10 Iron.   This is a mineral element which the body needs to make blood. There is iron in meat and in dark green, leafy vegetables and legumes. If there is not enough iron in the food the body cannot make enough blood, and so the blood becomes thin and weak and anaemic. Women are especially likely to lack iron and often become anaemic. This is because there is iron in blood, and each month a woman loses some blood in her period. A pregnant mother may also lack iron because iron is needed by the child in her womb.

4.11 Iodine.   This mineral element is found in very small amounts in water and in some foods. If someone does not have enough iodine, his thyroid gland may swell in his neck and he may get a swelling called a **goitre**. In some districts there is so little iodine in the ground that very little can get into the food. Goitres may therefore be so common that the local people have a name for them. The Bemba call them *chibukulo*. One way of preventing goitres in districts where there is very little iodine is to add some iodine to the salt that is sold. Iodized salt can thus prevent goitres in districts where they are common.

4.12 Calcium.   This mineral element is needed by the body to make bones. Pregnant and nursing mothers need calcium to make their child's bones. Many foods, especially milk, millet and dried fish, contain calcium. People get more calcium from eating dried fish than fresh fish because, when they

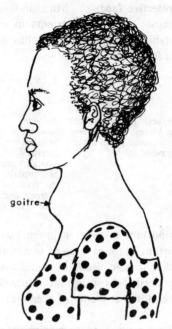

4-5,   A goitre

eat dried fish, they usually eat the bones as well. It is the bones that have the calcium. Some rocks contain calcium, and a little of it gets into water, such as well-water which has come through the ground. There is almost always enough calcium in the food, so disease caused by lack of calcium is rare.

4.13 Fluorine.   This mineral element is found in water and helps to build strong teeth. When there is no fluorine in the water of a district, many people get **caries** (holes in their teeth). When there is a little fluorine in the water—about one part of fluorine in a million parts of water—people's teeth become stronger, and there is little caries. However, too much fluorine in the water causes brown patches in the teeth. Just enough fluorine should therefore be added to water that has too little, so that it can help to stop people getting holes in their teeth. This is very easy and cheap, and in some countries many towns are adding a little fluorine to their water supply. There are other things which help to cause caries besides lack of fluorine. Sugar and fizzy drinks are just two of them but putting the right amount of fluorine in the water is a great help in making strong teeth.

4.14 Protective foods. Minerals and vitamins are the most important nutrients in many fruits and vegetables. These foods are thus often called protective foods.

TABLE 8
Protective Foods

cassava leaves, pumpkin and pumpkin leaves, sweet potato leaves and many green leaves from the bush	mangoes
	pawpaw
	oranges
tomatoes	guavas
peppers	avocado pears
carrots	pineapples
	the fruit of the *mpundu* tree, and wild fruits of many kinds

The important mineral in green leaves is iron. The important vitamins in green leaves are vitamins A, C and folic acid. Both iron and folic acid are especially needed by pregnant mothers. Mothers should therefore eat plenty of green leaves.

EVERYONE SHOULD EAT SOME PROTECTIVE FOOD EVERY DAY

Most people think of vegetables as a way of eating minerals and vitamins, but, as you have read, there is also a *little* protein in vegetables, especially in those with *dark* green leaves. Dark green leaves contain 5 per cent protein, whereas pale vegetables contain only 1 per cent. Dark green, leafy vegetables are thus useful both for providing minerals and vitamins and also for providing a little protein. By dark green, leafy vegetables we mean pumpkin leaves, spinach and cassava leaves and not cabbage, which is pale. A good rule when thinking about protective foods is to remember that the darker they are the more vitamins and proteins they are likely to contain.

The avocado pear is both a protective food and an energy food because it contains much oil, which provides 690 kilojoules (kJ) in 100 g. It is thus a good food for young children.

Some foods, such as onions, peppers, chillies and mushrooms, make food taste good, so that people want to eat more of them. They may thus be more important in helping people to eat more of other foods than they are as foods themselves.

NON-FOODS

4.15 'Fizzy drinks', beer and tea. Many families spend much money on fizzy drinks which contain nothing but water, gas and a very little sugar. Apart from the sugar and the water, they contain no nutrients at all. We cannot give you the names of these foods, because these are what are called **brand names,** and if we said anything bad about them, the makers would take us to court for saying that their drinks are not good! But you surely know their names very well. They are advertised on the radio and in the newspapers, and many people think that they are buying useful food when they are buying a bottle of one of these drinks. Children are sometimes given a bottle of fizzy drink for their meals, when they should be given some energy and body-building foods instead. This is sad, because fizzy drinks cost more than milk. These drinks are a block in the food-path (see Chapter 9) and are one of the important causes of malnutrition in many countries. This is why we have called them **non-foods.** 'Non' means no or not—they are *not* foods!

Fizzy drinks also help to cause caries or holes in the teeth. This is one of the reasons why the teeth of many town children are not so healthy as the teeth of their fathers, who did not have these drinks when they were young.

FIZZY DRINKS ARE NOT FOOD AND ARE A WASTE OF SCARCE MONEY

Beer is another non-food. Beer contains alcohol which makes people drunk and gives some joules of energy. Even so, beer is a bad food for children, and no child should be given beer. It should be a rule that beer is a man's drink, and that a child should not drink beer until he has become a man. In many places beer is an even more important cause of malnutrition than fizzy drinks. Read in Section 9.11 how beer blocks the food-path and causes malnutrition.

Tea and coffee are two more drinks that contain no food of any kind, except the milk or sugar that are added to them. But tea and coffee are not bad, they are not expensive, and they do not make you drunk. They are nice drinks, but they are not foods. One of the useful things about tea, coffee and fizzy drinks is that they are unlikely to contain any harmful micro-organisms (germs) because boiling kills them.

4.16   The food groups.   There are many kinds of food, and we have seen that most of them are mixtures of nutrients. Even so, it is sometimes useful to put foods of the same kind together into groups, especially for teaching. A group is several things of the same kind together. Foods are usually put into three food groups according to their main nutrient. These groups are the **body-building or protein foods,** the **energy foods,** and the **protective foods.**

There are several difficulties with the food groups. Maize, for example, is put with the energy foods because it contains 78 per cent of carbohydrate. Yet maize also contains 8 per cent of protein; it should therefore go into the body-building group as well. This is especially so as maize eaters commonly eat so much maize that they get most of their protein in this way. Dark green leaves are in the group of protective foods, yet they also contain a useful amount of body-building protein.

WATER

4.17a   Water.   Water is a nutrient. It is needed for drinking, cooking, and washing, as well as in the fields and factories. People die if they do not have water, and if they do not have enough good, clean water they become sick. Food and water are the most important needs of any family, and to be able to turn on a tap inside the house and get plenty of clean, safe water is one of the greatest blessings anyone can enjoy. Many families are not so fortunate, and mothers may have to walk many miles each day carrying water. A study in East Africa showed that mothers there use about 12 per cent of their daily energy fetching water, and in hilly districts as much as 27 per cent! A worker in an African city may spend between 10 and 20 per cent of his wages in buying water. Plenty of good food and enough cheap, clean, safe water are therefore some of the greatest needs of most families.

By safe water we mean water without any harmful micro-organisms in it which can cause disease. Many micro-organisms can be spread by water, and some of the most dangerous are those which cause diarrhoea. These micro-organisms usually get into the water from the gut (stomach, bowels, intestines) of other people. Safe water is therefore water which cannot have been mixed with human **faeces** or **urine** (the waste water from the body). By human faeces we mean the stools or waste from the bowels of people. Animal faeces can also be harmful, but they are not nearly so dangerous as the faeces of man. *Human faeces must therefore be kept out of food and drinking water.* Even a very very little can be dangerous—much less than we can see with our eyes.

KEEP HUMAN FAECES OUT OF DRINKING WATER

Faeces get into food and drinking water in three main ways.

Through the ground or in streams and rivers.   If wells for drinking water and pit-latrines for faeces are too close together, harmful micro-organisms can get through the ground with water into the well. Latrines and wells must therefore be as far apart as possible, so that micro-organisms cannot get from the latrine into the water. Wells and latrines should never be less than 50 metres apart. The top of a well should also be well protected with cement, so that the only water that can get into it has to come deeply through the ground. No water should be able to get into the well from the top, where it may contain dirt, and perhaps faeces with harmful micro-organisms in them.

Everyone should always pass their faeces and urine into a latrine, where it will slowly be made harmless, and not into a river or stream from which drinking water is drawn. Springs should be protected, so that clean water can be taken from them easily and there is no chance of them being mixed with human faeces.

On fingers.   When someone passes his faeces or urine, it is always possible that micro-organisms from his faeces or urine will get onto his fingers.

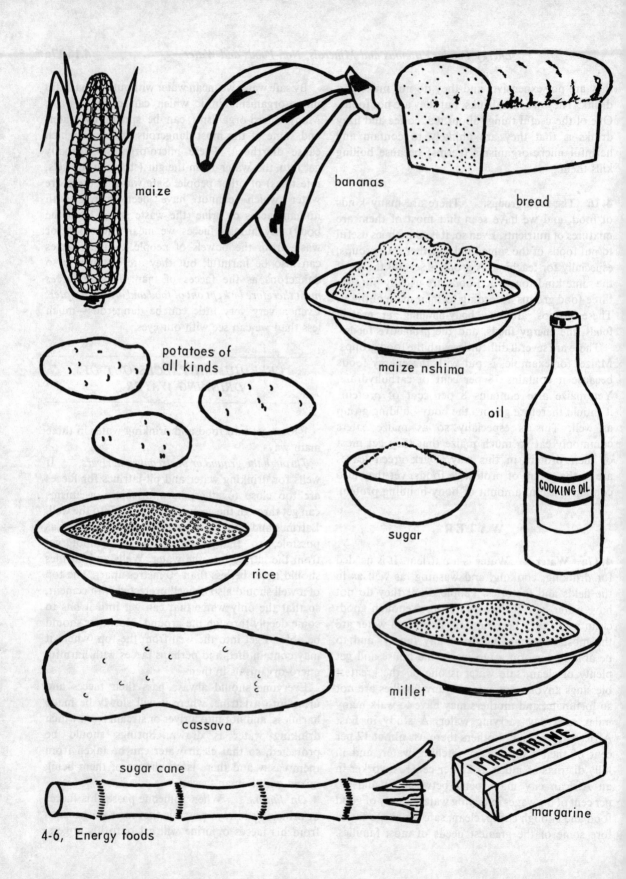

maize

bananas

bread

maize nshima

potatoes of all kinds

oil

sugar

COOKING OIL

rice

millet

cassava

sugar cane

MARGARINE

margarine

4-6, Energy foods

If he now goes and prepares food, these micro-organisms may get from his fingers into the food. They are not likely to harm the person from whom they came, but they may harm other people who eat the food. We must all wash our hands before cooking food, especially if we cook food for many people.

ALWAYS WASH YOUR HANDS AFTER GOING TO THE LATRINE

Through flies. It has been said that flies like two courses (parts) to their meal—a first course of faeces and a second course of our food! Micro-organisms from faeces stick onto a fly's feet and then fall off into our food. Faeces must thus always be passed into a latrine which is protected from flies, and flies must be kept away from food.

ALWAYS WASH YOUR HANDS BEFORE COOKING FOOD

4.17b Making water safe to drink. If you are not sure that water is safe, and it is possible for human faeces to have got into it, boil it. Boiling kills micro-organisms, and water which has been brought to the boil is safe to drink. There is no need to boil it for many minutes; all that needs to be done is to bring it to the boil, to make sure it is boiling well and then to let it cool. A good way to keep drinking water is to boil it and then put it into a clay pot with a lid, so that flies cannot get to it. A clay pot lets a little water through, so its outside is always slightly damp (wet). If the pot is in a place where the air is flowing past it well, some water will evaporate (go into the air) from the outside of the pot. The evaporation of this water cools the water in the pot, so that it is always cool to drink.

Everyone should drink safe water, but it is especially important that young children should always drink water that contains no harmful micro-organisms which may give them diarrhoea. This is why a young child should always be given boiled

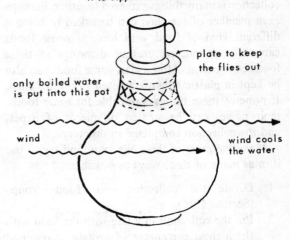

keep the cup on the plate so that it is clean when it is dipped into the water

plate to keep the flies out

only boiled water is put into this pot

wind

wind cools the water

4-7, Boiled water

water if he is thirsty, and why an *artificial feed should always be made with boiled water.*

A lot of fuel is needed to boil all the water a family drinks. But fuel is often so scarce that families cannot boil all their water. What can they do? As we saw in Section 2.3, underweight children get diarrhoea much more often than well-nourished ones. One thing that families *can* do is to keep their children well nourished, so that they will be less likely to get diarrhoea when they drink unboiled water. Also, when a well-nourished child does get diarrhoea, he is less likely to be harmed by it than he would if he were malnourished. Another thing that mothers can do is to make sure they breast-feed. As we shall soon see, there are no harmful micro-organisms in healthy breast milk.

IF A CHILD IS THIRSTY, GIVE HIM COLD BOILED WATER

The piped water of towns is made safe in another way. An element called **chlorine** is added to it which kills any harmful micro-organisms that may have got into it. Such water is said to be chlorinated.

4.18　　THINGS TO DO

(a) Making a food collection. Make a collection of as many different kinds of food as you can. A collection is many things gathered together. Perhaps each member of the class can be asked to bring a different kind of food with him. If some foods cannot be found, pictures or drawings of these foods can be used. After a class some foods can also be kept in plastic bags to be used in a later class. If none of these things is possible for some foods, their names can be written on pieces of paper, and the collection completed in this way.

Make the most of this collection, and try to use it in as many of these ways as possible.

1. Divide the collection into food groups (Section 4.16).
2. Put the collection in a line with the food with the highest percentage of protein at one end and the foods with no protein in them at the other end (Table 19, Section 6.6).
3. Put the plant proteins in one pile and the animal proteins in another pile (Sections 3.4 and 3.5).
4. Place foods together showing examples of two plant proteins and one animal protein (Section 5.2).
5. Put the foods in a line with those with the most joules in them at one end and those with the least joules in them at the other end (Section 4.2 and Table 19, Section 6.6).
6. Put the foods in a line with the most expensive foods at one end and the cheapest foods at the other end.
7. Put the foods in a line with the 'best buy' for protein (or reference protein) at one end and the most expensive buy at the other end (Section 6.4 and 6.6).
8. Put the foods in a line with the 'best buy' for joules at one end and the most expensive buy at the other end (Sections 6.5 and 6.6).
9. Use the food collection to make examples of balanced meals (Section 5.2).
10. Use the food collection to plan meals for people at different times of the year, for rich people and for poor people, for people in the town and for people in the country.
11. Ask members of the class which foods they would give to underweight children to make them grow. Do the rest of the class think that the right choice has been made? If mothers are there, ask them which food they would give to an underweight child.
12. Ask members of the class which foods they would give to a young child whose mother had not got enough breast milk (Section 7.2), a sick child (Section 7.19), a child with diarrhoea (Section 7.20) and to a child to take to school for lunch (Section 7.18).
13. In places where some foods are only grown at some seasons of the year, ask what foods could be used instead of these at other times of the year.

Several of these ways of using a food collection require you to know *the prices of food in your district—not those given in this book!* You will therefore have to have been shopping and to have made your own protein and joule best-buy list as described in Sections 6.6 and 6.10b. A food collection needs to be used in different ways for different kinds of class. For example, Nos. 1, 9, 10, 11 and 12 in the list above can be used in primary schools, but some of the others are too difficult.

(b) Collecting wild fruits and nuts. In rural areas families eat many kinds of fruits, roots and nuts from the bush. These often contain useful amounts of nutrients, and families should be encouraged to go on eating them. Make a list or a collection of these wild foods and the time of year when they are found.

(c) Measuring the vitamins A and C in foods. If you are a medical student you may be able to buy foods in the market and measure the vitamin A and C in them in your biochemistry practical classes. This is quite easy.

(d) Some exercises on joules. Here are some exercises, in case you are still not used to kilojoules and megajoules.

Change these into megajoules:

A child of two needs 5,300 kilojoules a day.
There are 10,000 kilojoules in 270 g of oil.
There are 71 kilojoules in 100 g of cabbage.

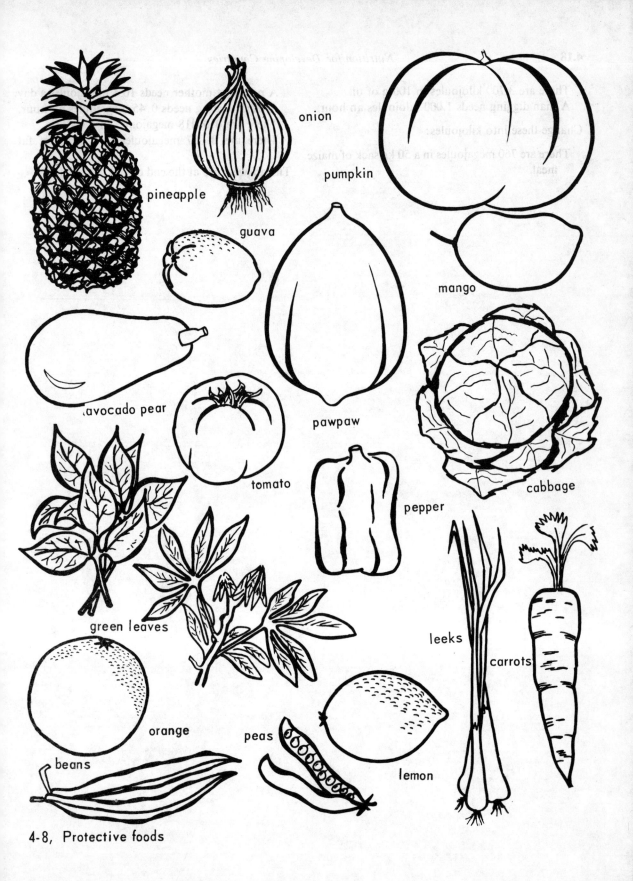

onion

pumpkin

pineapple

guava

mango

avocado pear

pawpaw

tomato

cabbage

pepper

green leaves

leeks

carrots

orange

peas

lemon

beans

4-8, Protective foods

There are 3,700 kilojoules in 100 g of oil.
A man digging needs 1,000 kilojoules an hour.

Change these into kilojoules:

There are 760 megajoules in a 50 kg sack of maize meal.

A pregnant mother needs 10.4 megajoules a day.
A clerk writing needs 0.45 megajoules an hour.
There are 0.00418 megajoules in a Calorie.
There are 0.037 megajoules in a gram of fat.

The answers are at the end of the next chapter.

Chapter Five

MORE ABOUT FOOD

5.1 Feeling hungry. Now that you know about nutrients it is time to think about hunger, and the meals we should eat.

Most people eat several times a day if they can, although adults usually want to eat less often than children. It may therefore seem a strange question to ask—why do we eat? Of course we eat to stop feeling hungry, but this is only part of the answer. The more important reason is that we eat because our bodies need food to keep alive and stay healthy; so eating is not only for stopping hunger. Hunger is the message that tells us our bodies need more food. But it is not a very good message, because it tells us to eat any food, and not food with the particular nutrients that we may need, such as protein, or a balanced meal. Also, if people have had too little food for a long time they may be malnourished, and yet feel less hungry than someone who usually has a lot to eat and misses one of his meals. It is true that people sometimes greatly want some special foods, like meat, and feel a great hunger for them. But they do not feel hungry for all protein foods just because they lack protein. Some malnourished children with kwashiorkor do not want to eat at all and have to be forced to eat, even though they are about to die from lack of protein. But children with marasmus are different—they are usually very hungry indeed, unless they also have some other disease.

---

*MALNOURISHED CHILDREN MAY
NOT FEEL HUNGRY*

A carbohydrate energy food like cassava will stop hunger and supply the body with the joules it needs without at the same time supplying enough protein. This is why our food must contain enough protein to give us the protein we need *before we have eaten so many joules that we no longer feel hungry*. This is also why meals, especially meals for young children, must not only contain enough joules, *but also enough protein in proportion to the joules they contain*. Most of Chapter 7 on feeding children is about how to make sure that a young child eats enough protein as well as enough joules.

What foods do we need to stop feeling hungry and stay healthy, and what foods does a child need to grow? First of all, *we must eat all three kinds of nutrients:* body-building proteins, energy-giving carbohydrates and fats, and protective vitamins and minerals. If possible, we must eat some of each of them at every meal.

Second, *we must eat enough of these nutrients.* How much of each nutrient we should eat will depend on what kind of person we are. Men, women and children all need different amounts. We shall say more about this in the next chapter. Meanwhile there is more to be said about the balanced meal, milk, sugar, food poisons and the food words.

5.2 The balanced meal. If adults are going to stay healthy and be able to work hard, and if children are going to grow, they need enough of each kind of nutrient. A meal that contains the right amount of body-building protein, energy-giving carbohydrate or fat, protective foods and minerals, is said to be a **balanced meal.** Not every meal need be balanced, but most of them should be.

Let us think about the protein first. In Section 3.9 we saw that animal proteins are expensive and that most families have to rely on plant proteins. We also saw that one plant protein by itself is not very good for body-building, and that plant proteins are made much better for body-building by mixing them. We also saw that if possible at least a little animal protein should be eaten as well. A balanced meal should never contain only one plant protein. It should contain two plant proteins, and a little animal protein if possible. It might also

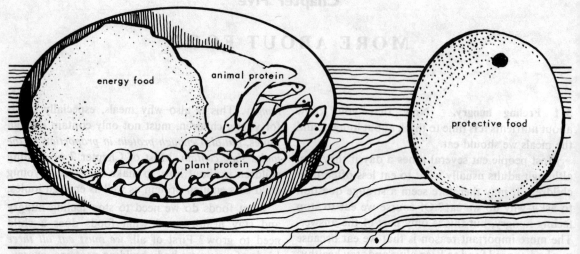

5-1, A balanced meal

contain one plant protein and some animal protein or, if the family is very rich and fortunate, animal protein alone.

ONE PLANT PROTEIN ALONE DOES NOT MAKE A BALANCED MEAL

Now for the carbohydrate. This is useful in two ways: it provides the energy that the body needs, and it stops the protein that is eaten being burnt to provide energy. As we have seen, protein can be burnt to provide energy, one gram of protein providing 17 kilojoules (kJ) of energy. If there is only protein at a meal and there is no carbohydrate or fat, this protein will be wasted. It will be burnt to provide energy and not used for body-building. This is a pity, because protein, especially animal protein, is more expensive than carbohydrate. By stopping protein being burnt wastefully, carbohydrate and fat save protein, and allow it to be used for its proper purpose, which is body-building. Because fat is expensive and too much of it can make people feel sick, there should be carbohydrate at every balanced meal. Fat is useful for cooking, it makes food taste nice, and it provides many joules of energy in a small space or bulk. Although it is not absolutely necessary, it is usually best if

about 15 per cent of the joules we need come from fat.

Protein and carbohydrate differ in a very important way. If a person eats more carbohydrate than he needs, his body makes it into fat and stores it. This is what makes fat people fat. The body cannot, however, store more than a little protein. If someone has a big meal of protein and eats much more than he needs, the amino acids from it are broken down and are either used for energy, or made into fat. This again is waste. If protein, especially animal protein, is scarce, it is better to eat only a little at each meal. Scarce protein should not all be eaten at once. It will be wasted because it cannot be stored.

The third part of a balanced meal is the protective foods—the vitamin and mineral foods. In every balanced meal there should be food such as green vegetables or fruit. The body is quite good at storing vitamins and minerals, and it is enough to eat fruit and vegetables once a day rather than at every meal.

Some balanced meals
(All these contain protein, carbohydrate and protective foods.)

Two plant proteins
    Maize *nshima*—beans—orange
    Cassava *nshima*—groundnuts—beans

Two plant proteins and a little animal protein
    Maize *nshima*—groundnuts—dried skim milk—
        pawpaw
    Cassava *nshima*—peas—beans—fish—mango
    Millet *nshima*—beans—egg—pineapple

One plant protein and some animal protein
    Cassava *nshima*—meat—beans—tomato
    Millet *nshima*—fish—banana
    Maize porridge—mother's milk—dark green
        leaves—**VERY IMPORTANT**

Animal protein alone—expensive!
    Cassava *nshima*—meat—orange
    Cassava *nshima*—eggs—carrots

Mother's milk—cheap!

Remember, when you make a balanced meal, that maize, bread and rice all contain about 8 per cent of plant protein as well as much carbohydrate, but that cassava contains almost no protein. One plant protein alone, such as beans, does not make a balanced meal when eaten with cassava, but it does when eaten with maize. In the list above we have taken dark green leaves to be a protective food, but, as we have already seen, they also contain about 5 per cent of protein, which is very useful.

You may be surprised to see maize porridge and mother's milk and dark green leaves listed as a balanced meal. This is one of the most important balanced meals there is, because mother's milk is the best animal protein of all for a young child. This is why the children of poor families, where there is little protein food, should go on breast-feeding until they are 18 months or two years old. Mother's milk is a balanced meal by itself, because it contains protein, joules of energy and protective foods. The only thing it does not contain is iron. But, as we shall see in Chapter 7, once a child is six months old, he is too big to live on breast milk alone. After that he must have plenty of porridge with added protein and protective foods as well, especially those containing some iron. Even so, the animal protein that a child can get from his mother's milk until he is 18 months or two years old is very important. It gives children of poor families a little animal protein which they may not be able to get from other foods.

Some village meals are well balanced. You will see that the Ugandan mother in the poem inside the front cover of this book used two stones to grind cassava with millet and sorghum. She was mixing two kinds of vegetable proteins, millet and sorghum, with cassava. She was making a good food for her family.

One of the important things about a balanced meal is that the foods are mixed—that is several different foods are eaten together. This balanced meal is unlike many village meals which contain two things only. Very often they are simply *nshima*, even plain cassava *nshima*, with perhaps a few wild green leaves. If a food is mixed it is almost certain to contain a mixture of proteins. This is why some people try to teach mothers that A GOOD FOOD IS A MIXED FOOD. This is a useful thing to teach, because a mixed food is likely to make a balanced meal.

A GOOD FOOD IS A MIXED FOOD

5.3 Milk. Cow's milk contains about 86 per cent water, 3.5 per cent protein, 4 per cent fat and 5 per cent carbohydrate. The carbohydrate in milk is a special kind of sugar called **lactose**. Human milk contains less protein and more carbohydrate than cow's milk. It contains 88 per cent water, 1.2 per cent protein, 3.8 per cent fat and 7 per cent carbohydrate. Some of us find these figures hard to remember, and if you want to remember them you may find it easier to do so like this: 'cow's milk 4–4–4' and 'breast milk 2–4–6'.

	Cow's milk	Breast milk
Protein	about 4%	about 2%
Fat	about 4%	about 4%
Carbohydrate	about 4%	about 6%

When milk straight from a cow is left to stand in a glass, the fat comes to the top as a yellow layer called **cream.** This is why milk straight from the cow is called **whole milk** or **full cream milk.** Sometimes, before it is sold, it is mixed in a special way so that the fat cannot come to the top. The cream is still there, however, and it is called 'homogenized' milk.

When the cream is taken away from whole milk,

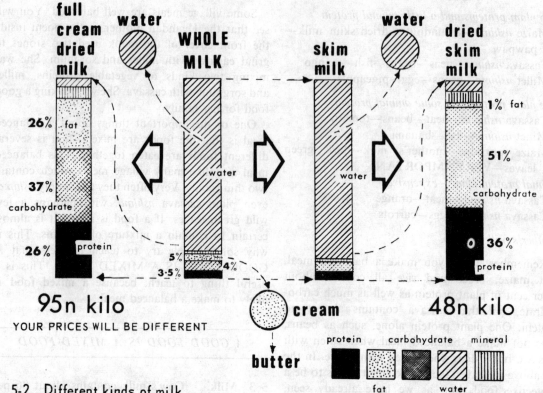

full cream dried milk   water   WHOLE MILK   skim milk   water   dried skim milk

26% fat

37% carbohydrate

26% protein

water

water

1% fat

51% carbohydrate

36% protein

5%
3.5%
4%

95n kilo

YOUR PRICES WILL BE DIFFERENT

cream

48n kilo

butter

protein   carbohydrate   mineral

fat   water

5-2, Different kinds of milk

the milk that is left behind is called skimmed milk or **skim milk.** Skimming means taking away the cream, which is either sold as it is, or else made into butter by being shaken for some hours. Water can be taken away from milk to leave a powder called **dried milk.** If water is taken away from full cream milk, **full cream dried milk powder** is made. This contains 26 per cent protein and 26 per cent fat or cream. If water is taken away from skim milk, **dried skim milk powder** is made. This contains 36 per cent protein and almost no cream.

Thus you will see that dried skim milk powder contains more protein (36%) than dried full cream milk powder (26%). This is because, when dried skim milk is made, water *and fat* are both taken away. So, when you buy one kilo of dried skim milk more of what you buy is protein. But, when full cream milk powder is made only the water is taken away, and both the protein *and the fat* are left behind. So, when you buy one kilo of full cream milk powder some of it is fat and less of it is protein. (See also Section 3.6, where we explained

why dried fish has more protein in it than fresh fish.)

Dried skim milk powder also contains about 51 per cent of lactose. It is thus about half lactose. This is important because if dried skim milk is not used in the right way the lactose in it sometimes gives children diarrhoea—see Section 7.20.

Butter and cream are expensive, so when milk is skimmed a farmer can make most of his profit by selling these two expensive foods. This means he can sell skim milk very cheaply. In Lusaka a kilo of dried skim milk costs 48n and a kilo of full cream dried milk costs 95n. *Not only does dried skim milk contain more protein than full cream milk, but it is about half the price!*

SKIM MILK IS A CHEAPER WAY OF BUYING PROTEIN THAN FULL CREAM MILK

After mother's milk; which has an NPU of 100 per cent and is 100 per cent used for body-building, cow's milk is one of the next best foods

Prices from Lusaka
in 1971

all these prices are per litre

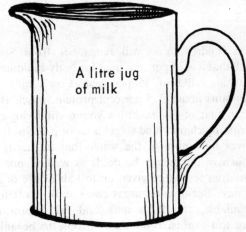

A litre jug
of milk

16n

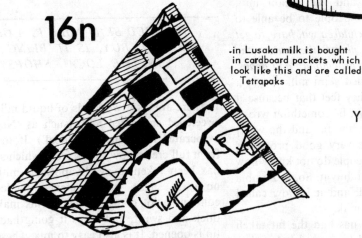

.in Lusaka milk is bought
in cardboard packets which
look like this and are called
Tetrapaks

YOUR PRICES WILL
BE DIFFERENT

This is what you would have had to have paid to have filled
up a litre jug with milk, if you had bought it in these ways.
You would have needed about $5\frac{1}{2}$ of the small tins and only
a little more than one of the large tins. Fresh milk would
have been the cheapest way of filling the jug.

21n

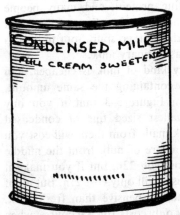

CONDENSED MILK
FULL CREAM SWEETENED

22n

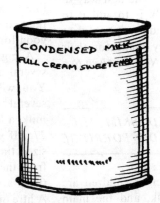

CONDENSED MILK
FULL CREAM SWEETENED

27n

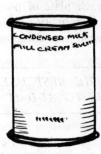

CONDENSED MILK
FULL CREAM SWEET

for children. You will remember from Section 3.8 that it is 75 per cent used for body-building and has an NPU of 75 per cent. Cow's milk only contains about 3.5 per cent protein, which is less than that of maize, but a young child can easily drink much milk and so get a lot of protein. It also gives him most of the water that he needs and much of the energy he needs as well. If possible, children should be given up to half a litre of milk a day. But in rural areas cow's milk is often not available, and fresh milk and full cream milk are too expensive for many people to be able to buy enough of them. *Most children will have to get most of their protein from plants like maize, and especially from legumes like groundnuts and beans.*

Some people feel that dried skim milk is not a very good kind of food. They feel that because it has been skimmed there must be something wrong with it. This is not so. Only the fat and the water have been taken away; the very good protein is still there. It is a pity that people do not know how good it is and do not want to buy it. So, in Zambia its name has been changed, and it is now called 'Proto' brand, high protein milk.

Because dried skim milk has had the fat taken away, it is not a good food for young babies less than four months old. It has too much protein and not enough joules for them. Sometimes it does not have enough vitamins either. If young babies have to be fed on cow's milk, it should be full cream cow's milk, and should be given to them in the ways described in Chapter 8. But dried skim milk is a very good food for babies older than four months who have started eating porridge. The best way to give these babies dried skim milk is to add it to their porridge. Tell mothers to add a spoonful to each plate of porridge that they make for their children. *Dried skim milk should NOT be given to a child from a feeding bottle.*

THE BEST USE FOR DRIED SKIM MILK IS TO ADD IT TO A CHILD'S PORRIDGE

At under-fives clinics underweight children are often given free dried skim milk, and the main reason why some mothers come to a clinic is to get it. If it is given to mothers, they must be taught how to use it—that is, they must add it to their children's porridge. *The giving away of dried skim milk must never stop clinic workers from trying to help and teach mothers how they can feed their children on the foods that they can themselves buy and grow.* Giving away dried skim milk will never do instead of the right nutrition education—see Section 9.24. Mothers should also be taught to buy dried skim milk in the shops, if it is there for them to buy.

IF DRIED SKIM MILK IS A GOOD PROTEIN BUY, IS IT BEING SOLD IN THE LOCAL SHOPS?

There are also two kinds of liquid milk in tins—**sweetened condensed milk** (such as 'Nestlés') and **evaporated milk** (such as 'Ideal'). Both are made from full cream cow's milk from which some water has been taken away. Evaporated milk contains no extra sugar, but sweetened condensed milk contains a lot of extra sugar. This makes it very thick and sweet, and stops it going bad when the tin is opened. It is also easy to mix. These are some of the reasons why mothers like it. Condensed milk is *not* a good food for children. It is expensive and contains too much sugar, and too little protein. Encourage mothers to buy other kinds of milk.

In Zambia a special kind of milk is on sale. It is called 'Lacto', and is liquid skimmed milk which has been made sour in a special way. It is a good, cheap way of eating protein, and many people like to add it to their porridge. Some tribes milk their cows and let the milk go sour. Sour milk is as good for children as ordinary milk.

A big tin of any kind of milk is cheaper than several small tins containing the same amount. You will see from Figure 5–3 that if you buy several of the smallest sized tins of condensed milk, a litre of milk made from them will cost you 27n. If you make a litre of milk from the middle sized tins it will cost you 22n, but if you make it from the largest tins it will only cost you 21n. But all of these are much more expensive than fresh milk. A litre of fresh milk only costs 16n. Of course, when you buy sweetened condensed milk you are buying sugar as well, but it is cheaper to buy sugar and to add it to fresh milk. A kilogram of sugar only costs 18n and will sweeten a lot of milk. The cheapest kind of milk is different in different districts. You can find out which is the cheapest milk in your district by turning to Section 5.7b. With food of any kind you will find that it is cheaper to buy one big tin rather than several small ones.

BIG TINS ARE A CHEAPER WAY OF BUYING FOOD THAN SMALL TINS

Although cow's milk is a good food for children, we cannot think of it as being a usual food for them, because so many mothers cannot get it. Although many villagers keep cows, they seldom milk them, and the kind of cow they keep does not often give much milk. Even in Zambia so little fresh milk is sold that only three people in every hundred can have a pint of fresh milk every day. Fresh milk has to be kept in a fridge, or it goes sour. Dried milk is cheaper and easier to transport, and more of it is sold. But most women in the villages have no money, and few rural shops keep any kind of milk except expensive brands of infant dried milks and small tins of sweetened condensed milk. *Most mothers will not therefore be able to give their children milk and will have to use mixtures of plant proteins, with a little animal protein if they are fortunate.* This is why we have said so much about plant proteins and the importance of mixing them.

There are other difficulties with dried and tinned milks. They have often to be brought from other countries, so they use precious foreign money, and it may not always be possible to pay for them. Until 1970 dried skim milk from Europe was cheap. But in that year the governments of some European countries stopped subsidizing (helping) their farmers to keep cows for milk, so the price of dried skim milk went up a lot, and it may go up still more. This is one good reason why it is much better for people living in a district to grow as much as possible of their own food, and to be self-supporting as is described in Section 11.2.

Goat's milk is also good for young children. If the villagers have goats, they should milk them to feed their children. Many local goats, like many local cows, are not good for milking, and better varieties are needed.

5.4 Sugar. Sugar is a new food that people are eating more and more. As you have read, it is pure carbohydrate, or pure energy food. Energy can be got quite as easily and much more cheaply from maize or cassava. Sugar is not, therefore, a necessary food, and is not one that we should encourage mothers to buy. Sugar helps to cause caries or holes in the teeth. Mothers can add sugar to their children's porridge, but it is much more important that they should add some kind of protein instead.

5.5 Two food poisons. There are two food poisons you should know about—**aflatoxin** in groundnuts and **cyanide** in some kinds of cassava.

When some foods are not properly dried, moulds grow in them. A mould is a very small plant which covers whatever it is growing on with very thin hairs. One common mould makes a poison in groundnuts called aflatoxin, which harms animals and men. Take care, therefore, to dry stored foods as much as possible, and don't let them get damp (slightly wet). Dampness will help the mould to grow. In the wet weather powdered groundnuts grow mouldy very easily.

KEEP YOUR GROUNDNUTS DRY

There is a poison in some kinds of cassava root. It is a kind of cyanide. This may be useful to the cassava plant because it stops the roots being eaten by animals and insects in the ground, but it is harmful to man. Before it is eaten this kind of cassava root should always be peeled and soaked very carefully. Peeling a food means taking the skin off it. By soaking we mean here that the cassava root is left in water for some hours.

5.6 The local food words. So far we have talked about food using the names from science. You have learned about things like protein, amino acids, joules and folic acid. It is now time to think

some kinds of cassava are poisonous
until they have been washed in a stream

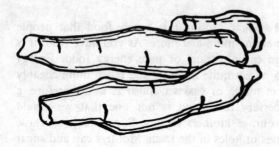

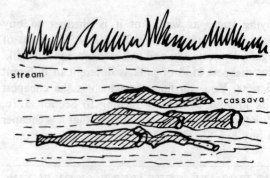

stream

cassava

the poison is removed by washing
in a stream

if groundnuts are allowed to grow mouldy the mould
may make a poison in them - keep groundnuts dry

groundnuts

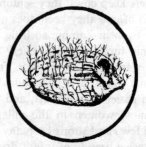

the mould that makes aflatoxin in
groundnuts makes them go yellow, it
cannot be seen without a microscope

5-4, Food poisons

about the food words villagers use. These are important for teaching.

Very often there may be no local word which means quite the same as the English word. There will certainly be no local word for such things as protein or vaccine. If you are going to talk about protein you will have to use the English word and explain what it means. Another thing you can do is to take some local word and widen or extend its meaning. Sometimes there will be many local words which mean the same as an English word, but are different from one another. There will probably be several local words for the various kinds of dried fish, for example. Be careful to find the right words.

The most important word is the one the local people use for 'food' itself. Some tribes have the same word for the staple food, such as maize, or cassava, and for food of any kind. In English the word 'bread' is sometimes used in this way. Thus the sentence, 'Can I have some butter on my bread?' uses the word bread to mean bread only. The sentence, from the Lord's prayer, 'Give us this day our daily bread', uses the English word bread to mean food of any kind. It is important to know if the local word for food has this double meaning.

Some tribes have a special word for the food that is eaten with the staple food. There is no good English word for food of this kind, and the word which is usually used is **relish.** In West Africa the word 'soup' is used. In Nyanja the word for relish is *ndiwo*, in Bemba *umunani*. By relish we mean the *cooked* meat, fish, beans or vegetables that are eaten with the staple food. In some languages there are different words for relishes made of meat or fish and those made from leaves. Some tribes do not think of the relish as food, but only as something which tastes good. These people think that only the staple of maize or cassava is proper food, because it fills you up. There is a story about a chief who went to Russia, and who came back saying that there was no food there, only relish! The only thing he thought of as food was his staple, cassava!

LEARN THE LOCAL FOOD LANGUAGE

Another important word is that for the thick porridge made of boiled maize, millet or cassava flour, that the Lunda and Nyanja call *nshima*. This is thick enough to be rolled into a ball and eaten with the fingers. There is no English word for this food, so we will call it **nshima.**

There is an English word **porridge**. This is made of a grain called oats boiled in water. It is eaten by men and women as well as children. Porridge is much too thin to be rolled into a ball with the fingers, so it is eaten with a spoon, usually with milk and sugar. Porridge used to be the staple food of people from Scotland. In this book we use the word porridge to mean *thin* maize or cassava food that is given to children with a spoon. In Bemba this is *umusunga*, and in Nyanja it is *phala*. There are two English words, gruel and pap, that mean porridge specially for children. They are old words and are not much used now. It is interesting that the word 'pap' is still used in Nigeria, long after it has stopped being used in England.

5.7   THINGS TO DO

(a)   Your own nutrition words.   Here is a list of the five most important food words in some African languages. There is space for you to put in the words in your local languages, if it is not one of these.

TABLE 9
Food Words

	The staple food of the country	Anything which is eaten	The food eaten with the staple	Maize, millet, cassava nshima	Thin children's porridge
English	bread (in England)	food	no word, 'relish' is best	no word	gruel or pap
Bemba	ubwali	fyakulya	umunani	bwali	umusunga
Swahili	wali	chakula	kitoweo	ugali	uji
Nyanja	chimanga	chakudya	ndiwo	nshima	phala
Your local language(s)					
	....	....	....	....	....
	....	....	....	....	....
	....	....	....	....	....
	....	....	....	....	....
	....	....	....	....	....
	....	....	....	....	....

Many other words are important; here are a few of them with spaces to fill in others. You know the importance of some of them now. You will learn the importance of the others later on. Take great care to find the right local words for healthy, fat, well and badly nourished. You may find that there are no local words for some of those in the list below.

TABLE 10
Some Important Nutrition Words in the Local Language

beans	milk, condensed..........
cabbage	milk, dried skim ....
cassava.................	milk, evaporated ....
chicken	milk, fresh ....
colostrum	millet ....
dark green leaves	oil ....
eggs	peas ....
energy.................	pestle and mortar........
fat	road to health..........
fish, dried	salt ....
fish, fresh	sugar ....
fizzy drink.............	dessertspoon ....
germs.................	teaspoon...............
groundnuts	fat ....
groundnut butter	well nourished ....
healthy	badly nourished..........
meal or flour	kwashiorkor.............
meat.................	marasmus..............
....	....
....	....
....	....
....	....

(b) The cost of milk. There are several kinds of milk, and most shops have more than one brand in several sizes of tin. If we are to teach mothers how to buy the cheapest kind of milk, we must go to the shops and find out which they are. Although we will tell you how to work out the cost of a litre of milk of each kind, *the best way to use dried skim milk is to add the powder to a child's porridge.* Mothers should breast-feed their children, but if they are going to bottle-feed them, they will need to know the cheapest kind of *full cream dried milk* to buy. A litre is about $1\frac{3}{4}$ pints (1.75 pints).

TABLE 11
The Cost of a Litre of Cow's Milk

As fresh milk		per litre	....
Brand	Size	Cost	Cost per litre

Made from full cream powdered milk
130 g of powder make a litre of milk

....	....	....	....
....	....	....	....
....	....	....	....

Made from dried skim milk powder
100 g of powder make a litre of milk

....	....	....	....
....	....	....	....
....	....	....	....

Made from evaporated milk
460 g make a litre of milk

....	....	....	....
....	....	....	....
....	....	....	....

Made from sweetened condensed milk
430 g make a litre of milk

....	....	....	....
....	....	....	....
....	....	....	....

Here is an example of how to work out these costs. In a Lusaka shop a tin of 'Ideal' evaporated milk costs 16n, and on the tin was written that it contained 410 g. This 410 g cost 16n, so 1 g cost $\frac{16}{410}$n. The amount needed to make one litre of milk, that is 460 g, therefore cost $460 \times \frac{16}{410} = 18$n.

Only the protein in the milk has been thought about in working out how much milk or milk powder should be used to make 1 litre of milk. Milk has been worked out to contain 3.5 per cent of protein, and 1 millilitre has been used as equal to 1 gram. This means that 1 litre (1,000 cc) of milk will contain 35 grams of protein. If some tins are still marked in ounces, pounds and pints, you may need to turn to the Appendix at the end of this book to help you to change them into grams and millilitres.

Some milk foods for children contain added carbohydrate, which is usually maize flour. They therefore contain less protein than full cream milk powder and are often a very bad buy. The percentage of protein they contain will be written on the tin. Work out how many grams are needed to make a litre of milk in the following way.

Grams of food needed to make a litre of milk=

$$35 \times \frac{100}{\% \text{ of protein in the food}}.$$

Once you have done your shopping you will be able to work out a best buy list like the one below. This has the cheapest litre of milk at the top, and the most expensive one at the bottom.

BUY MILK IN THE CHEAPEST WAY

TABLE 12
Best Buy List for Milk

Kind	CHEAPEST LITRE OF MILK Brand	Size	Cost
....	....	....	....
....	....	....	....
....	....	....	....
....	....	....	....
....	....	....	....
....	....	....	....
....	....	....	....

MOST EXPENSIVE LITRE OF MILK

(c) The cost of infant foods. This is a good place to show you how to work out the cost of the protein and joules in infant foods. You will read about this in Sections 6.4 and 6.5. When you look at a tin of infant food, it will usually tell you the number of calories in 100 g, and the percentage of protein. Take the NPU to be 75 per cent, which is the NPU of cow's milk. Calories are changed into joules by multiplying the calories by 4.2. We choose 40 g of protein and 10 megajoules so that we can compare them with other foods.

40 g of protein cost . . .

$$\frac{100 \times \text{cost of the tin of food} \times 40}{\% \text{ of protein in the food} \times \text{weight in grams of the food bought}}$$

Protein equal to 40 g of reference protein cost . . .
the cost of 40 g of protein, as above, $\times \frac{100}{75}$

10 megajoules cost . . .

$$\frac{100 \times 10,000 \times \text{cost of the tin of food}}{\text{calories in } 100 \text{ g} \times 4.2 \times \text{weight in grams of food bought}}$$

You will find that these foods are a very expensive way of buying both protein and joules!

(d) Answers from the last chapter. Here are the answers to the exercises that you did at the end of the last chapter.

Answers in megajoules	Answers in kilojoules
5.3 MJ	760,000 kJ
10 MJ	10,400 kJ
0.071 MJ	450 kJ
3.7 MJ	4.18 kJ
1.0 MJ	37 kJ

Chapter Six

THE NEED FOR FOOD AND ITS COST

THE NEED FOR FOOD

6.1 Protein needs.   In Chapter 3 we learnt that children need protein for growing and that pregnant and breast-feeding mothers need extra food to give to their growing children. We learnt that everyone needs protein for repairing his body, and also energy foods, so that they can work and keep warm. In this chapter we shall learn how much body-building protein and how many joules of energy each kind of person needs. We shall also work out how much they cost.

The amount of protein a person needs each day depends partly on how he is growing and partly on how heavy he is. Thus a growing child needs more protein for each kilo of his weight than an adult. A large person needs more protein for the daily repair of his body than a small person. As we shall see later, how hard a person works makes no difference to the amount of protein he needs.

Table 13 shows different kinds of people in Column 1. In Column 2 it shows us how much healthy people of each of these kinds should weigh. Column 3 shows us how many grams of egg or reference protein they need each day for each kilo of their weight. Column 4 shows us how many grams of egg or reference protein each kind of person needs altogether each day.

Table 13 is interesting in many ways. You will see that Column 2 shows that a child between the ages of 6 and 11 months weighs 9 kg. This is an average weight for children between these ages, because children are getting heavier all the time. The weights for the other ages of person are also average weights for the ages shown.

TABLE 13
Daily Protein Needs

Kind of person	Average weight in kg	Grams of egg or reference protein needed each day		Grams of maize protein needed per person per day
		per kilo per day	per person per day	
1	**2**	**3**	**4**	**5**
Infants				
6–11 mths	9.0 kg	1.53 g	14 g	25 g
Young children				
1–3 yrs.	13.4 kg	1.19 g	16 g	29 g
4–6	20.2 kg	1.01 g	20 g	37 g
7–9	28.1 kg	0.88 g	25 g	45 g
Older boys				
10–12	36.9 kg	0.81 g	30 g	54 g
13–15	51.3 kg	0.72 g	37 g	67 g
16–19	62.9 kg	0.60 g	38 g	69 g
Older girls				
10–12	38.0 kg	0.76 g	29 g	54 g
13–15	49.9 kg	0.63 g	31 g	57 g
16–19	54.4 kg	0.55 g	30 g	55 g
Reference adult man	**65.0 kg**	0.57 g	37 g	68 g
Reference adult woman	**55.0 kg**	0.52 g	29 g	52 g

Extra grams of protein needed each day for pregnancy and breast-feeding

{ Pregnancy   5.5 g

{ Breast-feeding 17.0 g

Just as it is useful for us to study and refer to one kind of protein, reference protein, it is often useful for us to study and refer to men and women of the same weight doing the same sort of job. We need what we call a **reference man** and a **reference woman.** At the bottom of Column 2 you will see that our reference man weighs 65 kg and our reference woman 55 kg. When we come to see how many joules they need, we shall see that they are doing fairly hard jobs.

From Column 3 you will see that from 6 to 11 months a child needs about one and a half (1.53) grams of protein each day for each kilo he weighs. But, when he is an adult and has stopped growing he only needs about half a gram of protein each day for each kilo he weighs (0.57 grams per kilo for a man and 0.52 grams per kilo for a woman). *A child in his first year thus needs about three times more protein for each kilo of his weight than an adult* ($3 \times \frac{1}{2} = 1\frac{1}{2}$). You will see that because older boys and girls are growing they also need more protein per kilo of their weight than adults. The only figures to remember in this table are that an adult man needs about 40 g (more exactly 37.0 g) reference protein daily and an adult woman about 30 g (more exactly 29.0 g). It is also useful to remember that adults need about half a gram of reference protein for each kilo and infants about one and a half grams of protein for each kilo they weigh.

AN ADULT MAN NEEDS NEARLY 40 g OF REFERENCE PROTEIN DAILY AND AN ADULT WOMAN NEARLY 30 g

---

You will see that a woman needs 5.5 g of *extra* reference protein when she is pregnant and 17.0 g *extra* when she is breast-feeding. A breast-feeding mother needs more protein than a pregnant mother because her child is larger. She needs 29.0 + 17.0 = 46.0 grams of protein. The 5.5 g of extra protein needed by a pregnant mother is the average for pregnancy. Early in pregnancy, when her child is small, she needs less. Later on, when he is large, she needs more. If we divide the nine months of pregnancy into four we can say that 1, 4, 8, and 9 g

of extra protein are needed daily during each of the four quarters of pregnancy.

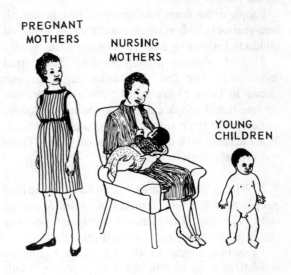

6-1, People who specially need protein

Columns 3 and 4 in Table 13 show the grams of egg or reference protein that are needed. But nobody lives on eggs alone, and, as we have already seen, most of the protein people eat, such as maize protein, is not so good for body-building as egg protein. Thus, when less completely used proteins with a lower NPU are eaten, more of them are needed. As an example of a less completely used protein with a lower NPU we shall take maize. This has an NPU of only 55 per cent and is only 55 per cent used for body-building. Column 5 shows the weight of maize protein needed by each kind of person. The figures in Column 5 were found by multiplying those in Column 4 by $\frac{100}{55}$. This comes to nearly two, so the figures in Column 5 are nearly twice as large as those in Column 4.

It may be easier to think of the weight of maize protein we need if we think of handfuls instead of grams. A handful of maize meal weighs about 50 g and contains 4 g of protein. Our reference adult man thus needs 17 handfuls of maize meal to give him the protein he needs ($68 \div 4$). If you think that this is rather a lot you should remember that, when other proteins are eaten with maize, we have a better chance of getting the essential amino acids we need. The NPU of the mixture goes up, and a smaller weight of food will give us the protein we need.

People differ from one another. Just as not all one-year-old children weigh exactly 10 kg, so not all children between 6 and 11 months need exactly 1.53 g of reference protein per kilo. Some need more and some less. The amounts of protein shown in Table 13 are called 'safe levels'. We can be sure that if people eat these amounts of protein, almost all of them will have the protein they need. It is the same with the next tables on joules. These too are safe levels.

6.2 The joules we need. Different kinds of people need different numbers of joules of energy food each day. This depends partly on how big they are and partly on how hard they work.

Table 14 has much to tell us. Column 2 gives the weights of boys of different ages. Column 3 tells us how many kilojoules they want for each kilo of their weight. At the top of Column 3 you will see that a boy in his first year needs 470 kJ for each kilo he weighs. At the bottom of this table you will see that a man only needs 192 kJ for each kilo of his weight. *Per kilo a child in his first year thus needs more than twice as many joules as an adult.* However, because adults weigh more than children, a child in his first year needs 3.4 MJ and an adult man 12.5 MJ.

YOUNG CHILDREN NEED PLENTY OF JOULES

Columns 5, 6 and 7 tell us that women and older girls need fewer joules than men and boys, except when they are pregnant or breast-feeding. This is partly because they weigh less and partly because they need fewer joules for each kilo they weigh. You will see that our 65 kg reference man needs 12.5 MJ each day and our 55 kg reference woman needs 9.2 MJ. Our reference man and woman do fairly hard jobs. If we want easier figures to remember, we can think of ordinary men doing very light jobs as needing 10 MJ a day. As we shall soon see they need much more if they are working hard. A breast-feeding mother needs many more joules because she must give many joules of energy to feed the child at her breast. Milk contains fat or cream which is a good energy food. If a mother is to give these joules to her child, she must first eat them herself. She needs 11.5 MJ, or 2.3 MJ more than she would do if she were not breast-feeding. When a mother is pregnant she needs 1.2 extra megajoules to give to the child in her womb, or 10.4 MJ altogether.

Our bodies are using joules of energy even when we are asleep. This energy is used for keeping our bodies warm, for breathing and for the beating of our heart. When an adult man is asleep in bed he

TABLE 14
Daily Joule Needs

Kind of person	Average weight in kg	Joules needed each day per kilo per day kJ	Joules needed each day per person per day MJ	Average weight in kg	Joules needed each day per kilo per day kJ	Joules needed each day per person per day MJ
	Boys and Men			Girls and Women		
1	2	3	4	5	6	7
less than 1 yr	7.3 kg	470 kJ	3.4 MJ	7.3 kg	470 kJ	3.4 MJ
1–3 yrs	13.4 kg	424 kJ	5.7 MJ	13.4 kg	424 kJ	5.7 MJ
4–6 yrs	20.2 kg	382 kJ	7.6 MJ	20.2 kg	382 kJ	7.6 MJ
7–9 yrs	28.1 kg	326 kJ	9.2 MJ	28.1 kg	326 kJ	9.2 MJ
10–12 yrs	36.9 kg	297 kJ	10.9 MJ	38.0 kg	259 kJ	10.9 MJ
13–15 yrs	51.3 kg	238 kJ	12.1 MJ	49.9 kg	209 kJ	12.1 MJ
16–19 yrs	62.9 kg	205 kJ	12.8 MJ	54.4 kg	179 kJ	12.8 MJ
Adult	65.0 kg	192 kJ	12.5 MJ	55.0 kg	167 kJ	9.2 MJ

Extra joules needed each day for pregnancy and breast-feeding   { Pregnancy   1.2 MJ   { Breast-feeding   2.3 MJ

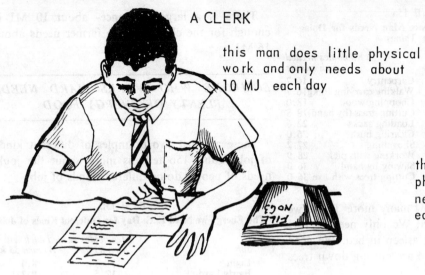

A CLERK

this man does little physical work and only needs about 10 MJ each day

A FARMER

this man does much physical work and needs about 16 MJ each day

6-2, The energy needs of a farmer and a clerk

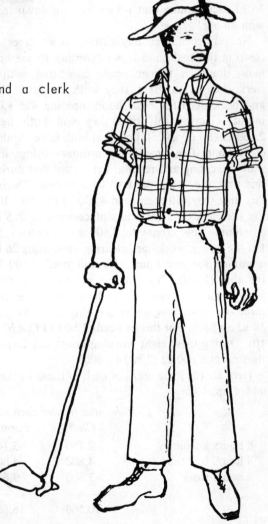

uses about 4.5 kJ every minute. When he gets up and starts working, he needs many more joules. The harder he works, the more joules he would need. We only need more joules when we work with our hands. *Brain work needs no extra joules!* Office workers and people who work with their brains need no more joules than if they were sitting doing nothing. Neither kind of worker needs extra protein because protein is only needed for building and repairing the body and is not needed to provide joules of energy for hard work. It is growing children and pregnant and breast-feeding mothers who need extra protein.

ADULTS DOING A VERY LIGHT JOB NEED ABOUT 10 MEGAJOULES A DAY. THEY NEED MORE IF THEY ARE WORKING HARD, PREGNANT OR BREAST-FEEDING

Table 15a shows the joules needed by a 65 kg reference man for different kinds of work.

TABLE 15a
The Joules a 65 kg Reference Man Needs for Doing Different Things

Kilojoules needed each minute		Kilojoules needed each minute	
Sleeping in bed	4.5	Carpentry	16.7
Sitting quietly	5.8	Walking carrying 10 kg	16.7
Driving lorry	6.7	Chopping wood	18.0
Standing quietly	7.3	Cutting grass (by hand)	18.8
Office work (sitting)	7.5	Loading sacks	22.6
Cooking	8.8	Clearing bush	26.0
Tailoring	12.1	Shovelling	27.2
Planting	15.1	Working with pick	28.9
Walking	15.5	Sawing by hand	36.0
Bricklaying	15.9	Cutting trees with axe	36.0

The table shows us how many more joules we need when we work hard. We only need 4.5 kJ each minute while we are asleep in bed. We need 36 kJ each minute that we are cutting down trees with an axe!

Nobody spends all day cutting down trees or clearing the bush, and it is interesting to see how many joules a farmer needs compared with a clerk. Let us say that they both weigh 65 kg, and both sleep for eight hours needing 4.5 kJ a minute. During this time they will both need 2,160 kJ ($8 \times 60 \times 4.5$). Let them both have another eight hours free time doing ordinary things like walking, eating and resting. Let us say that during this time they both need 10 kJ a minute. During this time they will each need 4,800 kJ ($8 \times 60 \times 10$). Let the clerk do eight hours office work at 7.5 kJ a minute. This comes to 3,600 kJ ($8 \times 60 \times 7.5$). Let the farmer work hard clearing bush using 26 kJ a minute for five hours. He will need 7,800 kJ for this ($5 \times 60 \times 26$). He cannot work as hard as this all the time, so let him spend the last three of his working hours standing or walking at 10 kJ an hour. For this he needs 1,800 kJ ($3 \times 60 \times 10$). During these eight working hours our farmer thus needs 9,600 kJ ($7,800 + 1,800$).

Here are the joule needs of each of these workers added up.

	Kilojoules needed each day	
	Clerk	Farmer
8 hours sleeping	2,160	2,160
8 hours free time	4,800	4,800
8 hours work	3,600	9,600
	10,560	16,560

There is a large difference—about 10 MJ is enough for the clerk, but the farmer needs about 16 MJ.

SOMEONE WHO WORKS HARD NEEDS PLENTY OF ENERGY FOOD

These are just two examples of different kinds of job. Table 15b tells us more about the joule needs of people doing different kinds of job.

TABLE 15b
The Energy we Need Each Day for Different Kinds of Job

Job	Megajoules needed each day	
	Men 65 kg	Women 55 kg
Light	11.3	8.4
Fairly hard	12.5	9.2
Very hard	14.6	10.9
Very hard indeed	16.7	12.5

Thus we see that our clerk was doing a very light job and our farmer a very hard job indeed.

The number of joules we need for a job depends on how hard the work is (cutting down trees requires more joules than writing) and how much we weigh. Big heavy men and big fat women need more joules for doing a job than small light men and women. This is partly because they can do more work such as cutting down more trees, and partly because their bodies weigh more and so need more energy to move. Here are the joules that different weights of men need for doing different jobs.

TABLE 15c
How the Joules a Man Needs for a Job Depends Upon his Weight

Weight kg	Kind of job, MJ needed daily			
	Light	Fairly hard	Very hard	Very hard indeed
50	8.8	9.6	11.3	13.0
55	9.7	10.6	12.4	14.3
60	10.5	11.5	13.6	15.6
65	11.3	12.5	14.6	16.7
70	12.3	13.5	15.8	18.2

We see that our 65 kg reference man does a fairly hard job and needs 12.5 MJ daily. Our reference woman also does a fairly hard job, but partly because she is lighter she only needs 9.2 MJ each day.

HEAVY PEOPLE NEED MORE JOULES THAN LIGHT ONES

Much of this book is about feeding children, because children are usually the most malnourished part of the community. But adults are also important, especially if they should be working hard. Many of them are malnourished and do not get the joules that we have just seen they need. If they are farmers, they are unable to work hard and grow more food. They therefore stay malnourished. This is a vicious circle and is explained more fully in Section 9.2. Food is so important for hard work that in some factories workers are given cheap meals or even free meals so that they can work harder. We shall say more about this in Section 7.21.

Now that we know how much protein and how many joules each member of a family needs, we must think about the best ways in which these joules can be bought. We shall start with some rules for good shopping.

THE COST OF FOOD

6.3 Buying wisely.   In the rural areas almost everyone grows their own food, but in towns most people buy it. The rural areas are therefore different from towns, and these next sections are mostly for people in towns who buy their food in shops. They will, however, help people in rural areas to know what foods they should grow.

The cost of food is important, and costs change. In writing this book costs had to be taken from somewhere, so they were taken from Lusaka in 1971. They will be different in other places and will have changed by the time that you read this book. So you must go to your own market and find out how much food costs there. From this you can work out for yourself the various figures that you will read about. Because prices change so much you may get very different answers.

The cost of food depends upon how much food you buy and where you buy it. If you buy a very small tin of milk or a little tinful of groundnuts, you may pay only five ngwee or a few cents, but

you will get *very* little food for your money. If, however, you buy larger amounts of food you will have to pay more money, but you will get *much* more food. You have already read about the cost of milk in Section 5.3, so let us take the small dried fish that the Zambians call *kapenta* as an example. On the shore of Lake Tanganyika *kapenta* costs 15n a kilo, but if you buy it in Lusaka in large quantities, say a sackful at a time, it costs 37n a kilo. If, however, you buy small quantities from a small shop *kapenta* costs about 9n for only 100 g. Like this a kilo of *kapenta* costs 90n!

6-3,   The cost of a kilo of kapenta

This means that a shopkeeper in Lusaka has bought *kapenta* wholesale by the sackful at 37n a kilo, and sold it retail in 100 g handfuls at 90n a kilo. We say that he has made a **mark-up** of 53n on each kilo of *kapenta* (90−37=53). This is also called a mark-up of 143 per cent; $\frac{53}{37} \times 100 = 143\%$.

Such a shopkeeper will not be able to keep all the 53n profit for himself, because he will have to pay for the running of his shop, but he will probably be able to keep most of it. 143 per cent is a lot of profit, and 30 per cent would be fair, so the *kapenta* should have been sold at about 48n a kilo, or 5n for 100 g. Small shops sell so few things that they have to make a lot of profit on each thing they sell. This is the main reason why it is better to go to bigger shops which sell more things, and thus need to make less profit on each of them. This is, however, very hard on the small shopkeeper, whose only way to make a living may be to sell a very little food at a big mark-up.

BUY FOODS WHICH KEEP IN AS LARGE QUANTITIES AS YOU CAN

This shows how important it is to tell mothers how to get the best value for their money. It usually means persuading them to buy foods in quantities of not less than a kilogram *in the bigger shops*. Other foods have a similar mark-up to *kapenta*, and on groundnuts in Lusaka the mark-up is often 400 per cent. Prices will be different in your district; so you must go round the shops carefully to find the best prices before you start teaching.

Because of this, it is important to persuade women to buy all their food in the largest quantities at the best prices they can. Especially persuade women to buy foods by weight, such as a kilogram or half a kilogram, and not by small tinfuls of only a few grams. This is why girls in school must learn the arithmetic of shopping by weight and volume, and why all food shops must have scales. Big shops are usually cheaper than small ones, and shops nearer to the middle of town are usually cheaper than those far out. Mothers may have further to walk if they go to the better shops, but if they buy in larger quantities they will not have to shop so often. But if food is bought in larger amounts families must be able to store it; so talk to mothers about the best ways in which they can do this. One of the difficulties of buying food in large amounts is that, if a family's relatives know there is plenty of food, they will come and eat it! A woman's friends know how much she buys, and often want to share it. This is why she may walk several miles every day just to buy a few spoonfuls of oil each time.

TEACH FAMILIES TO BUY FOOD BY THE KILOGRAM

All over the world poor people get less good value for their money, but in many African towns poor people often get almost nothing for their money. Mothers must therefore know what to buy and buy wisely.

Because most foods, such as maize, are mixtures of nutrients, a mother buys both protein and joules of energy when she buys maize. To make the cost of food easier to understand, we shall think first about the cost of protein and then about the cost of joules.

6.4 The cost of 40 g of protein, and the 'best protein buy'.   By now you will know that one of the most important nutrients in a food is protein. You will also know that some foods contain a lot of protein, and some foods only a little. Some protein foods are expensive, and others are cheap. How can we tell families with only a little money how to buy the most protein with the money they have? The easiest way to do this is to find out what weight of food we have to buy to get 40 g of protein, and then to find out how much this weight of food costs. 40 g is the weight of about one small handful of maize meal, so it is not a big weight. *We have chosen 40 g because this is about the weight of reference protein needed by an adult man.* Here is what we found that 40 g of protein cost in Matero market in Lusaka in 1971.

TABLE 16
The Cost of 40 g of Protein in Matero Market in July 1971

	Food	Cost of 40 g of protein
1	Maize meal	2.8 n
2	Dry *kapenta* (fish)	4.6 n
3	Beans	8.3 n
4	Groundnuts	9.0 n
5	Dried skim milk	9.3 n
6	Fresh milk	11.0 n
7	Bread	12.0 n
8	Meat (cheap cuts)	20.0 n
9	Eggs	25.0 n
10	'A well-known infant food'	30.0 n

You will see that maize meal, which contains 8 per cent of protein, is the cheapest way of buying this nutrient. Eggs and 'a well-known kind of infant food', on the other hand, are an expensive way of buying protein. But this is not a fair way of comparing the costs of these proteins because, as you read in Section 3.8, egg protein has an NPU of 100 per cent and is 100 per cent used for body-building. Maize, on the other hand, has an NPU of only 55 per cent and so is only 55 per cent used for body-building.

We have, therefore, to make another table which tells us how much it costs to buy a weight of each of our food proteins that will be equal to 40 g of egg or reference protein. There are about 40 g of protein in five eggs. For example, because maize is only 55 per cent used for body-building we shall have to buy $\frac{100}{55}$ times more of it than we would if it were perfectly used for body-building. $\frac{100}{55}$ is about two, so we have to buy about twice as much maize protein to get protein equal to 40 g of reference protein.

there are about 40 g of reference protein in five eggs

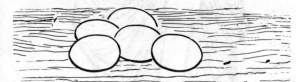

6-4, 40 grams of reference protein

Here then is our table altered in this way. You will see that the foods are now in a different order, and that some have become a better buy than others.

TABLE 17

The Cost of Various Kinds of Protein in Weights Equal to 40 g of Egg or Reference Protein in Matero Market in July 1971

BEST PROTEIN BUY

	Food	Cost of 40 g of reference protein
1	{ Maize meal	5.1 n
	{ Dry *kapenta*	5.1 n
3	Dried skim milk	12.8 n
4	Fresh milk	15.0 n
5	Beans	17.7 n
6	Groundnuts	19.0 n
7	Bread	23.0 n
8	Eggs	25.0 n
9	Meat	29.0 n
10	'A well-known infant food'	40.0 n

MOST EXPENSIVE PROTEIN BUY

You will see that the only protein of which we want the *same* weight as before, and for which we pay the same price, is egg protein. This is because it has an NPU of 100 per cent and is 100 per cent used for body-building. We have to buy *more* of all the other proteins. We need about twice as much maize, and only about 20 per cent more *kapenta*. Maize and *kapenta* are thus equal best buys at the top of the list. The infant food is still the most

expensive buy. Eggs have beaten meat. Groundnuts have been beaten by both kinds of milk.

6.5 The cost of 10 megajoules, and the 'best joule buy'.   The cost of energy food is even easier to work out than that of protein. A good way of doing this is to work out the cost of 10 megajoules. *We chose 10 megajoules because this is a useful number of joules to work with. It is the number of joules needed by a man doing a very light job.* You will remember that our reference man doing a fairly hard job needed 12.5 MJ, and that our reference woman, also doing a fairly hard job, needed 9.2 MJ.

DON'T TALK TO MOTHERS ABOUT JOULES —TELL THEM THE BEST FOODS TO BUY

At the same time as we worked out the cost of protein foods, we worked out the cost of 10 megajoules. We bought some joule-containing foods and weighed them. We noted how much we paid for them, and then worked out how much it would cost to get 10 megajoules from each kind of food. Here is what we found.

TABLE 18

The Cost of 10 Megajoules in Matero Market in July 1971

BEST JOULE BUY

	Food	Cost of 10 MJ
1	Maize meal (whole)	3.2 n
2	Maize meal (refined)	6.6 n
3	Beans	11.0 n
4	Sugar	14.0 n
5	Margarine	18.0 n
6	Bread	19.0 n
7	Groundnuts	23.0 n
8	Cassava flour	23.0 n
9	Oil	34.0 n
10	'A well-known infant food'	59.0 n

MOST EXPENSIVE JOULE BUY

You will see that even though there are many joules in cooking oil, it is an expensive way of buying energy. In this market dried cassava was also quite expensive. Maize meal is seen to be the cheapest joule food of all, and to be the best joule buy. You will remember that it was also one of the best protein buys. It is thus a very good cheap food. One of its disadvantages or difficulties is its

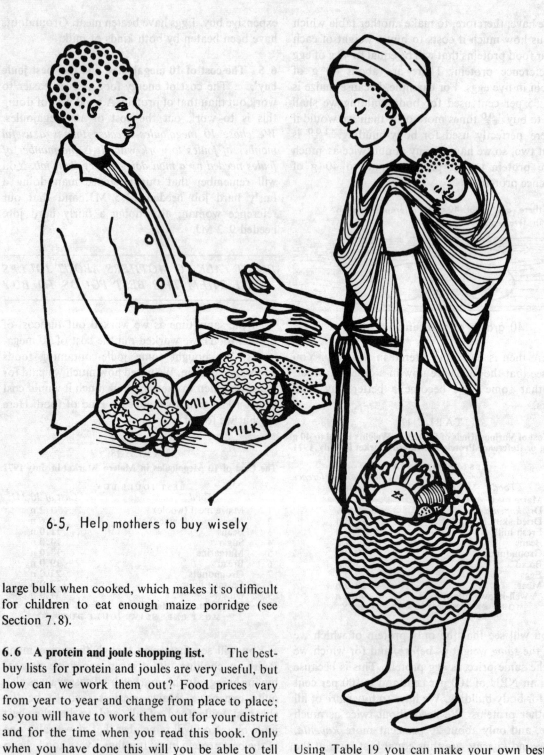

6-5, Help mothers to buy wisely

large bulk when cooked, which makes it so difficult for children to eat enough maize porridge (see Section 7.8).

6.6   A protein and joule shopping list.   The best-buy lists for protein and joules are very useful, but how can we work them out? Food prices vary from year to year and change from place to place; so you will have to work them out for your district and for the time when you read this book. Only when you have done this will you be able to tell the women you are teaching how to shop wisely.

Using Table 19 you can make your own best-buy list very easily.

TABLE 19
A Food Table

(1) Food	(2) Weight of food containing 40 g of protein	(3) Weight of food containing protein equal to 40 g of reference protein	(4) Weight of food containing 10 MJ
Dried fish (63%, 83%, 1,300)	63 g	76 g	770 g
Dried skim milk powder (36%, 75%, 1,500)	110 g	150 g	660 g
Soya beans (34%, 56%, 1,690)	120 g	210 g	590 g
Full cream milk powder (26%, 75%, 2,090)	150 g	210 g	480 g
Shelled groundnuts (23%, 48%, 2,290)	170 g	360 g	440 g
Peas (dry) (22%, 44%, 1,450)	180 g	410 g	690 g
Beans (dry) (20%, 47%, 1,420)	200 g	430 g	700 g
Fresh fish (fillet) (18%, 83%, 550)	220 g	270 g	1,800 g
Meat (beef) (18%, 70%, 920)	220 g	320 g	1,100 g
Liver (offal) (16%, 65%, 598)	250 g	390 g	1,700 g
Termites (15%, ?, 585)	270 g	—	1,700 g
Chicken (dressed) (12%, 65%, 510)	330 g	510 g	2,000 g
Eggs (12%, 100%, 602)	330 g	330 g	1,700 g
Wheat flour (white) (10%, 52%, 1,520)	400 g	770 g	660 g
Millet (10%, 56%, 1,421)	400 g	710 g	700 g
Maize meal (whole) (8%, 55%, 1,500)	500 g	910 g	660 g
Condensed milk (8%, 75%, 1,340)	500 g	670 g	750 g
Maize meal (refined) (7%, 55%, 1,500)	570 g	1,000 g	660 g
Evaporated milk (7%, 75%, 577)	570 g	760 g	1,730 g
Rice (polished) (7%, 57%, 1,500)	570 g	1,000 g	660 g
Bread (white) (7%, 52%, 1,090)	570 g	1,100 g	920 g
Cow's milk (3.5%, 75%, 272)	1,100 g	1,500 g	3,700 g
Dark green leaves (3%, ?, 92)	1,300 g	—	11 kg
Irish potatoes (2%, 71%, 290)	2 kg	2,800 g	3,400 g
Sweet potatoes (1%, —, 410)	4 kg	—	2,500 g
Cassava flour (1%, —, 1,410)	4 kg	—	700 g
Avocado pear (1%, —, 690)	4 kg	—	1,400 g
Cabbage (1%, —, 71)	4 kg	—	14 kg
Plantains, *matoke* (1%, —, 310)	4 kg	—	3,200 g
Honey (0%, —, 1,210)	—	—	830 g
Sugar (0%, —, 1,620)	—		620 g
Margarine or butter (0%, —, 3,010)	—		330 g
Cooking oil or fat (0%, —, 3,700)	—		270 g

(For the cost of infant foods see Section 5.7 c.)

Note: Under each kind of food you will see three figures in brackets. The first is the percentage of protein in that food, the second is the NPU of that protein, and the third is the number of kilojoules that there are in 100 g of food. Here is an example:

Dried fish

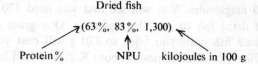

Protein%   NPU   kilojoules in 100 g

Columns (2), (3) and (4) are worked out like this:

$$\text{Weight of food needed to get 40 g of protein (column (2))} = \frac{40 \times 100}{\text{protein} \%}$$

$$\text{Weight of food needed to get protein equal to 40 g of reference protein (column (3))} = \frac{40 \times 100 \times 100}{\text{protein} \% \times \text{NPU} \%}$$

$$\text{Weight of food needed to get 10 megajoules (column (4))} = \frac{10,000 \times 100}{\text{number of kilojoules in 100 g of food}}$$

The figures in this table have been 'rounded' to (made or changed into) 'two significant figures', because this makes food costs easier to work out. Thus, when the table was first made the first figure came to 63.49 g of dried fish. This has been rounded to 63 g. The second figure came to 76.49 g. This has been rounded to 76 g.

Table 19 has four columns. On the left in the first column is a list of foods. The second column tells you how much of each kind of food is needed to get 40 g of protein. The third column tells you how much of a food to buy to get an amount of protein equal to 40 g of egg or reference protein (about five eggs). The fourth column tells you how much food to buy to get 10 megajoules. All you have to do is to work out how much each of these weights of food costs in your shops or market.

Let us say that you go to a market and buy a pile of fish which costs 10n. You take it home and weigh it and find that it weighs 30 g. This 30 g of fish will thus have cost you 10n. One gram of fish will therefore have cost you $\frac{10}{30}$n. From the second column in Table 19 you will see that you need 63 g of dried fish to give you 40 g of protein. These 63 grams of dried fish will therefore cost you $63 \times \frac{10}{30}$n. This comes to 21n.

Use the third column in Table 19 when you want to find out how much food to buy to get an amount of protein equal to 40 g of egg or reference protein. For dried fish this is 76 g. You will thus have to spend $\frac{10}{30} \times 76n$. This comes to about 25n. You will therefore have to buy 25n worth of dried fish to get an amount of protein equal to 40 g of egg or reference protein.

The cost of 10 megajoules is worked out in the same way. The figures in the fourth column tell you how much of each food you need to buy to get 10 megajoules. You will see that you need 770 g of dried fish to get 10 megajoules. One gram of dried fish costs you $\frac{10}{30}n$; so 770 g will cost you $770 \times \frac{10}{30}n$. This comes to about K 2.50. Dried fish is an expensive way of buying joules; so families get most of their joules from cheap foods like maize.

Table 19 is interesting in many ways. You will see that it starts with the foods that contain 40 g of protein in the smallest weight. This is only another way of saying that it starts with the foods that have the highest percentage of protein. We have just seen that there is 40 g of protein in 63 g of dried fish. But if you want to buy 40 g of protein as cow's milk, you will have to buy 1,100 g, which is more than a litre. This is because milk contains only 3.5 per cent of protein; so you have to buy a lot of it to get 40 g of protein. However, as we saw in Section 5.3, a child can easily drink a lot of milk.

You will see that cassava contains so little protein (1 %) that you have to buy 4 kg to get 40 g of protein. There is so little protein in cassava that its NPU has not been worked out!

At the bottom of Table 19 you will see that you only need 270 g of cooking oil to get 10 megajoules. This is because oils, like cooking oil, contain more joules than any of the other foods.

You will see that there are so few joules in cabbage (71 kJ in 100 g) that you have to eat about 14 kg to get 10 megajoules. Cabbage also contains very little protein and few vitamins or minerals, so it cannot be considered a useful food.

WORK OUT THE BEST PROTEIN AND JOULE BUYS FOR YOUR DISTRICT

6.7 How much money does a family need to buy food?   In Sections 6.1 and 6.2 we saw how much

protein and how many joules each kind of person needs. In Section 6.6 we saw how much of each kind of food a mother must buy to get an amount of protein equal to 40 g of reference protein or 10 megajoules. We can now work out how much food a family needs in a month, and how much it costs them. This is the money that a mother must have if she is to feed her family well.

Let us take a family with four children; one aged 3 months, one of 5, one of 8 and one of 11 years. The two-year-old child in this family has just died of measles! Let us say that the three-month-old child is being nursed by his mother. The father is doing a light job as a clerk. Here then is the number of joules and the weight of reference protein that each member of the family needs in one day. These figures come from Sections 6.1 and 6.2.

A family's daily needs for protein and joules

Person in the family	Mega-joules	Grams of reference protein
Father	12.5 MJ	37.0 g
Mother (breast-feeding)	11.5 MJ	46.0 g
Boy of 5 years	7.6 MJ	20.0 g
Girl of 8 years	9.2 MJ	25.0 g
Boy of 11 years	10.9 MJ	30.0 g
Total for the family each day	51.7 MJ	158.0 g

To make the figures easier to work out let us say our family needs 50 MJ and 160 g of protein each day. The total for a 30-day month is 30 times as much. It is $30 \times 50\text{MJ} = 1,500$ megajoules and $30 \times 160 = 4,800$ g of reference protein.

Let us say that the family eats maize and gets one-tenth of the joules it needs from cooking oil. A tenth of 1,500 is 150; so the family would get this number of megajoules from cooking oil. The family will therefore have to eat $1,500 - 150 = 1,350$ megajoules as maize.

This maize meal would also give the family some protein. We saw from Table 19 that 10 megajoules are contained in 660 g of maize meal. Maize meal is 8 per cent protein; so, when every 660 g of maize meal is bought containing 10 megajoules,

$\frac{8}{100} \times 660 = 52.8$ g of protein are bought as well. The family has bought enough maize meal to give them 1,350 megajoules, so they are getting $\frac{1,350}{10} \times 52.8 = 7,128$ g of protein at the same time.

However, this is only maize protein with an NPU of 55 per cent. 7,128 g of maize protein is therefore equal to

$7,128 \times \frac{55}{100} = 3,920$ g of reference protein.

But the family needs 4,800 g of reference protein; so they will have to get $4,800 - 3,920 = 880$ g of reference protein from some other food. Let us say they get it from *kapenta*. There is protein equal to 40 g of reference protein in 76 g of *kapenta*. The family will therefore have to buy

$880 \times \frac{76}{40} = 1,672$ g of *kapenta* to give them the rest of the protein they need.

This *kapenta* would also give them some more joules, for there are 10 megajoules in 770 g of *kapenta*. 1,672 g of *kapenta* would therefore give them

$\frac{1,672}{770} \times 10 = 21.8$ megajoules.

This is, however, such a small number of joules compared with the 1,500 megajoules that the family needs during the month, which they get from maize and oil, that we will not think about it any more.

It is not easy to work out a family's needs for minerals and protective foods, so we will make a guess and say that the family spends one kwacha a month on these foods for each person in the family. The family has therefore to spend K6 during the month.

Now let us add up the cost of all these foods. We will use the costs in Tables 17 and 18.

Maize	1,350 megajoules at 3.2 n for	
10 megajoules=		K4.32
Cooking oil	150 megajoules at 34 n for	
10 megajoules=		K5.10
Kapenta	equal to 880 g of reference	
protein at 5.1 n per 40 g=		K1.12
Protective foods, say,		K6.00
		K16.54

This is interesting in several ways. It shows us that a family which eats maize can get about 80 per cent of the protein it needs from maize. Families

eating maize which contains 8 per cent of protein are therefore much more fortunate than those which eat cassava containing only 1 per cent.

Many families buy their maize in 50 kg bags. Table 19 tells us that there are 10 MJ in 660 g of maize meal. A bag therefore contains:

$$\frac{50 \times 1,000 \times 10}{660} = 760 \text{ MJ}.$$

Our family wanted 1,500 megajoules from maize during the month. It therefore needs about two bags to give it the joules it needs. Many families try to live on a bag, or a bag and a half, which is not enough.

6.8 Budgeting. Planning to spend money wisely is called **budgeting**. Because this is a book about nutrition, we are interested in the money that is spent on food, but good budgeting also means planning to have the right money for rent, school fees and taxes and clothes. All families must budget their money carefully if they are going to be able to feed their children well. Food is thus the most important part of the family budget. Here is an example.

Let us say that a family of three adults and three children wanted to eat porridge with dried skim milk in the morning, *nshima* with green leaves and groundnuts in the middle of the day, and *nshima* with *kapenta* or beans in the evening. It would cost them about K20 per month, and it would have to be spent like this:

Food	Amount to buy	Cost in Lusaka in 1969
Maize meal	100 kg	K6.30
Sugar	2 kg	0.35
Margarine	12 × 300 g tins	2.16
Spinach or	2 × 250 g	3.00
cassava leaves	bunches daily	
Groundnuts	4 kg	1.60
Kapenta	2 kg	1.80
Beans	4 kg	1.80
Salt	1 kg	0.06
Dried skim milk	6 kg	2.88
Total		K19.95

MONEY FOR FOOD IS THE MOST IMPORTANT PART OF THE FAMILY BUDGET

Families often budget badly. On a farm the money that is earned from selling crops is used for buying clothes, a bicycle, or a radio. It is not used for buying food, because food is grown, and does not need to be bought. When farmers move to town they may not understand how much money has now got to be spent on food for their families. They may buy a sack of maize meal at the end of the month and give their wives only about 5 kwacha for buying relish. They may keep the rest of the money to buy beer for themselves. An important part of nutrition teaching is thus to try to persuade men to give their wives more of the money they earn each month. The family can then buy several kilograms of beans and groundnuts, or dried skim milk, as well as maize meal at the end of the month.

Many women budget badly and only buy small amounts of food which are only enough for one day's meals at a time. This is an expensive way of buying foods such as beans and groundnuts which can be stored. We must thus try to teach mothers to buy larger amounts of these foods less often, to buy them by the kilo, and to keep them until they are wanted. This is a much cheaper way of buying food. Foods which cannot be stored, such as green vegetables, have to be bought each day, if a mother cannot grow them herself.

THE WAY TO SPEND MONEY WISELY HAS TO BE TAUGHT AND LEARNT

A month is a long time, and it would be easier for families to budget if men were paid each week instead of each month. This might make it easier for them to buy the food their children need.

You will see that in this section and the last one we have found that a family of five people needs between K16 and K20 each month to buy food. Let us say K20 to be on the safe side. The foods

that were used to work this out are those that people eat in Lusaka, and the prices were those of 1969–71. In other places people eat different foods, and prices change. From what you have learnt in this chapter and from the prices in your market, you will be able to work out how much a family in your district needs to buy enough food for good health. If you like, you can use the family in Section 6.7 as an example. We will call the least sum of money that an ordinary-sized family needs to buy enough food each month the **minimum family food budget.** Minimum means least.

WORK OUT THE MINIMUM FAMILY FOOD BUDGET FOR YOUR DISTRICT

The minimum family food budget has to be compared with **the basic wage.** Basic means bottom, simplest or least. The basic wage is thus the lowest wage that anyone should earn who has a full time paid job. People who have no job, or who work part of the time, or who work for themselves, may earn much less than this. In Lusaka at the time this book was written the basic wage was about K1 each day, or about K30 per month. *Thus two thirds of the basic wage has to be spent on food to feed a family of six people.* The K10 that is left is hardly enough to pay for rent, clothes, fuel, and perhaps transport to work that a family has to have to live. We see that in Lusaka the basic wage has to be spent very carefully indeed, if a family is to be well nourished, and is to have something to wear, and somewhere to live. Even so, it is hardly enough. No money is left over for beer, or for anything that is not really necessary!

What is the basic wage in your district? What percentage of it is taken by the minimum family food budget?

6.9 Selling wisely. Many families sell too much of the food they grow, and do not store enough to eat later in the year. Later on they may have to buy some back when it is more expensive, so that they get back less than they sold. They may not have enough money and may thus go hungry for several months in the year. We have to teach people that the most important use for the food they grow is to feed their families. The only food that should be sold is the food that the family does not need to eat. Farmers need money; so they must learn to grow more food, so that there is some to sell as well as enough to eat all through the year. If village families are always to have enough food to eat, it has to be stored from one harvest until the next. As you will read in Sections 9.5 and 9.6, better ways of storing food are important in preventing malnutrition.

DON'T SELL FOOD THE FAMILY SHOULD BE EATING

6.10   THINGS TO DO

(a) Your own best buy.   Go to your own shops or markets. Buy food, weigh it and work out the best protein and best joule buy for your district. For this you will need a balance weighing up to about 500 g. If you have not got enough money to buy food, the retailer may let you weigh it in the shop. Take a letter with you saying who you are and what you are doing. These best-buy lists are of the greatest importance in helping families to learn how to spend their money wisely. When you have made your lists fill them in here. Fill in the name of your district and the date you went shopping, because prices change. Find the costs of the quantities that mothers usually buy. If they buy

maize by the sack, find out the cost and weight of a sack. If they buy oil by the half cupful, find out how much this costs and how much it weighs.

Best-buy list for................District; Date ....

BEST BUY

40 g protein		Protein equal to 40 g of reference protein		10 megajoules	
Food	Cost	Food	Cost	Food	Cost
....	....	....	....	....	....
....	....	....	....	....	....
....	....	....	....	....	....
....	....	....	....	....	....
....	....	....	....	....	....
....	....	....	....	....	....
....	....	....	....	....	....
....	....	....	....	....	....
....	....	....	....	....	....
....	....	....	....	....	....
....	....	....	....	....	....
....	....	....	....	....	....

WORST BUY

Best-buy lists like this are very easy. Make a list like this in your notebook. The (2), (3), and (4) that you see here are the figures for each food that you will find in columns (2), (3) and (4) in Table 19. Fill in the best-buy list above when you have worked it out in your notebook like this.

A PAGE FROM YOUR NOTEBOOK

Food	Price paid (a)	Weight in grams (b)	Cost per gram (c) = (a)/(b)	Cost of 40 g of protein (c) × (2)	Cost of protein equal to 40 g of reference protein (c) × (3)	Cost of 10 MJ (c) × (4)
....	....	....	....	....	....	....
....	....	....	....	....	....	....
....	....	....	....	....	....	....

(b) A shopping guide. Some shops are much cheaper than others. Which are the cheapest shops in your district? Which are the most expensive? Which shops sell food by the kilo? Which shops sell foods in expensive little handfuls? What are the cheapest shops in your district for buying each kind of food? We will call a list of shops like this a **shopping guide.** Make your own shopping guide and fill it in below.

Shopping guide for .... *District; Date* ....

Food	Cheapest shop	Most expensive shop
....	....	....
....	....	....
....	....	....
....	....	....
....	....	....
....	....	....
....	....	....
....	....	....
....	....	....
....	....	....

(c) Piles of food of equal value. See if you can buy or borrow enough foods to make piles of each kind of food that will give 10 megajoules or 40 g of protein or protein equal to 40 g of reference protein. You will then see for yourself how much of each food is needed to give these amounts of protein and joules.

(d) Your own minimum family food budget. Take the family in Section 6.7 and the foods and prices in your market to work out the least amount of money that this family needs to spend on food. You will be able to work out the cost of the protein and joules very well, but you will have to guess how much they need to spend on protective foods, because to make an accurate measure needs more knowledge than there is space to tell you about here.

Sometimes families will tell you that they only have, say, K15, or even less, to buy food each month. From what you have read in this chapter, you will be able to tell them the best way to spend it, even if it is less than the minimum family food budget. One way to make a little money go further is not to buy protective foods, but to gather green leaves from the fields and the bush.

Find out the basic wage in your district. How does the minimum family food budget compare with this? What percentage of the basic wage is taken up by the minimum family food budget?

(e) Best buys for meat. In Table 19 you saw that we have said that beef contains 18 per cent of protein. This is for beef which contains little fat and no bones. Some cuts (kinds) of meat look quite cheap in the shops and yet contain much bone and fat. There may be so little real meat in these cuts that they are an expensive way of buying meat. The only way to see which cuts of meat are the best buy is to go to the butcher and to find out. Buy some meat of each of the different cuts. Take away the meat from the bone and the fat with a knife. Weigh the meat that you have bought with each cut and find out how much a kilo of it would cost. You may find that 'shin', 'ribs' or 'brisket' are expensive ways of buying meat, and that 'mince' or 'gravy beef' are better. Liver and kidneys may also be good buys.

(f) How much food can you buy for 10n? Many families have little money to buy food and spend only 5 or 10n at a time. Find out how much food you can buy for, say, 10n, in your district, and make a collection of piles of food, each costing this amount.

(g) A food-consumption survey and some food budgets. Visit some families earning different amounts of money, some poor and some rich. Try to find out what they eat and how much they spend on food. This is not easy, but you may be able to find out something. A survey of this kind is called a food-consumption survey. Work out a food budget for each kind of family, and see if you can work out how many grams of protein and how many joules they are eating.

Chapter Seven

FEEDING THE FAMILY

YOUNG CHILDREN AND THEIR MOTHERS

7.1 Breast-feeding. Breast milk is the perfect food for a baby. It has the right amount of body-building protein that the young child needs to grow. It also has plenty of energy-giving carbohydrate and fat, as well as all the vitamins, minerals and water that a young child needs. Breast milk is always ready and does not have to be cooked. Breast milk is safe and contains none of the harmful micro-organisms (germs) that are so often found in dirty feeding bottles. Breast milk never goes sour or bad—*even when a mother is pregnant.* It is never too hot or too cold. Mothers who breast-feed their babies have no feeding bottles to clean. When a mother is travelling with her child, breast milk is always there for him on the journey, and there are no feeding bottles to be carried and washed, which may be very difficult.

Much of this chapter is about how important it is that all mothers should breast-feed their children for as long as they can and stop breast-feeding them as *slowly* as possible. By slowly we mean that a mother should give a child less and less milk over several weeks until she is finally giving him none at all. At the same time she must increase the other foods she gives him.

BREAST-FEEDING IS BEST

Breast-feeding is the *natural* way young children should be fed. All other kinds of feeding are called **artificial feeding**. The common kind of artificial feeding is bottle-feeding. In the next chapter you will read how dangerous bottle-feeding is and also why it is so dangerous. Because breast-feeding is so good and bottle-feeding can be so bad, one of the most useful things that we can do is to encourage mothers to breast-feed their children.

At the start of suckling the child opens his mouth and feels the nipple placed inside it. His tongue goes underneath the nipple and pulls it right inside his mouth. Once the nipple is well inside the mouth, the baby's gums (part of the mouth where teeth will grow) press onto the sides of the nipple and press the milk out of it into his mouth. Sucking is much less important than the pressing on the sides of the nipple by the baby's gums. Farmers who keep cows know this and press the milk out of the sides of a cow's nipple in the same way. If breast-feeding is going to be successful, a mother's nipples have got to be able to get right into her baby's mouth. During her first pregnancy a woman's nipples grow in such a way that they can do this.

7.2 Feeding a child from birth until he is four months old. The milk that comes from a mother's breast for the first few days is thin and watery and is called **colostrum.** It is very good for babies; so they should be put to their mother's breast as soon as they are born. Many babies start sucking almost at once, but if a baby does not start sucking for a few hours, wet the inside of his mouth with a spoonful of cold boiled water. This will often start him sucking.

Most mothers feed their children well during the day, but what about the night? Tell them to take their young babies to bed with them. As we shall soon see, a breast that is suckled from often makes more milk, and the night is as important for suckling as the day. The fear that some people have that a baby may be harmed by his mother lying on top of him ('overlying' him) is not true. One of the reasons why so many women in Europe and America are not successful in breast-feeding their children, is that they do not take them to bed and feed them during the night.

Breast-feeding alone is enough for the first four months of a child's life, and there is seldom

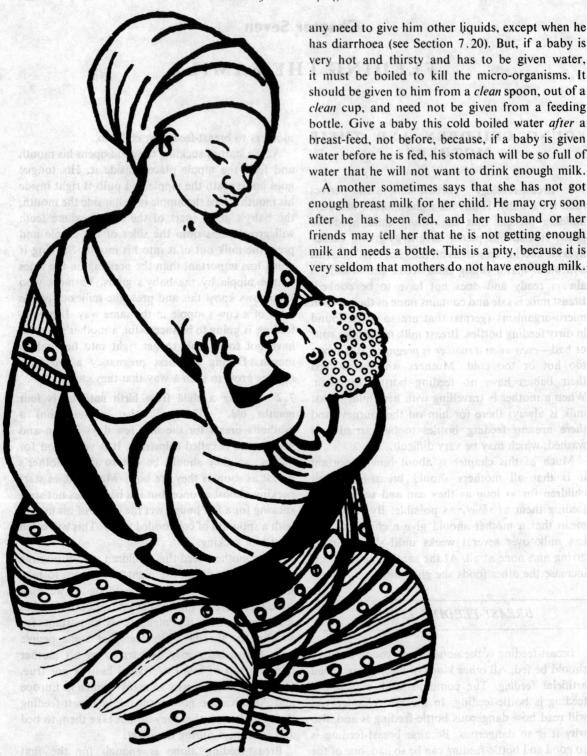

any need to give him other liquids, except when he has diarrhoea (see Section 7.20). But, if a baby is very hot and thirsty and has to be given water, it must be boiled to kill the micro-organisms. It should be given to him from a *clean* spoon, out of a *clean* cup, and need not be given from a feeding bottle. Give a baby this cold boiled water *after* a breast-feed, not before, because, if a baby is given water before he is fed, his stomach will be so full of water that he will not want to drink enough milk.

A mother sometimes says that she has not got enough breast milk for her child. He may cry soon after he has been fed, and her husband or her friends may tell her that he is not getting enough milk and needs a bottle. This is a pity, because it is very seldom that mothers do not have enough milk.

7-1, Breast milk is the best food for a young child

The baby who cries is nearly always just a baby who cries more than other babies. He may have stomach pains, but these pains do not mean that he is ill. It is difficult for a family to live with a baby who is always crying, and it is often easy for them to give him a feeding bottle full of milk. This may stop him crying, even though he does not need it. A mother must not start bottle-feeding for this reason, because it may kill him in the end! In Zambia and in some other countries it is the custom to put something belonging to a child on his grave when he dies. It is sad to see so many children with the feeding bottle that may well have killed them put on their graves!

DON'T START BOTTLE-FEEDING JUST BECAUSE THE BABY CRIES

A child's sucking is the best way of making milk come in his mother's breast. If he sucks well and takes all the milk from her breast, it will make more milk. If he does not suck well and leaves some milk behind, the breast may 'think' that it is making too much milk, and start making less. Giving a child a feeding bottle does two things. It fills his stomach and makes him less hungry, so that he sucks less well from his mother. He may also find that it is easier to suck from a bottle than from the breast, and he may get lazy about sucking from the breast. Both these things may make him suck less hard, so that the breast will make less milk. When this has been happening for a few weeks there will be so little milk in his mother's breasts that he really will need his bottle, which may kill him. *A baby must not therefore be given a feeding bottle just because he cries too much when he is a few weeks old.* A baby seldom cries because his mother is not giving him enough milk.

A BABY'S SUCKING MAKES MILK COME IN HIS MOTHER'S BREASTS

What should you tell a mother who says that her young baby cries because she has not got enough milk in her breasts and who wants to start bottle-feeding? Tell her that many babies cry, and that it is usually becasue they are more lively than other babies. Tell her to breast-feed him whenever he seems to want it and that the more he sucks the more milk will come. Persuade her *not* to give him a bottle! Weigh him, and weigh him again in a week's time. If he is now heavier and has grown, he must have been getting enough milk. Tell her that he will stop crying in a few weeks, when he is about three months old, and that it is better for her to wait until then.

Most babies will have gained weight. But a baby who has not, and who seems otherwise well, should still not be given milk from a bottle. Instead he can start to take a little porridge from a cup and spoon. You will remember from Section 5.6 that by porridge we mean the *thin* food for young children that is made by boiling maize, millet or cassava flour in water, and which is so thin that it must be eaten from a spoon or cup. It is usually quite safe to give a baby porridge when he is about six weeks old. Add some protein food to this porridge, such as dried skim milk, egg or well-mashed skinned beans. Unless groundnuts are very well pounded they may give a young baby diarrhoea. The Rhodesians have a good custom of making a food for babies by pounding groundnuts in water, and mixing this with their porridge.

A baby may get slight diarrhoea from any of these foods. If he does, try giving him porridge without added protein for a week or two. He could also be given some boiled cow's milk, with water and sugar added, as in Section 8.7. *He must go on breast-feeding*, and he need only be given these extra foods once a day, or later on twice a day. Give him these foods *after* breast-feeding, and after he has taken all the milk he can get from the breast.

Sometimes, when a mother really has no milk, one of her friends or relatives may be breast-feeding a child and may be able to give the child some milk. It is quite safe for a child to suck from another mother, and if there is difficulty in breast-feeding a child, it is often useful to ask if this is possible.

Last of all, do not forget to tell a mother who is having difficulty breast-feeding that she must feed herself well. If she is malnourished herself, she will probably have less milk for her child. Some women think that beer makes more milk come in their breasts, but food is more important for making good milk.

Provided babies are breast-fed, most of them grow well until they are five or six months old. This first six months is the only time in many people's lives when they are properly fed. It is usually after the age of six months, when babies should be getting protein foods and don't get them, that they become malnourished.

7.3 A child's first porridge.   A mother's breast milk usually gives a child all the food he needs until he is about six months old. But, when he is six months old, he has become so big that breast milk is not enough by itself. If a child is to continue to grow well he must therefore be eating plenty of porridge, as well as breast milk, before he is six months old. *His mother should start giving him plain maize porridge when he is about four months old.* He will then be well used to it by the time that he needs it. Most children get their first tooth when they are about six months old, *so a child must be eating porridge well before he gets his first tooth.* Some mothers wait to give a child his first porridge until he reaches out for her food with his hand. Most children start to do this at about six months. This is too late, and they should be having porridge well before this.

START GIVING A CHILD PORRIDGE
WHEN HE IS FOUR MONTHS OLD

At first a child's mother should give him porridge once a day, when he is most hungry. When he is eating it well, he can have it two or three times. Because maize and millet both contain about 8 per cent of protein, they make much better porridge for young children than cassava, which only contains 1 per cent. As soon as a child is eating plain porridge well, some body-building protein foods must be added to it and mixed in well. These can be pounded groundnuts, groundnut butter, mashed skinned beans, dried skim milk, eggs,

minced meat, pounded fresh fish or something else. A very good porridge to give young children is the Likuni *phala* that you will read about in Section 7.13. A child needs these body-building foods, and he must be eating them well by the time he is six months old. If he is only eating plain porridge at this time he will not be getting enough body-building food.

When a child is first given porridge, most of it falls out of his mouth. This is partly because he does not like the taste, and partly because he has been sucking from a breast, and does not yet know how to get food into his mouth from a spoon. He has thus to get used to the taste of his new food and to learn how to get food from a spoon. His mother can teach him these things by giving him one or two small spoonfuls of the new food once a day for the first few days. She should only give him one new food at a time, and not try another until he is used to the first one. If a mother goes on trying, she can get her child to like most foods. *She should start by giving him these new foods when he is hungry, before he has had his breast milk.* Because he is hungry he is more likely to eat them and get used to them. *But once a child likes a food well, he should be given it after he has drunk all the milk he can from the breast.* This is important, because a child will not suck strongly if he is full of porridge when he is put to the breast. As we said earlier, if he does not suck well the supply of breast milk will get less. This is bad, because a child still needs all the breast milk he can get, even though he is having other foods.

AS SOON AS A CHILD IS EATING PORRIDGE
WELL ADD PROTEIN FOODS TO IT

A mother may say that some food, such as groundnuts, makes her child cough or choke. A child may get a whole groundnut stuck in his throat, but pounded groundnuts are quite safe. Any baby who is learning to eat may sometimes get a piece of *any* kind of food stuck in his throat. This may make him cough or choke, but it is not the fault of that kind of food. His mother must not stop giving it to him because she thinks it makes

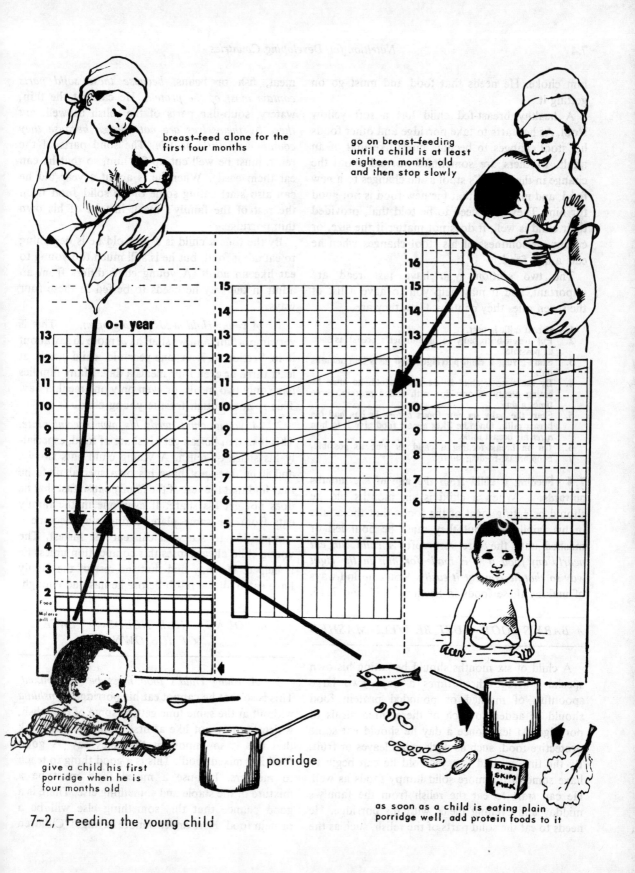

breast-feed alone for the
first four months

go on breast-feeding
until a child is at least
eighteen months old
and then stop slowly

o-1 year

give a child his first
porridge when he is
four months old

porridge

as soon as a child is eating plain
porridge well, add protein foods to it

DRIED
SKIM
MILK

7-2, Feeding the young child

him choke. He needs that food and must go on getting it.

A healthy breast-fed child has a soft yellow stool. As he starts to take porridge and other foods his stool changes to become more like that of an adult. Mothers are sometimes worried about the change in their child's stool as he changes to a new food, and may think that the new food is not good for him. They may need to be told that, provided their child is well, it does not matter if the size, or colour, or solidness of his stool changes when he eats a new food.

The two sections you have just read are important, and it may help you to have a list of the seven rules they contain. Here they are.

1. **Breast milk is best.**
2. **Put a new-born baby to his mother's breast as soon as possible.**
3. **Start giving a child porridge when he is four months old.**
4. **By the time a child is six months old, he must be eating plenty of porridge with added protein, three times a day.**
5. **Start the baby on new foods *before* he has had his breast milk. Once he likes a new food give it to him *after* his breast milk.**
6. **Go on breast-feeding a child as long as possible.**
7. **Stop breast-feeding slowly.**

7.4 Feeding a child from the age of six months onwards.   When a child is six months old he should be eating most of the foods that the adults in his family eat, but they must be pounded or mashed until they are very soft. *A child can eat nearly any food if it is made for him in the right way so that he can eat it easily.* You can find ways of making these foods in Sections 7.11 and 7.15.

A BABY'S FOOD MUST BE WELL MASHED

A child of six months should be eating his own special porridge three times a day. Two large spoonfuls of mashed or pounded protein food should be added to each of these three meals of porridge. At least once a day he should eat some protective food, such as dark green leaves or fruit. By the time a child is a year old he can begin to have some of the more solid lumpy foods as well. He can start to eat the relish from the family's midday and evening meals with his porridge. He needs to eat the solid parts of the relish, such as the

meat, fish or beans, *because these solid parts contain most of the protein.* He can eat the thin, watery, soup-like parts of the relish as well, *but these by themselves are not enough because they contain very little protein.* The solid parts of the relish must be well cut up for him, so that he can eat them easily. When he is about a year old he can also start eating some of the solid food from the rest of the family's meal, instead of his own thin porridge.

By the time a child is a year old he is beginning to eat adult food, but he is still much too young to eat like an adult. A young child differs from an adult in the way he needs to be fed in these four ways.

1. *A young child needs feeding often.*   This is very important, and we shall have more to say about it in Section 7.7. A one-year-old child needs at least three or even four meals a day. Many families have only two meals, or even only one meal, a day, This is not enough for the young child.

2. *A young child needs his own special plate.* This is so that he can get his share of food, especially his share of relish. A young child eats slowly, and if he does not have his own special plate he may find that the rest of the family eat so fast that he does not get his share. If everyone in the family eats from the same plate, eating may become a competition to see who can eat the fastest. The young child always loses this competition unless he is helped. He may find that the rest of the family have eaten all the relish before he has had enough.

A YOUNG CHILD NEEDS A PLATE OF HIS OWN

---

3. *A young child's food must be well mixed.* This is so that he cannot eat his porridge or *nshima* without at the same time getting some of the relish, which he may not like at first. Some people think that this is so important that they say 'A good food is a mixed food'. This is a good thing to teach to mothers, because a mixed food must be a mixture of the staple and something else. There is a good chance that this something else will be a protein food. Here are two more sayings: 'Children

need plenty of relish', and '*Nshima* fills the stomach, but relish makes you grow'. These are good sayings, because relish contains the proteins that children need to grow.

4. *A young child needs to be fed with a spoon.* Young children are bad at feeding themselves with their fingers, and need to be fed with a spoon. At first they need to be helped, but later on they can learn to feed themselves.

Most adults and older children eat *nshima* with their fingers. They take some *nshima* from a plate, roll it into a ball, make a hole for the relish with their thumb, use the lump of *nshima* like a spoon to pick up relish, and then eat it. A young child is very bad at doing this and puts food all over his face. It may be hot, and he is not so good at holding it as his brothers and sisters. Sometimes he may make a ball of *nshima*, or his elder sister may make it for him, but he just dips it into the watery part of the relish and does not get any of the solid part at all. He may therefore get little *nshima* and even less relish. In some families children are not allowed to make a hole in the *nshima* with their fingers in case they eat too much relish! A ball of *nshima* dipped into the watery part of the relish is not good enough for a young child. It does not give him enough protein.

HELP A YOUNG CHILD TO FEED HIMSELF WITH A SPOON

Some mothers do not give children body-building foods like meat and fish in case they get to like them too much! This is a pity because young children need these foods. Like all foods for young children, they should, if necessary, be well pounded or cut up, so that they can be eaten easily.

A young child will get more food if his family does these things for him:

> Give him a plate of his own;
> Give him plenty of relish;
> Mix his relish with his *nshima*;
> Let him eat with a spoon until he can use his fingers well;
> Help him to eat by feeding him with a spoon;
> Make sure that his food is well cut up for him.

All these things are *much* more important than you might think. Young children not getting their share of the family's food is one of the most important causes of malnutrition. It is one of the most serious 'blocks in the food-path' that you will read about in Section 9.18. Customs also block the food-path here, because it is not the custom to mix *nshima* and relish. It is also usually the custom for everyone to eat from the same plate, and for everyone in the family to eat with their fingers. There is no nutritional reason why the rest of the family should eat with a knife and fork, and they should not be persuaded to. As we have seen, there is, however, a very good nutritional reason why the young child should be helped to feed himself with a spoon until he is old enough to use his fingers well. We see therefore that *some* customs are bad for child feeding and need to be changed. Other customs are much better left as they are.

7.5 When should breast-feeding end? Because mother's milk is such an important way in which a child gets protein, a mother should go on breast-feeding her child until he is eighteen months or two years old. If she wants to go on longer, she can. A mother must stop breast-feeding slowly. When a child is very young he needs to be fed very often, but, by the time he is a year old, his mother can breast-feed him in the morning, go out to work, and then breast-feed him again in the evening. If she can, she should also breast-feed him in the middle of the day. When her child is eighteen months old, a mother can stop the earlier breast-feeds, so that in the end he is only being breast-fed at night.

BREAST-FEED A CHILD UNTIL HE IS EIGHTEEN MONTHS OR TWO YEARS OLD

Breast-feeding must stop slowly, for the health of both a mother and her child.

For a mother. If the mother of a very young child stops breast-feeding suddenly, her breasts may swell with milk and become painful. She may also get abscesses (sore places) in them.

For her child. Breast-feeding is very important in a child's life and makes him feel happy. He goes to the breast when he is hurt. If he suddenly cannot do this, he may become very unhappy, and may not eat any food at all.

BREAST-FEEDING MUST END SLOWLY

Some mothers put hot peppers or the juice of trees on their breasts when they want to stop breast-feeding. This is a bad thing to do. It is sad for a child who has got used to his mother's breast to suddenly find his mouth full of red-hot pepper!

A child should be eating plenty of porridge and protein food by the time breast-feeding stops. If he is not eating plenty of these foods when breast-feeding ends, he may not get enough to eat and may become thin and malnourished. He may even die. If he is eating porridge only, without added protein, when breast-feeding suddenly stops, he may get kwashiorkor. A child should be eating all kinds of food by the time he is eighteen months old. If he is doing this, he will not miss his breast-feeds when they slowly finish, and he will not become malnourished.

A CHILD MUST BE EATING RELISH WELL BEFORE HE STOPS BREAST FEEDING

Some mothers start bottle-feeding as soon as they stop breast-feeding! This is not necessary and can be harmful. When a baby stops breast-feeding he should already be having at least three good protein meals a day, and he should also be drinking well from a cup. Other mothers do not start giving their child relish until they stop breast-feeding. This again is bad. A child should have been eating relish with his porridge for several months before he stops breast-feeding.

Breast-feeding is sometimes stopped because a mother says her child's stomach is 'too fat'. Many children have fat stomachs, especially if they are malnourished, so this is a bad reason for stopping breast-feeding.

Breast-feeding is sometimes stopped because a child has diarrhoea. This is bad and a mother should continue to breast-feed her child with diarrhoea. He may have diarrhoea because he is already malnourished, so stopping breast-feeding will make his malnutrition worse.

7.6 Breast-feeding in pregnancy.   Many women stop breast-feeding as soon as they get pregnant, or even when they start sleeping with their husbands again, and think they might get pregnant. They do this because they think that the milk from a pregnant mother harms a baby, and may become 'sour'. A mother's breasts make less milk when she is pregnant, but there is nothing wrong with the little milk that they do make.

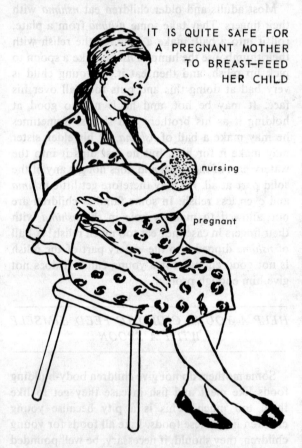

IT IS QUITE SAFE FOR A PREGNANT MOTHER TO BREAST-FEED HER CHILD

nursing

pregnant

7-3, A pregnant breast-feeding mother needs plenty of extra protein and joules

Some tribes have a special word for the disease a breast-feeding child gets when his mother becomes pregnant again (see Section 2.5). The Bemba call it *ulunse*, which is the same as kwashiorkor. It is interesting that people know this disease, because, as we have said, children may get kwashiorkor *because they stop breast-feeding, and not because*

they are breast-fed while their mother is pregnant.
When a mother finds she is pregnant, she is worried
because she thinks she has already harmed the
child at her breast. She need not worry, for she
will only harm him if she suddenly takes him away
from her breast, and stops him from drinking the
protein in her milk. This is what makes him malnourished. But if she goes on breast-feeding, she
will do no harm to the older child at her breast, to
the younger one in her womb, or to herself.

PREGNANT MOTHERS CAN BREAST-FEED; THEIR MILK IS NOT 'SOUR'

Although a mother can go on breast-feeding
while she is pregnant, she now has three people
to feed—herself, the baby sucking at her breast
and the baby growing in her womb. She will
therefore need plenty of extra protein foods. In
Section 6.1 we saw that a woman needs 5.5 g more
reference protein when she is pregnant and 17.0 g
more when she is breast-feeding. So, when she is
both pregnant and breast-feeding, she needs
5.5+17.0=22.5 g more reference protein, or larger
amounts of other proteins which are not so good
for body-building.

Many mothers will not go on breast-feeding
when they are pregnant. Try hard to persuade them,
but, if a mother still wants to stop breast-feeding,
make sure she stops *slowly*. She should slowly
breast-feed her child less and less often until,
at the end of a month, she has stopped breast-
feeding him altogether.

In some tribes it is the custom for a young child
to be sent away to his grandmother or some
other relative when his mother becomes pregnant.
A young child needs his mother's care; so this may
make him very unhappy. One of the first things an
unhappy child does is to eat less. Children who
are sent away from the family are sometimes badly
fed and may get kwashiorkor. It is thus usually
better for young children to stay at home with their
parents and brothers and sisters.

A mother who is breast-feeding is a little less
likely to become pregnant than a mother who is not
breast-feeding. But breast-feeding is not the best
way of preventing pregnancy. There are much
better ways, which are called 'family planning', and
which are so easy and safe that they should be
provided at every health centre—see Section
11.22. Family planning tries to make sure that
babies are not born too close together. It tries to
prevent mothers becoming pregnant again, when
they are still breast-feeding. The time between
two children is called the **birth interval.** An interval
is a gap or space. A short birth interval of a year
is bad, both for the nutrition of children and their
mother, especially if the family is poor and there is
little food to eat. The poorer the family, the longer
the birth interval should be. In the poorest families
it should not be less than two and a half years.

TOO SHORT A BIRTH INTERVAL HELPS TO CAUSE MALNUTRITION

7.7 How often to feed children. When a breast-
fed child is being carried on his mother's back he
can easily be fed very often. Women usually do this
well, and breast-fed children usually grow well.
But many mothers do not give their children enough
meals as they grow older. An adult can eat enough
food in one meal to last him all day. A child cannot
do this. His stomach is too small to get enough
food for a whole day in one, or even two meals.
Children, especially very young children, need
at least three meals a day. Four meals a day are
even better. Many families only eat a proper meal
in the evening; so if children only eat at this meal,
they only eat once a day, which is not nearly
enough. Children must therefore have at least two
other meals specially made for them. Give them any
of the meals that are described in Section 7.15.

CHILDREN MUST NOT MISS THEIR MEALS

If a child is going to have three meals a day,
the fire has got to be lit three times, water boiled
and porridge made. Some protein food has then to
be added to the porridge. This is hard work for a
busy mother, and it means that more fuel has to be
carried or bought. However, only a little water

needs to be boiled, and other children may be able to help. The 'convenience baby foods' described in Section 7.11 make it easy to add protein once porridge has been made. Children can also be given cold food when fuel is scarce. This is not so good, but it is better than nothing.

Too few meals a day is one of the most serious blocks in the food-path in many districts. It should also be one of the easiest to put right. Many families have no money to buy protein foods by the middle of the month. But, most of them have enough maize meal during most of the time, and they could feed their children more often. We must teach them how important this is. The meal that children most often lack is breakfast.

MOST MOTHERS COULD FEED THEIR CHILDREN MORE OFTEN

Some countries have this saying; 'Children, like chickens, should always be pecking (eating)'. This is a good saying to tell parents when they ask how often they should feed their children.

7.8   How much to feed children and the difficulty of 'bulk'.   In Sections 6.1 and 6.2 we saw how much protein and how many joules a young child needs to grow. We saw that a child of two needs 1.19 g of reference protein and 424 kJ each day for each kilo he weighs. A healthy two-year-old child weighs $12\frac{1}{2}$ kg, so he needs $12\frac{1}{2}\times1.19=14.8$ g, say 15 g of reference protein each day. Because maize protein has an NPU of 55 per cent, he needs $15\times\frac{100}{55}=27$ g of maize protein. Because maize is about 8 per cent of protein, our young child could get the protein he needs in $27\times\frac{100}{8}=340$ g of maize meal.

As for energy food, he needs $12\frac{1}{2}\times424=5{,}300$ kJ, or say 5.4 MJ each day. We saw in Table 19 that there are 1.5 MJ in 100 g of maize meal. If our child of two is to eat these 5.3 MJ, he must eat $100\times\frac{5.3}{1.5}=353$ g of maize meal. This is nearly the same amount of maize meal that he has to eat to

A two-year old child needs to eat four large platefuls of maize porridge a day if he is to get all the joules and protein he needs

... but this is more than a child can eat, so what should a mother do?

She should feed her child often

She should add protein foods to his porridge

If she can, she should add some high-joule food such as margerine or cooking oil

A TWO-YEAR OLD CHILD

this child needs 5.3 megajoules and 15 g of reference protein each day

maize porridge

7-4, Maize porridge is a very bulky food

give him the protein he needs. So let us say that he needs about 350 g of maize meal to give him both the protein and the joules he needs.

How much porridge does 350 g of maize meal make? It makes about 2,000 g of porridge. This is two kilos or four very large platefuls. This is more than a child of two can possibly eat, even if he has four meals a day! Because so much porridge contains so little maize meal, we say it is a very bulky food. By this we mean that the food containing the necessary nutrients takes up a lot of space.

What can a mother do to give her child the protein and joules he needs if maize is to be his staple food?

First, she must feed him often. A child has a small stomach and can only eat a little porridge at one meal. If he is to eat as much porridge as he can during the day, he must have at least three, or better still, four meals a day.

YOUNG CHILDREN NEED FEEDING OFTEN

Second, she must add extra protein food to his porridge. She can add groundnuts, which have 23 per cent of protein, or beans, which have 20 per cent, or dried skim milk, which has 36 per cent, or some other protein food. When these foods are cooked with water, they do not swell up as much as maize meal does. They are thus less bulky than maize porridge. They give more nutrients in the same weight of porridge, and so a child can eat more of them.

When we add beans and groundnuts or dried skim milk to maize porridge, we are mixing proteins. We saw in Section 3.7 how good this is, and how mixtures of proteins are much better for body-building than one protein alone.

Third, she should add some extra joule-food to her child's porridge. Groundnuts contain 45 per cent fat, and each 100 g of groundnuts contain 2.29 megajoules, so when a mother adds groundnuts to her child's porridge, she is adding protein *and joules*. Another way to add extra joules to a child's porridge is to add some margarine, or a spoonful of cooking oil. There are 3 megajoules in 100 g of margarine. Cooking oil, you will remember has

more joules than any other food—3.7 megajoules in 100 g. But oil and margarine are expensive, and many families cannot buy much of them. They must thus feed their children *often*—and add protein foods.

7.9 When to feed children. This does not matter greatly, provided that children are fed *often* and have *enough of the right food to eat*. It is, however, important that children should have one meal early in the morning. In towns many mothers give their children bread and tea in the morning. This is not a good breakfast, but it is better than nothing. A slice of bread only gives a child about 520 kilojoules, so one or two slices of bread are not going to supply many of the joules he needs. In the rural areas, where bread is scarce, children can be given some groundnuts, and some cold boiled sweet potatoes, or some sweet cassava, or cold *nshima* for one of their meals.

Sleeping children are often not fed when they should be. If a child is asleep when it is time for his food, wake him up. He can easily go to sleep again after he has eaten, but if he misses one meal he may have to wait quite a long time for the next one. Children need at least three meals a day and must not miss them. If a mother is away from the house or on a journey, she must see that her children always have something to eat.

Children are often hungry in between meals, and when they want food, they should be given it. Food that is eaten between meals is often called a **snack.** Snacks can be groundnuts, cold *nshima*, bread, or anything else that the family may have. The best snacks, such as groundnuts, contain protein and joules. Fizzy drinks, you will remember, are non-foods, and are thus useless as snacks.

MEALS FOR YOUNG CHILDREN

7.10 Maize porridge is better than cassava. Even though maize porridge is more bulky than cassava, maize porridge has 8 per cent of protein instead of only 1 per cent. Maize or millet meal is therefore a much better food than cassava. Try therefore to persuade mothers to use maize or millet meal, instead of cassava, for their children's

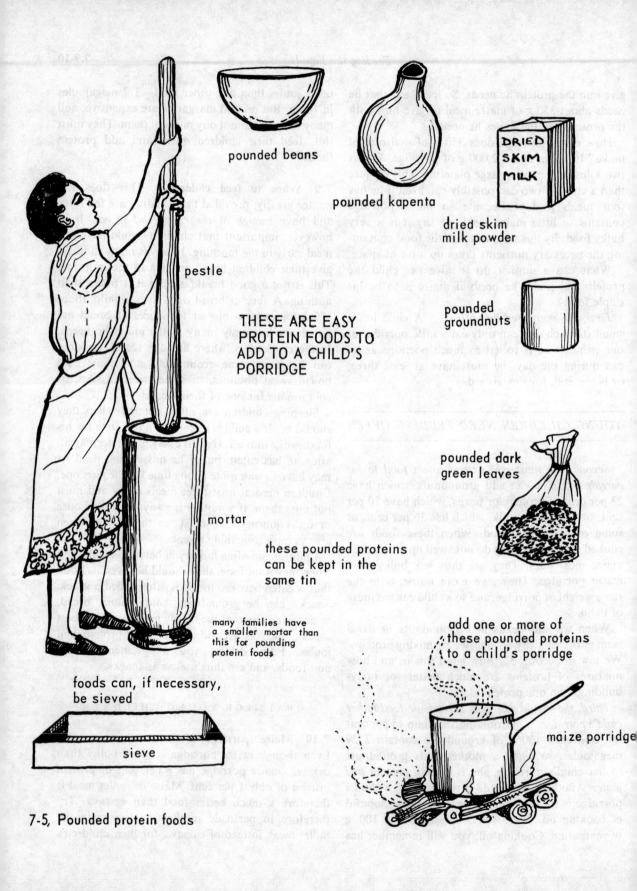

pounded beans

pounded kapenta

dried skim milk powder

DRIED SKIM MILK

pounded groundnuts

THESE ARE EASY
PROTEIN FOODS TO
ADD TO A CHILD'S
PORRIDGE

pestle

mortar

many families have
a smaller mortar than
this for pounding
protein foods

foods can, if necessary,
be sieved

sieve

pounded dark
green leaves

these pounded proteins
can be kept in the
same tin

add one or more of
these pounded proteins
to a child's porridge

maize porridge

7-5, Pounded protein foods

food. If they will not use maize meal alone, see if they will use a mixture of cassava and maize meal. Cassava mixed with millet meal is even better. Some families live mostly on cassava and have only a little maize or millet. These families should keep what maize or millet they have for their children, and not make all their millet into beer.

Soft boiled rice makes quite a good infant food, but rice is more expensive than maize meal. Money is much better spent on protein foods than on buying rice.

This book has several important things to tell mothers. The first is that breast-feeding is better than bottle-feeding. The next message is that plain porridge by itself is not enough for an infant. This is true even if it is maize porridge which contains 8 per cent protein. Maize protein is plant protein, and it has an NPU of 55 per cent, which means that only about half of it is used for body-building. *Some other protein must therefore always be added as well.* It is not enough for a mother to add a high protein food to her child's porridge *sometimes*. She should try to add something to his porridge *every time*. Most mothers should be able to add another plant protein, groundnuts for example, and at least a little animal protein. If cassava porridge is being used, it is even more important to add two different proteins. The next section tells you how you can make special powdered protein foods which make it easy to add protein to the child's porridge.

PLAIN PORRIDGE IS NOT ENOUGH

7.11 'Convenience baby foods'—pounded proteins. In the evening a young child's food can often be part of the family meal. He can have some of the maize or cassava nshima that his parents eat, and also some of their protein relish, such as beans or fish, if it is well minced or mashed. But this only gives a young child one meal a day. What is he to eat for the other two or three protein-containing meals that he needs each day? In Europe and America some mothers use what are called 'convenience baby foods'. These are small bottles or tins of special foods for babies, such as potato

and minced meat, or egg and porridge. These foods are expensive and no better than ordinary food which has been pounded well. A village mother has no money to buy this kind of convenience baby food, but she can quite easily make convenience baby foods of her own. The easiest and best foods for her to use are powdered protein foods which she can add to her child's porridge. These powdered protein foods are easy to make, because many women have a pestle and mortar with which they pound some foods, such as maize or groundnuts. If mothers do not have a pestle and mortar they can usually borrow one. In Bemba and Nyanja a pestle and mortar are called *bende* while in Swahili the mortar is called *kinu* and the pestle is *mchi*.

Some tribes do not pound foods in a pestle and mortar, but grind them into a powder between two stones. There are several foods that families can pound or grind in this way. They are dried fish, groundnuts, cashew nuts, dried beans and dried green leaves, such as cassava leaves. These pounded powdered foods are sometimes called 'flours'—groundnut flour, bean flour and fish flour. Dried skim milk is another powdered food that can also be added to porridge. Powdered protein foods can easily be stored in tins, or plastic bags, or in pots or gourds, and can be added to cassava or maize meal *before it is made into porridge*. Make fresh pounded foods every few days and do not keep them too long. It is best if each mother can have a sieve as well as a pestle and mortar, so that the powder can be sieved and the large pieces taken out and then pounded smaller. Many families have sieves.

ALWAYS ADD SOME PROTEIN FOOD TO A YOUNG CHILD'S PORRIDGE

Pounded fish. Many kinds of dried fish can be easily pounded into powder, and the powder sieved to remove the bones. Mothers are sometimes worried about the bones sticking in their children's throats, but if the powder is sieved this will not happen. The easiest kind of dried fish to pound is the small dried fish that is called *kapenta* in Zambia, but many kinds can be used. Mothers should not pound too much dried fish at a time, *nor should they keep it for more than one or two days, or it will go bad.*

Kapenta can also be pounded when it is fresh, or when dried *kapenta* has been made wet with water. As we shall see in the next section, *kapenta* must be cooked, so it should be added to the maize meal *before* it is made into porridge.

Even though *kapenta* is a good food for young children, many of them will not begin to eat it until they are about two or three years old, and many mothers are unwilling to give them *kapenta* until they are this age. So don't try to force a mother to give her child *kapenta* before she thinks he is old enough. He should be given some other protein food which he likes and will eat.

Pounded beans. Beans of many kinds can also be made into a powder and added to the maize meal from which a child's porridge is made. Powdered beans need cooking; so they must be cooked with the maize meal. Dry beans are hard to pound, and it is usually easier to add mashed cooked beans to porridge.

Pounded groundnuts. These can also be pounded in a pestle and mortar and kept in a tin. If ordinary groundnuts are used they make a powder. This powder can be sieved and the larger pieces pounded smaller. If there are enough groundnuts, groundnut flour can be made into porridge by itself. This is a very high-protein and high-joule porridge. If the groundnuts are fried first, and then pounded, they make a soft oily butter—groundnut butter. In Bemba groundnut butter is called *chinkonko* and in Nyanja *chimande*. Pounded fresh groundnuts must be cooked with the porridge, but groundnut butter can be added to maize porridge after it has been cooked. If the baby is going to get his groundnut butter, it may have to be hidden from father and the rest of the family! Roasted groundnuts can also be pounded into a powder. This tastes good and does not need cooking. Some children get diarrhoea if they are given a lot of groundnuts all at once, especially when they are very young. If this happens, do not give them groundnuts for a few days, and then try again with a smaller amount.

Both pounded groundnuts and groundnut butter should be kept in a tin and used as needed. Pounded groundnuts must not get damp, or they will go mouldy. Do you remember what you read in Section 5.5?

Pounded cashew nuts. In parts of Tanzania many cashew nuts are grown. Cashew nuts grow on trees outside a fruit. Like groundnuts they contain much protein and oil and can be pounded to make a good infant food, which can be cooked with porridge.

Pounded dark green leaves. You have read that dark green leaves contain 3 per cent of protein. Some leaves contain even more and may contain as much as 7 per cent. Leaves can be pounded fresh or when they have been dried. When leaves are dried they lose water, and the light, dry leaves contain quite a lot of protein. When dried leaves are pounded in a mortar they make a green powder, which can be added to the meal from which an infant's porridge is made. Dark green leaves can be found almost everywhere, and if only mothers would gather and dry more leaves children would have more protein. They are best used with other protein foods.

Dried skimmed milk. You read about this in Section 5.3. It is a very good food, but it will probably be only town mothers who can buy it. Sometimes it is given out at clinics. As you have read, *the best way to use dried skimmed milk is to add it to a child's porridge.* NEVER give dried skimmed milk to a child through a feeding bottle.

If dried skim milk is given to a child without any joules of energy food being given at the same time, his body will burn the protein in it to give him energy. If dried skim milk is eaten with porridge, porridge gives joules of energy, and the skim milk protein can be used for body-building.

THE BEST WAY TO USE DRIED SKIM MILK IS TO ADD IT TO PORRIDGE

Pounded caterpillars. Caterpillars are common at some times of the year. They can be pounded to make a good convenience baby food.

A convenience baby food made from roasted

maize meal. Women in Botswana make a convenience baby food by roasting maize or millet meal in a thick black iron pot until it is just brown. They stir it well to stop it burning, and add a little salt and some sugar. For use it is stirred into milk or water, and some pounded protein food added. A child's porridge can be made in this way without lighting the fire to boil water every time. This is useful when fuel is scarce.

7.12 Using pounded protein foods. Pounded dried fish, pounded groundnuts, pounded cashew nuts, pounded beans and pounded dark green leaves all need cooking; *so they should be added to maize or cassava meal before it is cooked.* Added like this they will be cooked with the porridge, and after they are cooked they will be easier to digest. Dried skim milk, however, needs no cooking and can be added to maize or cassava meal, either before it is cooked, or just before it is eaten. There will be no lumps if it is well mixed with maize meal before it is cooked. But if dried skim milk is added to porridge after it is cooked, there may be some white lumps. These do not matter, but if a mother wants to stop them, and still add dried skim milk to hot porridge, she should first of all mix the dried skim milk with a little boiled water in a cup. This thick liquid milk can then be added to the porridge without making any lumps. Once again, dried skim milk should be added to a child's porridge, and *not* given to him in a feeding bottle!

ADD ONE OR TWO LARGE SPOONFULS OF PROTEIN FOOD TO EVERY PLATE OF PORRIDGE

Try very hard to persuade mothers to add one or two large spoonfuls of one or more of these protein foods to the maize or cassava meal from which they make all their child's porridge. Ask them to do this *every time* they feed their child with porridge. A

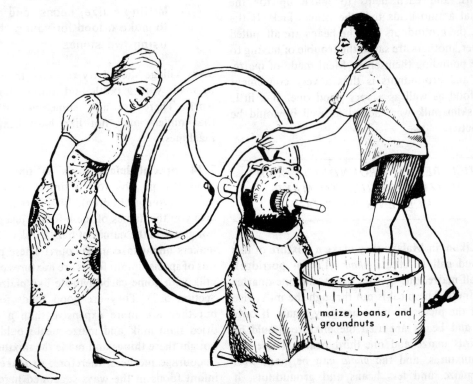

7-6, Using a hand-mill to make a food for young children from maize, beans, and groundnuts

spoonful of each of two different pounded proteins is better than two spoonfuls of the same one. As we have seen, 'a good food is a mixed food'. A child should not be fed plain porridge except when he is learning to eat it for the first time. After he has learnt to eat plain porridge, always give him porridge to which some protein food has been added. And, as you will remember, a young child needs feeding at least three or four times a day. A young child cannot eat much porridge at once, so *a mother need only make a little porridge at a time*. If she makes too much the protein foods she adds to it may be wasted.

7.13 Milling maize with groundnuts and beans. Many villages have a mill which makes maize into meal or flour. A good food for young children can be made by milling a mixture of maize with beans. If groundnuts are added as well this makes a better mixture. As we saw in Section 3.7, this is because maize, beans and groundnuts are plant proteins, and each helps to make up for the essential amino acids that the others lack. If the maize, the groundnuts and the beans are all milled together, mothers are saved the trouble of having to do the pounding themselves. Meal made of maize, beans and groundnuts is thus a very convenient baby food as well as a very good one. If a little dried skim milk were added as well it would be even better.

MILL BEANS, GROUNDNUTS AND MAIZE TOGETHER TO MAKE CHILDREN'S PORRIDGE

At Likuni in Malawi they make a mixture of this kind and call it Likuni *phala* (Likuni porridge). It is half maize, one-quarter beans and one-quarter groundnuts. The meal is put through the mill twice so that the pieces of meal are very small. If only maize and beans are used the mixture should be two-thirds maize and one-third beans. These are 'rich' mixtures, and the *phala* can be made with more maize, and less beans and groundnuts, if these are scarce.

These are good foods for young children, and

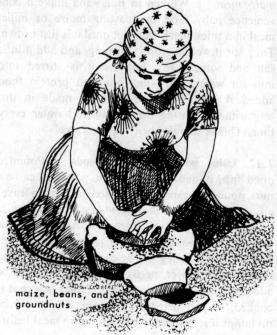

maize, beans, and groundnuts

7-7, Milling maize, beans, and groundnuts to make a food for young children using two stones

every village should try to make them. They can be made with a pestle and mortar, but it is hard work. There are also sometimes difficulties in that millers may not like hard beans in their machines.

7.14 Special infant foods in tins. In some shops it is possible to buy tins of special foods for infants (young children). In this book we cannot give you the names of these foods, just as we could not give you the names of fizzy drinks. If we did the makers might take us to court! These packets and tins of special infant foods are mixtures of powdered milk with some carbohydrate like maize meal (see Section 5.7). They are good foods for children, but they are more expensive than a mixture of dried skim milk and maize meal would be, if you bought these things and made the mixture yourself. Encourage mothers, therefore, to make their own infant foods in the ways suggested here. Persuade them not to buy the expensive infant foods some shopkeepers will try to make them buy.

7.15 Some more meals for children. plain maize porridge that is not eaten at the evening meal is often kept and eaten cold the next day. In Bemba cold food of any kind is called *fyakulya yatalala* and in Nyanja *yosisira*. These cold foods are very useful, and are usually quite safe to eat the morning after they have been cooked. *Cold food containing powdered kapenta should however be eaten immediately or thrown away.* Don't keep it until the next day because it can make you ill.

Here are some more infant foods that mothers may like to use. Teach them to use the foods that you find they like, and leave the others.

Porridge with beans. Cook some beans until they are soft. Mash them with a spoon, and mix some of these soft, mashed beans into the child's porridge. The skins of some legumes make them hard to digest, so if the skins are thick take them off. In some villages bean porridge is thought to be a good food for old people without any teeth. It is also a good food for young children.

Porridge with hard boiled egg. Boil an egg until it is hard, and then take off the shell and cut the egg into small pieces. If the egg is put into cold water as soon as it has been boiled it will peel easily. Add these chopped pieces to the child's porridge.

Porridge with fresh milk. The best way of making this is to use milk instead of water when the porridge is made. Another way is to add the milk to thick porridge after it has been cooked.

Porridge with egg. Make the child's porridge. While the porridge is still hot add an egg. Stir the egg well into the porridge. The heat of the porridge will cook the egg. Most children like this porridge with egg.

Milk and egg. An egg can be well mixed into milk. This is a very good food, and the egg is not cooked but eaten raw. Raw eggs are not poisonous as is sometimes thought. A 'fertile' egg, from a hen who has been running with a cock, is also just as good as the egg from a hen which has not been with a cock.

Mashed sweet potato and pounded groundnuts. Add some cooked pounded groundnuts to mashed sweet potato. This is a recipe from the Luapula Province of Zambia.

Porridge with minced meat. Mothers may be able to buy minced meat for a child, or they can cut up larger pieces of meat with a knife. Meat can also be scraped (rubbed) with a knife off soft boiled meat and can be added to a child's porridge. But, however it is cooked, the meat must be given to a child in small pieces.

Porridge with fish. Add some boiled fish to the child's porridge. Make sure you take out the bones first. Tinned fish such as pilchards can be bought in many shops. They are also good food for children, even though they are expensive.

Protective foods. Young children can also have boiled green vegetables with any of these meals. They can also have mashed pawpaw, ripe mango, banana or avocado pear. Mashed avocado pear is especially useful, because it also contains much energy-giving oil. By the time they are five months old they must be having these protective foods.

Some other foods. Insects and caterpillars make good protein foods for children. So don't forget to tell mothers to use them when they are available. Small children can eat most foods, but don't give them hot peppery foods.

Animal protein of any kind is likely to be scarce. The best way to use it is to use it with vegetable proteins, and to give a child at least a little animal protein with every meal. If this is not possible, he should have a little at least once a day. So try hard to persuade mothers to give their children some animal protein every day, and certainly every time they buy it from the market.

7.16 Meals to be careful about. Some meals are not as good as they might be. Here are some to be careful about.

Porridge with margarine. This is a good food for children, because margarine contains many joules in a small bulk. Children need plenty of joules. But margarine does not contain any body-building protein. If margarine is added to porridge, some protein food must therefore be added as well. *Porridge with margarine is good, but it is not enough.*

Porridge with sugar. Sugar can be added to porridge and will also give the child some joules, but margarine is better. Once again, sugar is not enough, and *protein foods must be added as well.*

7.17 How should a working mother feed her young child? Some mothers have jobs in offices and shops, and want to go to work as soon as their baby is born. What should they do? How can they avoid bottle-feeding? If they can, they should take their baby to work with them. Village mothers always do this and take their baby with them to the fields where they work. A secretary working in an office should do the same. She should keep her baby on her back or leave him in a basket in a corner of the office. Better still, she should leave him in a **crèche** (spoken 'cresh') or a **day care centre.**

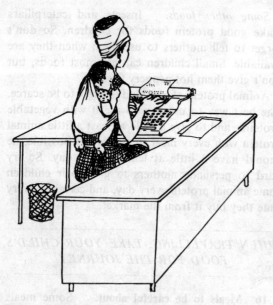

7-8, How should a working mother look after her young child ?

These are places where mothers can leave their young children and where there is someone to look after them. Offices and factories where there are many women workers should try to provide a crèche, or a day care centre.

DON'T STOP BREAST-FEEDING WHEN YOU GO TO WORK

A working mother should feed her young child early in the morning before work starts, at about five in the evening when it is finished, and again late at night. She need only feed him twice during working hours—during the morning tea break, and again at lunch time. This is certainly best for her baby. Her boss may not like it, but if she is a good secretary, he will probably not mind too much, because he will not want to lose her. As soon as her child is five months old, she can leave him at home with someone to look after him carefully. Village mothers are not ashamed to breast-feed their babies at work. Town mothers who work in offices should not be ashamed to feed them either. Breast-feeding is the best way to feed children, so why should anyone be ashamed about it? Being ashamed about breast-feeding is one of the worst things that has come with town life.

If a mother has to leave her baby at home, she should continue to breast-feed him before and after she goes to work, and in the night. *She should not stop breast-feeding.* While she is at work she must see that someone else feeds him by cup-and-spoon, and *not* with a feeding bottle. The best person to do this will probably be another mother, who is staying at home. Many mothers leave their babies with older children or girls who do not know how to look after them well. These mothers should not be surprised when their children get diarrhoea and die. When a mother goes to work, she should leave the things ready for the three feeds that her child will need. She should also make sure that the person who is looking after her child can make up a *safe* cup-and-spoon feed. She should not make up the feed herself, unless she has a fridge in which she can safely leave it. See Section 8.6.

TRY TO TAKE YOUR YOUNG BABY TO WORK WITH YOU

FEEDING THE SCHOOL CHILD

7.18 Something to take to school. Children often have to leave home for school very early in the morning and it is difficult to light a fire and cook breakfast for them before they go. So we must not be surprised when many children come to school without any breakfast. This is very bad because hungry children do not learn well, and are more likely to fail their exams than well fed ones. Thus children who are going to learn well must be well fed. A school child needs breakfast before he goes to school, and also something to take with him to eat for lunch in the middle of the day. Many parents do not have breakfast themselves, so that they do not think that their children need breakfast either. School children are growing and need plenty of joules for their walk to school. Their parents would also be able to work harder, if they had breakfast too.

SCHOOL CHILDREN NEED BREAKFAST AND A MEAL IN THE MIDDLE OF THE DAY

Ask mothers to give their children food to take to school, rather than money, because children may buy fizzy drinks which have no food value. Fizzy

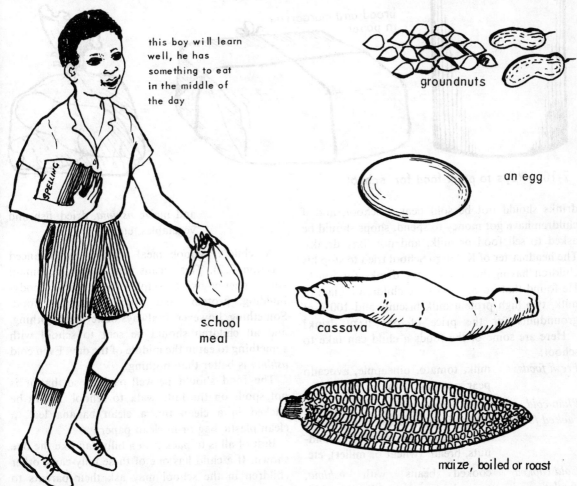

this boy will learn well, he has something to eat in the middle of the day

school meal

groundnuts

an egg

cassava

maize, boiled or roast

7-9, Food for school

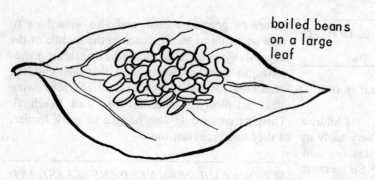

boiled beans
on a large
leaf

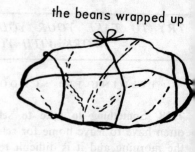

the beans wrapped up

maize porridge
and groundnuts
in a tin

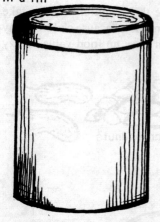

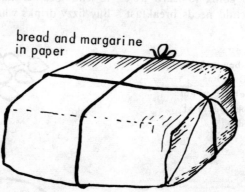

bread and margarine
in paper

boiled cassava
in a plastic bag

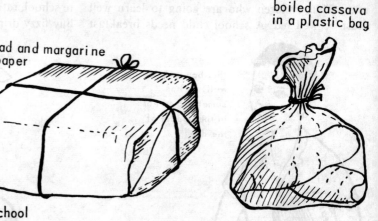

7-10, Ways to pack food for school

drinks should not be sold near a school, and if children have got money to spend, shops should be asked to sell food or milk, and not fizzy drinks. The headmaster of Kalongo School tried to stop his children having buns and fizzy drinks for lunch. He found that he could sell the children a glass of milk, two high protein milk biscuits and 100 g of groundnuts for the price of one fizzy drink!

Here are some of the foods a child can take to school:

Fresh foods: milk, tomato, pineapple, avocado pear, pawpaw, banana, etc.

Plain cold cooked foods: beans, sweet potato, maize cob (roasted or boiled), hard boiled egg, roast cassava, roasted groundnuts, bread (wheat or millet), etc.

Cold cooked meals: cooked beans with *nshima*, groundnut sauce with vegetables and maize *nshima*, dried fish and vegetables, etc.

A child's school meal should be balanced (Section 5.2). This means that it should contain some energy-giving staple food, some body-building protein, and some protective food. Something, however, is always better than nothing, and all children should be sent to school with something to eat in the middle of the day. Even cold *nshima* is better than nothing.

The food should be well packed, so that it is not spoilt on the long walk to school. It can be packed in a clean tin, a clean banana leaf, a clean plastic bag or in clean paper.

Best of all is to pack it in a billy-can like the one shown. If a child has one of these billy-cans, other children in the school may ask their parents to give them one also. Figure 7–12 shows several billy-cans hanging on a tree while the children are having their morning lessons. If you cannot get these billy-cans in the shops, ask the shopkeeper to get them for you.

SEND YOUR CHILD TO SCHOOL WITH A BILLY-CAN OF FOOD FOR HIS LUNCH

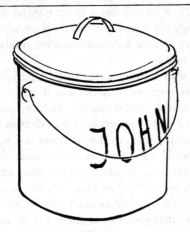

7-11, A billy-can is a good way to take food to school

In many schools children are expected to share their food with their friends. A child who does not share his food may find that he has no friends. But, if he does share his food he may find that he has very little left for himself. Every child must therefore take some food to school. Teachers should try to persuade the parents of all children to send them to school with food. The best place to discuss this is at the Parent Teachers Association (PTA). Parents can also be sent letters about the importance of feeding schoolchildren.

It is so difficult to cook food in many schools that 'milk biscuits' are starting to be given to children in some schools. Each biscuit weighs about 10 g, and four biscuits give a child 8 g of protein and 790 kilojoules. These biscuits cost 1n each and can be given to younger children also. Children like them, and they make a good porridge when they are made soft with a little boiled water. They are, however, much more expensive than maize porridge and dried skim milk.

Perhaps the worst fed school children of all are the primary boarders. These children live in

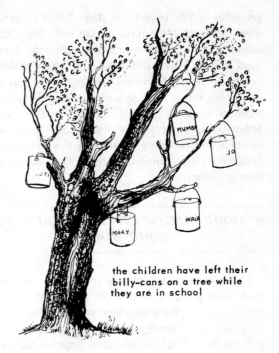

the children have left their billy-cans on a tree while they are in school

7-12, Billy-cans on a tree

villages some miles away from the school, and walk there each week, bringing a week's food with them. They often bring too little food of the wrong kind, and are very hungry indeed. Can school teachers look at the food their primary boarders bring, and try to see that parents send them with enough food of the right kind?

School children sometimes eat only after the older members of the family have finished, and may only

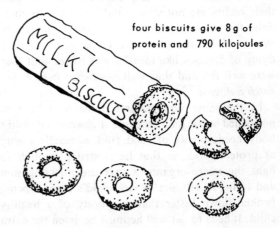

four biscuits give 8 g of protein and 790 kilojoules

7-13, Milk biscuits

get what is left over from their father's evening meal. Some children have a long walk back from school and so arrive home late, after the family meal is over. This is not good, and school children must be properly fed in the evenings. This may not matter so much with schoolgirls who help their mothers to cook and often eat while cooking. Schoolboys, however, do not usually help their mothers and therefore do not get this extra food. Schoolboys are therefore more likely to go hungry than schoolgirls.

A GOOD BREAKFAST IS NEEDED FOR GOOD WORK

In the earlier parts of this book much has been said about people's food needs at special times in their lives. You have read how young children, and pregnant and nursing mothers, need plenty of protein food. There is one other time we must not forget. This is the time of puberty, when boys become men and girls become women. Both boys and girls grow faster at this time and need plenty of food. The child between eleven and thirteen, who keeps saying he is hungry, is not just greedy, he is growing fast and needs more food.

7.19 Sick children need feeding. We read earlier how underweight children are often killed by measles and other diseases which seldom kill healthy children. We saw that they die because their bodies are not strong and healthy enough to fight the micro-organisms that try to kill them. We found that the way to prevent so many children dying of diseases like measles was to see that they were well fed and thus well nourished *before they catch a disease.*

In the same way children must also be well nourished *when they have got a disease.* A child's body needs plenty of food, and especially plenty of protein food, so that he is strong enough to fight the micro-organisms that are infecting him and trying to kill him. A sick child's body is being broken down faster than the body of a healthy child. If he is to get well he must be given the extra food that his body needs to repair itself.

Milk is the best food for a sick child, and mother's milk is the best food for a sick baby. So, when a baby is sick, don't stop breast-feeding him. Mother's milk is often the best medicine that a sick baby can get!

When an older child is sick, don't stop trying to feed him when he won't eat. He may not like his usual food, so make something special for him that he likes. Often he will eat a more babyish food—like porridge, or bread and milk—if he won't eat nshima. Try to give him some protein foods, such as eggs or milk.

A child with measles needs to be especially well fed. This is even more important if he is under-weight, because underweight children may get kwashiorkor when they get measles. Measles makes a child's mouth sore, so that he does not want to eat. He should thus be given soft foods that he likes and are easy to eat. Measles also harms a child's eyes, especially if he lacks vitamin A, so give him plenty of foods that contain this vitamin, such as pawpaw, mangoes (when these are in season), tomatoes, carrots and eggs. Most important of all, measles also harms a child's gut and gives him diarrhoea so he does not absorb food well, and so needs to be particularly well fed.

SICK CHILDREN NEED PLENTY OF PROTEIN FOOD

7.20 Diarrhoea. Many children have diarrhoea, and it often kills them. It can be caused by many things, but two of the most common are mal-nutrition and infection, which often happen together. By infection causing diarrhoea we mean harmful micro-organisms getting into a child, and growing in his gut to cause diarrhoea. These harmful micro-organisms usually get into him in his food or his drinking water *from the gut of another person.* This is why it is so important that human faeces should not get into drinking water. We saw how this could be prevented in Section 4.17.

But, how does malnutrition give a child diarrhoea? We have seen that food is digested in the gut by special substances called enzymes, which are themselves proteins which the body puts into the gut. If the body is malnourished and lacks essential amino acids, it cannot make these digestive enzymes as it should. Malnutrition also harms the gut in other ways. If enzymes are partly lacking and the gut is harmed, food is not digested and absorbed well, so diarrhoea results. Harmful micro-organisms also grow more easily in a malnourished gut, which also helps to cause diarrhoea. Thus we see that malnutrition causes diarrhoea.

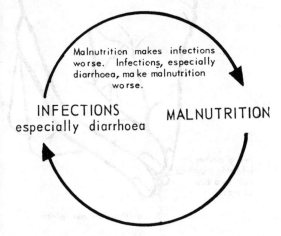

Malnutrition makes infections worse. Infections, especially diarrhoea, make malnutrition worse.

INFECTIONS
especially diarrhoea

MALNUTRITION

7-14, A vicious circle

Diarrhoea also causes malnutrition by preventing food being digested and absorbed properly. Thus diarrhoea helps to cause malnutrition and malnutrition helps to cause diarrhoea! When two things help to cause one another we say we have a **vicious circle**. This is the vicious circle of malnutrition and diarrhoea. Figure 9–2 shows another vicious circle—the vicious circle of malnourished farmers and less food production.

We have seen that diarrhoea is an infection, and that it causes malnutrition. Other infections can also help to cause malnutrition. They do this by causing a child's body to be broken down faster than usual, and measles, for example, also makes a child's mouth sore, besides giving him a special kind of diarrhoea. Other infections besides diarrhoea, especially whooping cough and tuberculosis (TB) are also made worse by malnutrition. *Thus the vicious circle of malnutrition and diarrhoea is only an example of a more general vicious circle—the vicious circle of malnutrition and infections of many kinds.*

MALNUTRITION MAKES INFECTIONS WORSE AND INFECTIONS MAKE MALNUTRITION WORSE

The only way to break the vicious circle caused by malnutrition and infection, and especially that caused by malnutrition and diarrhoea, is to feed a child well with protein foods. This will give him the best possible chance of digesting and absorbing enough protein to cure both his malnutrition and his diarrhoea. This is not easy, because giving a child more food may make his diarrhoea worse for a time, before it makes it better. His stools may be larger when he is given more food, but even so, he will still be getting well. A child must be given this extra food, because this is the only way in which he will be cured. He may take several weeks to get well, so don't stop trying.

Because the diarrhoea of malnutrition sometimes lasts for some weeks or months, we say it is **chronic**. A chronic disease is one which lasts for a long time, and from which the patient dies or gets better slowly. The diarrhoea of malnutrition is not usually very bad, and a child may only pass three or four stools a day. *Protein food is much more important than medicine in curing this kind of diarrhoea.* This is well shown by the story of Hariet in Section 9.30.

PROTEIN FOOD IS THE BEST 'MEDICINE' FOR CHRONIC DIARRHOEA IN UNDERWEIGHT CHILDREN

Diarrhoea and dehydration. When a child gets diarrhoea his body loses water in his stools. Other things are also lost, but it is the water that matters most. When children die from diarrhoea, they die usually because their bodies have got dry and run out of water. When children have lost water in this way, we say they are *dehydrated*. Diarrhoea may come on very quickly, and a child may die in a few days or even hours from **acute** dehydration. An acute disease is one which lasts a short time, and from which the patient dies or gets better quickly.

When a child loses water in his diarrhoea stools and becomes dehydrated, *this water must be put back*. When it is put back most children get better quickly. In looking after a child with diarrhoea the most important thing to do is to put water back into his body. The easiest way to do this is to give him plenty of water to drink by cup and spoon. He may not want to drink, but his mother should go on making him drink little by little. The body loses salt as well as water in diarrhoea stools. She should thus add a quarter of a teaspoonful of salt (not more!) and two teaspoonfuls of sugar to each cup of water she gives her child. Only a *little* salt is needed in this 'salt-and-sugar water'—a quarter of a teaspoonful to a cup of water. More salt or more sugar than this will not help the child—they may make him worse because he will vomit (be sick). It may help a mother to know how much salt to add, if you tell her that she should add as much as she can pinch in three fingers. Show her what you mean by this. She may find this easier than measuring salt in a teaspoon. Most children soon get well again if they are given plenty of this salt-and-sugar water as soon as they start to get diarrhoea.

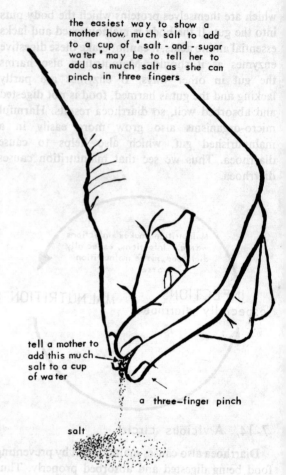

the easiest way to show a mother how much salt to add to a cup of 'salt - and - sugar water' may be to tell her to add as much salt as she can pinch in three fingers

tell a mother to add this much salt to a cup of water

a three-finger pinch

salt

7 - 15, A three-finger pinch of salt

SALT-AND-SUGAR WATER IS THE BEST 'MEDICINE' FOR ACUTE DIARRHOEA

So many children with diarrhoea come to a health centre that it is important to treat them properly. They must start their oral (by mouth) rehydration ('filling up with water') *before they go home*. It is no good telling the mother of a dehydrated child to give him plenty of fluid when she gets home. He is already dehydrated, and needs his fluids *now*! He may have a long walk home, and he may be worse by the time he gets there. Besides, a mother may not understand what she has to do unless she has herself first done it in a health centre. So she must be shown how to start the rehydration of her child in the health centre before she goes home.

The best way to do this is to have a 'diarrhoea corner' in a quiet part of the health centre where

two or three mothers can sit and rehydrate their children with salt-and-sugar water from a cup and spoon. Hand the mothers a cup and spoon, fill it with water, and then offer them a bowl of sugar and a bowl of salt. Let them take a spoonful of sugar and a 'three-finger pinch' of salt and make the mixture themselves. They will then know how to do it when they get home. Many dehydrated children are very thirsty, and it is wonderful to see them getting better while you watch them taking their mixture. Let the mothers of all dehydrated children, and all children with diarrhoea, give them salt-and-sugar mixture in this way. It may be necessary to give a child medicine, but salt-and-sugar water by mouth is usually more important, and is often all that is needed.

GIVE A CHILD SALT-AND-SUGAR WATER AS SOON AS HIS DIARRHOEA STARTS

Not all dehydrated children can be treated successfully with salt-and-sugar water by mouth. A few get worse, especially when they are vomiting as well as having diarrhoea. When a child is very dehydrated, his eyes start to go back into his head. Also, if you pinch up the skin over his stomach, it may stay pinched up for a while, instead of going back smooth straight away. His mouth may be very dry. These are signs that his body is very short of water and that he is severely dehydrated. Doctors or medical assistants, in a hospital or health centre, can quickly give a child the water he needs from a bottle through a tube into one of his veins.

This kind of bottle and tube is called a 'drip'. If a child is given a drip before he is too dehydrated he soon gets well again. Many mothers bring their children to hospital too late, so that even a drip cannot save the child's life. They have therefore come to think that a child who is given a drip is going to die, and they take their children away from the hospital. If children with diarrhoea are

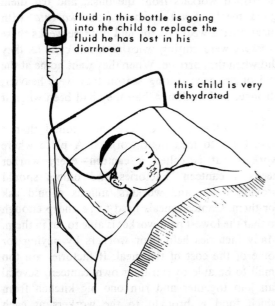

fluid in this bottle is going into the child to replace the fluid he has lost in his diarrhoea

this child is very dehydrated

7 - 16, A very dehydrated child needs a ' drip '

going to live, they must be given plenty of water to drink as soon as they start to get diarrhoea, and they must be brought to a health centre or hospital before they get too dehydrated. One of the most useful things we can do is to teach mothers to give their children weak salty water *as soon as they pass a loose stool and start to get diarrhoea.* If every mother did this, few children would need to go to hospital and few would die.

Drugs and medicines may also be needed for curing diarrhoea, but many children can be cured with plenty of good protein food, if they are under-weight and have chronic diarrhoea, or plenty of salty water, if they are dehydrated. In Section 9.30 we shall see how Hariet's diarrhoea was cured with dried skim milk.

Breast-feeding and diarrhoea. As you will read in the next chapter, bottle-fed children often get diarrhoea. They get it badly and many die, but even breast-fed children get it sometimes. They do not get diarrhoea because of breast-feeding. They get diarrhoea because micro-organisms get into the body in other ways. *Breast-feeding itself never causes diarrhoea.* When a breast-fed child has diarrhoea, his mother must go on breast-feeding him. The very worst thing that she can do is to stop breast-feeding him and start bottle-feeding. *If she stops breast-feeding him and giving him fluids he may die.* Breast-fed babies do not usually get diarrhoea badly, and if a mother looks after her child carefully, he will soon get well again.

Other foods and diarrhoea. Mothers often say that some other foods, such as millet or beans, give their children diarrhoea. Children often get diarrhoea, but it is usually caused by germs in dirty food or unboiled water, and especially by badly managed bottle-feeding. Good, clean, well-cooked food does not cause diarrhoea, unless a large amount is given to a young baby who is not used to it. Give new foods to a baby a little at a time, so that he gets used to them and does not get diarrhoea. If beans have thick skins they may be hard to digest, so take off the skins after the beans have been left in water to make them soft. It is sad if mothers stop giving children good protein foods, such as beans, because they fear diarrhoea.

If mothers do not believe what you say about foods not causing diarrhoea, make some food and give it to some of the babies at the clinic. Next month, when these mothers come again, ask them if their children have had diarrhoea. They will probably not have had diarrhoea, and mothers may come to believe what you say.

Lactose and diarrhoea. In Section 5.3 we saw that dried skim milk contains 51 per cent of a carbohydrate called milk sugar or lactose. This means that it is about half lactose. Some children beyond the breast-feeding age, and especially malnourished ones, may not have enough of the right enzyme (called lactase) in their gut to digest all this lactose. This undigested lactose may give a child diarrhoea if he is given large quantities of milk, especially dried skim milk. If mothers say that their children get diarrhoea with dried skim milk they may be right. Ask them to add a little less dried skim milk to all their child's porridge and to add other protein foods, such as beans or groundnuts, as well. In this way they are adding a little animal protein to a mixture of plant proteins, which is very good. It uses foods in the best way for body-building, and it is less likely to cause diarrhoea.

FEEDING FATHER

7.21 Feeding the workers. Most of this chapter has been about feeding children and their mother, but we must not forget father. Fathers work, and if a country is to develop and go forward, all the workers in farms, factories and offices need to work hard. Only if this happens will farms grow good crops and factories produce the things that everyone needs. This making and growing things is called **productivity.** Productivity needs hard work, and hard work requires the right food. You will remember from Table 15 and Section 6.2 that a man who is working hard with his hands needs many extra joules of energy food to give him the energy that he needs for his work. Lack of enough energy food is one of the reasons why many workers do not and cannot work as hard as they might. It is an important cause of low productivity, and thus of the slow development of a country.

Workers, like school children, need a good breakfast before they go to work, and a good meal in the middle of the day—a bottle of fizzy drink is not enough! Most workers live too far away from their work to be able to go home for lunch. They have too little time, and the transport would cost too much. They must thus bring food with them, or get food at work. Any of the meals for school children described in Section 7.18 can also be taken by fathers to work.

PRODUCTIVITY REQUIRES HARD WORK AND HARD WORK REQUIRES PLENTY OF ENERGY FOOD

It is difficult to teach workers to bring food with them to work, and few do so. Many workers have no breakfast. Yet well-fed workers are so much more productive than badly-fed ones. They are also likely to change their jobs less often, to have fewer accidents, and to be less often sick. This is so important that it often pays a factory to feed its workers free. For example, one sugar plantation (farm) needed workers for six months each year to cut the sugar cane. It took thin, badly-nourished workers from the bush, and fed them good meals of *nshima*, beans, and *kapenta*, with meat once a week. At the end of three weeks these workers were cutting twice as much cane as they did when they arrived. When they went home at the end of the cane-cutting season they were heavier, stronger and healthier than they had been when it began.

Many other factories have also found that it pays them to feed their workers. A place where workers eat is called a **canteen**—every worker needs a canteen. Factories and offices should provide them, and workers' unions should ask for them. Canteen meals need to be cheap enough so that the lowest paid worker is able to eat in them. Many factories help their workers by paying for some of the cost of the meal. If factories are too small to be able to run their own canteen, several can join together and run one big kitchen from which food is brought to the workers at each factory. Sometimes food sellers can be asked to visit a factory and sell food. It is so necessary to feed workers that some countries have laws about providing canteens in factories, just as they have laws about safety in the factory.

EVERY WORKER NEEDS A CANTEEN

7.22   T H I N G S T O D O

(a) Cooking foods for children. Try to make *all* the foods for young children that you read about here. If you are learning domestic science in school, these are much the most important meals that you can learn to make. You may later on be able to give your own children better meals than these, but if you can make them you can teach other people how to make them, which is what matters. A domestic science kitchen must have the pots and stoves that the people use as well as smart electric and gas stoves that only rich families can buy. Is there a pestle and mortar in your domestic science classroom? Are there any grinding stones if these are used in the district?

Can you teach families in the under-fives clinics how to make these meals? Can you cook eggs in the ways that are described here?

Can you teach the mother of a child with diarrhoea how to give her child salt-and-sugar-water with a cup and spoon?

(b) Feeding rats on different foods. Get some young rats or mice. Divide them into two groups so that the rats in each group are as nearly the same in weight and age as possible. Feed one group of rats on an unbalanced diet of the staple food alone. Feed a balanced diet to the other group of rats. Make a weight chart for the rats in each group. Look after the rats very carefully. Which group of rats grow best?

(c) Making a pan of porridge to give 5.3 megajoules. We saw in Section 7.8 that one of the difficulties in feeding young children is the large bulk of maize porridge. Try this for yourself. Make thin porridge for a child out of 350 g of maize meal. This would give a two-year-old child the 5.3 megajoules he needs. Do you think he could eat it?

Chapter Eight

ARTIFICIAL FEEDING

8.1 Why bottle-feeding is so bad. In the last chapter you read about what a good food for babies breast milk is, and how important it is that mothers should breast-feed their children. This chapter tells you how dangerous bottle-feeding can be, and how difficult it is for a village mother to make a good, clean, safe bottle-feed.

Bottle-feeding is one of the worst things that have come to Africa from Europe and America. So try hard to persuade mothers to breast-feed their children. Some people feel so strongly about the dangers of bottle-feeding that they do not think that a book of this kind should say anything about it. However, when you know how bottle-feeding should be done, you will understand more easily why it goes wrong so often. Also, there are some mothers who are going to bottle-feed their children however hard we try to teach them not to. Some of them will have already started using feeding bottles before we see them, and all we may be able to do is to teach them how to use their bottles better, so that they are less dangerous to their children. There are also a very few mothers, perhaps one in a hundred, who really cannot breast-feed their children and will have to feed them artificially. If a mother dies in childbirth, her baby may also need artificial feeding, unless another woman can be found who will feed the child.

Bottle-feeding is not as good as breast-feeding for these reasons.

Bottle-feeding is dangerous. It is dangerous because it makes babies sick and often kills them. It does this in two ways:

1. STARVATION. A young baby needs a lot of milk. Powdered milk is expensive, and many mothers do not have the money to buy enough milk. They do not put enough milk powder into each bottle of water, and do not give their children enough feeds each day. Their babies

thus have too little food and become thin and marasmic. Marasmus is often caused by children not getting enough milk in their bottles.

BOTTLE-FEEDING IS OFTEN BOTTLE-STARVATION

---

2. INFECTION. Micro-organisms (germs) like growing in milk and grow quickly in warm, dirty, feeding bottles. If even a little milk is left in a feeding bottle after a feed, micro-organisms will grow in it. When more milk is put in the bottle, they will grow in this milk also. If a baby is given a feed of dirty milk with many micro-organisms in it, he will get diarrhoea and may die.

When harmful micro-organisms get into a child and grow in him we say he is infected. To prevent infection we have to kill the harmful micro-organisms in a feeding bottle *and on a cup and spoon* before they are used. The best way of doing this is usually to kill them with boiling water.

These are the reasons why many bottle-feeds contain so little milk that the baby starves, and so many micro-organisms that he gets diarrhoea. Mothers sometimes make a bottle-feed by putting a little powdered milk in water until it looks a bit white like milk. They try to make a tin of milk last longer by putting less of it into each bottle. They do not understand that a bottle of milk made like this is nothing like fresh milk or breast milk. There is not nearly as much food in thin, weak, watery milk of this kind as there is in properly made milk. No wonder bottle-fed babies often die. Starvation and diarrhoea are both dangerous, but starvation is usually the more common and thus the greater danger.

It is difficult to get rid of the dangers of bottle-feeding because:

Safe bottle-feeding needs much water and fuel. A feeding bottle is used several times a day. Each time it is used it must be washed in water and boiled to kill the micro-organisms inside it. Many mothers have neither enough water nor enough fuel to wash and boil their feeding bottles properly.

Safe bottle-feeding is expensive.   You will see in Section 8.5 just how expensive it is. It is expensive because a mother has to buy a lot of milk, and also fuel to boil the bottle. If a mother has no money to buy *enough* milk and fuel, she must *not* bottle-feed her child!

Safe bottle-feeding takes time.   Breast milk is always ready for a baby, but a bottle-feed takes time to make.

If a mother was fortunate enough to have the kind of kitchen shown in Figure 8–1, she could make a safe bottle-feed if she wanted to. But the mother in Figure 8–2 could not make a safe bottle-feed, however hard she tried. She has not got enough money to buy milk. She has a long way to walk for water. She has little fire-wood, no fridge and not enough time. She has never been to school and cannot work out measures of milk or remember numbers, even if she could get all the things she needed. Many mothers are more fortunate than the poor woman in Figure 8–2, but even so they have not got all the things in the expensive kitchen in

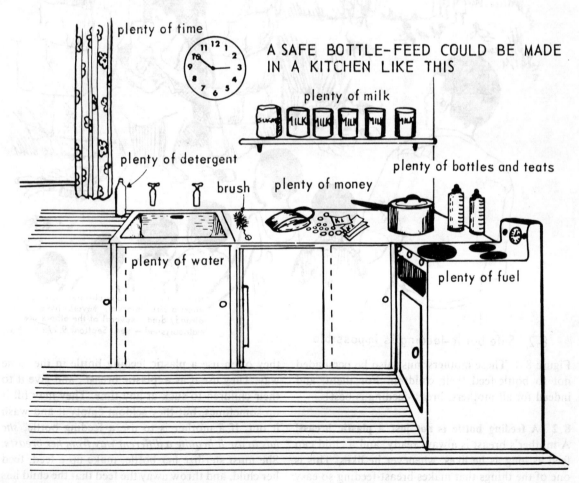

plenty of time

A SAFE BOTTLE–FEED COULD BE MADE IN A KITCHEN LIKE THIS

plenty of milk

plenty of detergent

plenty of bottles and teats

brush   plenty of money

plenty of water

plenty of fuel

8-1, Safe bottle-feeding is possible

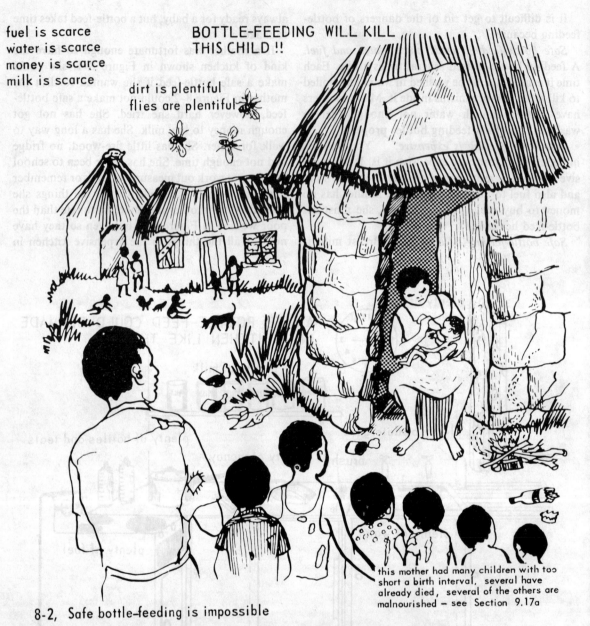

fuel is scarce
water is scarce
money is scarce
milk is scarce

BOTTLE-FEEDING WILL KILL
THIS CHILD !!

dirt is plentiful
flies are plentiful

this mother had many children with too
short a birth interval, several have
already died, several of the others are
malnourished — see Section 9.17a

8-2, Safe bottle-feeding is impossible

Figure 8–1. These mothers must also be persuaded not to bottle-feed their children. For them, and indeed for all mothers, breast-feeding is best!

8.2 A feeding bottle is not just a plastic breast!
A mother's breast is always ready, and a child can feed as long as he likes, whenever he likes. This is one of the things that makes breast-feeding so easy and safe. But, when mothers start bottle-feeding, they often use a plastic feeding bottle in the same way. They use it as a 'plastic breast', and give it to their children to suck at any time. They may fill it up sometimes, but they seldom empty it and wash it out. If a mother is to use a feeding bottle, *she has to use it in quite a different way from her breasts.* She must sterilize her bottle, make up a feed, feed her child, and throw away the feed that the child has not drunk, or give it to someone else in the family.

She must then wash the feeding bottle. At the next feed she must do the same things all over again! All this must happen five times a day.

A FEEDING BOTTLE IS NOT JUST A PLASTIC BREAST

8.3 When breast-feeding fails. We have seen how important it is that mothers should breast-feed their children. But say we have tried hard and failed, and a mother says she cannot or will not breast-feed her child. What are we going to do then? And what are we going to do about the one mother in every hundred who cannot breast-feed her child, either because she is ill, or because she has some disease of her breasts?

The first thing to do is to persuade her to go on giving her child at least some breast milk if she can. She may perhaps be able to breast-feed her child at night and in the morning. This will save her from making all the feeds, she will not have to buy so much milk, and her child will get at least some breast milk. If she does this, her breasts will go on making some milk, and she will be able to feed her child when she goes on a journey with him. This is the time when many women feel that they need to take a bottle for their child so that he can have a drink.

Perhaps some other mother can breast-feed the child? This is a good thing to do. In some tribes it is common for a child whose mother has no breast milk to be allowed to suck from the breasts of other mothers who have plenty of milk. In some tribes a grandmother or aunt may be able to feed the child.

The next thing to do is to give artificial feeds as safely as possible. The best way to do this is to teach her to feed her child with a cup and spoon. Cup-and-spoon feeding takes a little longer than bottle-feeding, but it is safer because a cup and spoon can be washed more easily than a feeding bottle. But even a cup and spoon are not perfectly safe, because harmful micro-organisms can live on them and give the baby diarrhoea. In Section 8.6 you will read how *these micro-organisms have to be killed with boiling water before a cup and spoon are used.*

If a mother is going to feed her child artificially, she must know what kind of milk to buy. She must know how much to buy, how to mix it up, and how much to give her child.

8.4 The best kind of milk to buy. After mother's milk, the next best food for a child is cow's milk. As you saw in Section 5.3, the main difference between mother's milk and cow's milk is that mother's milk contains more sugar and less protein than cow's milk. We can make cow's milk a little more like mother's milk by adding a *little* water (so that there is less protein) and some sugar (so that there is more sugar). Some people use fresh cow's milk in this way, but *it is probably best for most mothers to use the cheapest kind of FULL CREAM dried milk and to add sugar to it.*

Mothers should not use dried *skim* milk, because this has no fat and therefore contains too few joules for a young child. Many kinds of dried skim milk also contain too few vitamins. Mothers should not buy condensed milk, because this contains much too much sugar and therefore contains too many joules. Too much sugar may also cause diarrhoea. Even if a child drinks enough condensed milk to give him the joules he needs, he will not be getting enough protein and so will become malnourished. Babies who are bottle-fed with condensed milk may be fat from having plenty of joules, but they may also get kwashiorkor from getting too little protein. Babies can be fed with unsweetened evaporated milk, but we will not describe it here.

CONDENSED MILK IS BAD FOR BABIES

We thought about the cost of milk in Section 5.7. We saw that some kinds of special infant milk are more expensive than ordinary full cream milk and contain some added carbohydrate, so that there is no need to add extra sugar. These can be used, but the cheapest brand of ordinary full cream dried milk will be just as good if sugar is added to it. We dare not give the names of these special infant milks; so try to guess the ones we mean! In Zambia the cheapest kind of full cream milk is 'Dawn' brand full cream powdered milk.

BUY A MONTH'S SUPPLY OF MILK AT THE BEGINNING OF THE MONTH

8.5 How much full cream dried milk must a mother buy? At the end of the month, when mothers have money, they must buy enough full cream dried milk to last them the whole of the following month. If a mother does not buy a whole month's supply of milk at once, she will probably find herself without either milk or the money to buy any more before the end of the month, so her baby will starve. When this book was written full cream milk cost 95n a kilo in Lusaka, and dried skim milk 48n a kilo. Here is the amount of milk a mother needs and how much it will cost her.

TABLE 20
The Cost of Artificial Feeding

Age of baby	Kilos of full cream milk needed each month	Kwacha needed to buy milk each month
0–2 months	2 kg	K1.90
2–4 months	2½ kg	K2.38

At four months the baby must start eating porridge. As soon as he is eating this well, add some protein food to every meal.

4–7 months	3 kg	K2.85

By this time the baby should be well used to new foods; he should be eating three meals a day and should be drinking well from a cup. Some or all of his milk can now be dried skim milk, which is cheaper.

7–8 months	2½ kg	K2.38
8–10 months	2 kg	K1.90
10–12 months	1 kg	K0.95

You will see that a baby only needs 2 kg of milk in his first month. But as he grows older he needs more and more until he needs about 3 kg by the time he is four months old. This is the time that he must start to eat porridge, and as soon as he is eating it well, some protein food must be added to every meal. By the time he is seven months old he should be well used to new foods, and should be drinking easily from a cup. From now on he needs less milk each month, and some or all of his milk can be dried skim milk, which is cheaper than full cream milk and can be added to his porridge. However, it is better for a child to drink full cream milk, and a mother should try to give all her children half a litre (a pint) of full cream milk to drink every day,

if she can. If she cannot get fresh milk she should use powdered full cream milk.

HOW MUCH DOES ARTIFICIAL FEEDING COST IN YOUR DISTRICT?

If you add up the money that a mother must spend each month to artificially feed her child, you will see that it comes to about K25 which buys 26½ kg of full cream milk. If, after her child is seven months old, she buys only dried skim milk, she will only have to spend K21.20. She will also have to buy sugar, and if she uses a feeding bottle she will need plenty of fuel to boil the water to make it safe. Costs change, so find out how much dried milk costs in your district and how much it would cost a mother to feed her child artificially.

IF A CHILD IS TO BE ARTIFICIALLY FED HE MUST GET ENOUGH MILK

Breast-feeding is much cheaper than artificial feeding, but it does not cost nothing, because a breast-feeding mother should buy and eat plenty of extra food herself. You will remember from Section 6.1 that each day she needs *extra* protein food equal to 17.5 g of reference protein.

Mothers must understand that the full cream milk in Table 20 is the milk that the baby needs and is for him only. If other people in the family are going to have milk in their tea, a mother must buy more milk than this. Tell her also to keep the lid on the tin, so that dirt and micro-organisms do not get into it and harm her child.

CUP-AND-SPOON FEEDING

8.6 Making the feed. Besides plenty of full cream milk powder a mother needs a teaspoon and a cup. The cups used to measure here are ordinary teacups holding about 200 ml. Mothers often do not know the words for different sizes of spoon, so to be sure that they understand, it is a good idea to show them a real spoon of the size you are talking about. A *teaspoon* is a small spoon of the

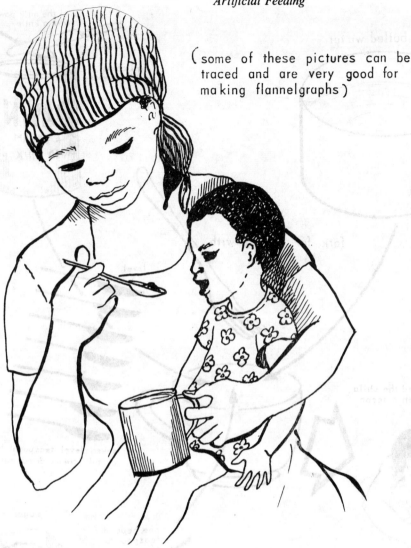

(some of these pictures can be traced and are very good for making flannelgraphs)

8-3, Cup-and-spoon feeding

kind used for stirring tea. All the measures given here are for teaspoons. A dessert spoon is the kind of spoon that adults use for eating food. Mothers will also need a fork with which to mix the milk.

Mothers will also need plenty of safe *clean* water. Water from wells may contain dangerous micro-organisms which cause diarrhoea, so *all water for bottle-feeding must be boiled*. The micro-organisms which cause diarrhoea are killed as soon as the water boils, so there is no need to boil it for very long. Ask mothers to keep some cold boiled water in a large jar or bottle, as described in Section 4.17.

This water should de fresh, so ask them to change it every few days.

There are usually fewer micro-organisms on a cup and spoon than there are in a feeding bottle, but even so there may be enough to give a child diarrhoea. A cup and spoon should therefore be boiled like a feeding bottle. If this is not possible, they should be washed clean, and boiling water poured over them to kill at least some of the micro-organisms. If there is no fuel with which to boil water, both the cup and the spoon must be made as clean as they can be with cold water. If boiling water is to be used to kill the micro-

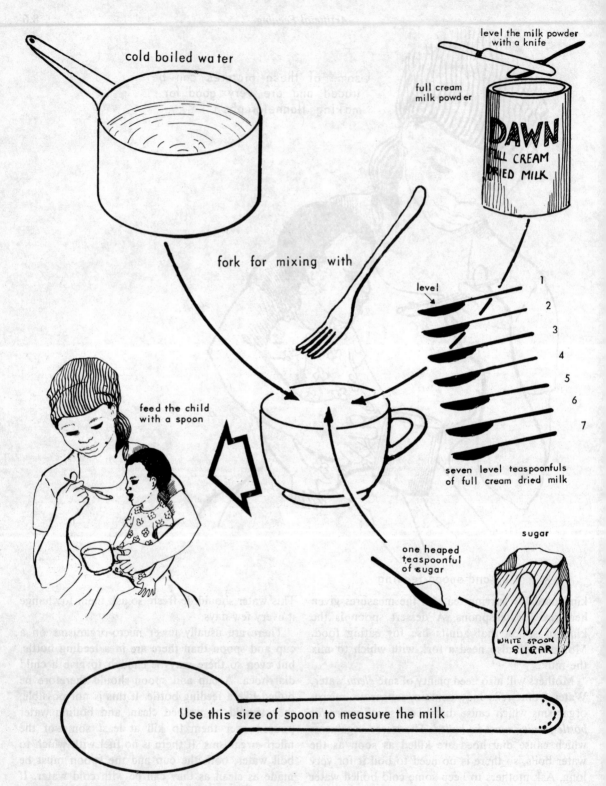

cold boiled water

level the milk powder
with a knife

full cream
milk powder

DAWN
FULL CREAM
DRIED MILK

fork for mixing with

level

1
2
3
4
5
6
7

seven level teaspoonfuls
of full cream dried milk

feed the child
with a spoon

one heaped
teaspoonful
of sugar

sugar

WHITE SPOON
SUGAR

Use this size of spoon to measure the milk

8 - 4, Making a cup - and - spoon feed

organisms on cups, they must be made of metal not plastic, or the hot water may harm them. Plastic feeding bottles are made so that they can be boiled without spoiling.

Cow's milk contains less sugar than breast milk, so some sugar is also needed, which makes it a little more like breast milk.

Tell a mother to make a feed like this:

1.   Boil her cup and spoon in boiling water. If this is impossible tell her to pour some boiling water over them. If fuel is very scarce, tell her to make them as clean as she can with cold water. She could also wash them and leave them in hypochlorite, as in Figure 8–7.

2.   Fill a cup half full of cold boiled water.

3.   Add *seven level teaspoonfuls* of full cream dried milk powder. You will see in the figure that the spoonfuls of milk powder are being made flat or level with a knife (Figure 8–4.)

4.   Add one heaped teaspoonful of sugar.

5.   Dissolve the milk in the water by beating with a fork.

6.   Fill the cup with cold boild water.

IF YOU HAVE TO TEACH ABOUT BOTTLE-FEEDING, SHOW MOTHERS HOW TO DO IT WELL

A mother should then carefully feed her baby with a teaspoon. Some babies will start to drink from a cup when they are three months old, or even younger, and no longer need to be fed with a spoon. Sometimes a child will drink very easily from the spout of a jug. The spout is the part of a jug from which the liquid is poured. Children should be encouraged to drink from a cup or a jug, because this saves their mothers much time. If a jug is used it should be washed and looked after with the same care that is described above for a cup and spoon.

8.7 Using fresh cow's milk.   This is often a little cheaper than dried full cream milk, but it is not so convenient and easy to use because it soon goes sour. Even so, some mothers may want to use it.

Teach a mother to add one part of water to three parts of milk, and to add one *heaped* teaspoonful of sugar to each cupful of milk.

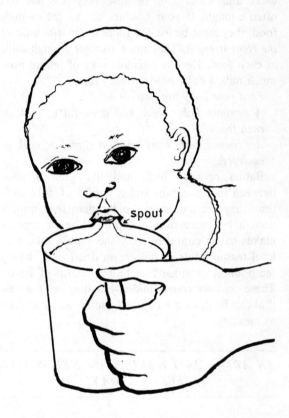

spout

8 - 5, Quite young children will often drink from the spout of a jug

By adding a little water and some sugar to cow's milk in this way, we are making it a little more like breast milk. By 'parts' we mean three cupfuls, or pints, or any other measure, of milk to one cupful, or pint, or other measure, of water. The measures must, of course, be the same—that is three *cupfuls* of milk to one *cupful* of water.

Cow's milk, like water, should always be boiled before it is given to a young child. Boiled milk is more easily digested, and boiling also kills any micro-organisms that there may be in the milk. Children should also be fed from a *clean* cup. It is no use boiling water or milk and then putting it in a dirty cup with many micro-organisms.

8.8   How much milk to give the baby.   Artificial feeding most often goes wrong because babies do not get enough milk, either because the milk is weak and watery, or because they are not fed often enough. If young babies are to get enough food, they must be fed *five times a day with milk of the right strength*. They must also get enough milk at each feed. Here is a simple way of telling how much milk a baby needs at each feed.

Feed your baby five times a day.

A newborn baby needs half a cupful of milk at each feed.

A five-month-old baby needs a cupful of milk at each feed.

Babies between birth and five months need between half a cupful and a cupful of milk each time they are fed. Babies older than five months need a bit more than a cupful. When a mother makes half a cupful of feed, she should take four level teaspoonfuls of full cream dried milk, half a teaspoonful of sugar and half a cupful of water. These are only rough guides, but they are the best that can be done if a cup and spoon are to be used as measures.

AN ARTIFICIALLY FED BABY NEEDS FIVE FEEDS A DAY

Babies older than five months should be getting maize or millet porridge with protein foods added to it. They can thus drink less milk as they grow older, *but only if they are getting enough porridge with added protein*. If a family is poor, the amount of full cream dried milk that a baby is given can get less, and he can be given cheaper dried skim milk instead. Give him this in his porridge; he may get diarrhoea if he drinks it. A child who has his milk powder added to his porridge will be getting less liquid than one who drinks his milk. He may be thirsty and should be given cold boiled water to drink.

After mother's milk, cow's milk is the best food for babies, and, as you have read, families who have enough money should give each of their older children half a litre (a pint) of milk each day.

8.9   If mothers will not use a cup and spoon. Many doctors hate bottle-feeding so much, because it kills so many children, that they think we should not talk about it in a book of this kind. But, however hard we try, some mothers are going to bottle-feed their children whatever we do to tell them not to. A few mothers cannot use a cup and spoon and will use a feeding bottle. This usually happens when a baby is very young, and it is more difficult for him to feed from a cup and spoon. What are we to tell them?

Teach them to use a *glass* feeding bottle which can be boiled and to buy several teats. Glass is much better than plastic because you can see more easily when it is clean. The feeding bottle must have a wide mouth so that it can be more easily cleaned. It should also have 'ml' written on its side. The hole in the teat must be big enough. When you hold a bottle of milk upside down the milk should just come out in fast drops. If the milk only comes out in slow drops, make the hole bigger. One way of doing this is to use a hot needle.

A fork and a teaspoon will also be needed. So will *plenty* of full cream milk powder and cold boiled water. Mothers must also have a bottle brush and some soap or washing powder, a pan with a lid, and plenty of fuel.

8.10   Washing and sterilizing the bottle.   The best way to kill the germs in a feeding bottle and on a teat is to wash and boil both of them carefully after *every feed*. A mother needs a pan with a lid. The boiled bottle and teat should stay in the covered pan until the next feed. In this way the micro-organisms in the bottle are killed, and no new ones will get into it before it is used again. A feeding bottle and its teat should not be allowed to lie around on the floor! Provided the pan has a lid, there need only be a little water in the bottom of the pan. The micro-organisms on the bottle will be killed by the hot steam when the water boils. When a bottle is boiled to kill the micro-organisms we say it is **sterilized**. Boiling is very important, and one of the reasons why bottle-feeding is so bad is that so few mothers boil their feeding bottles.

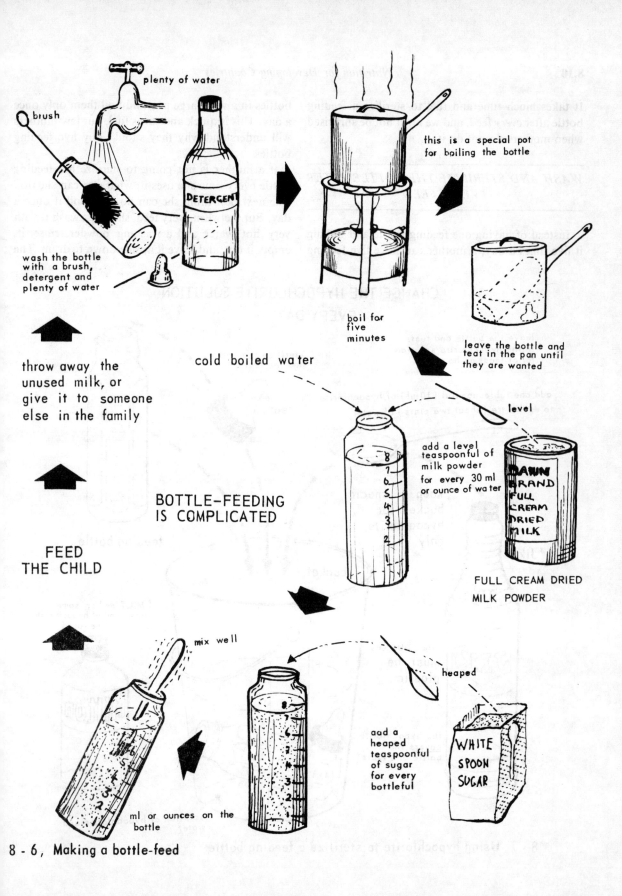

brush

plenty of water

DETERGENT

wash the bottle with a brush, detergent and plenty of water

this is a special pot for boiling the bottle

boil for five minutes

leave the bottle and teat in the pan until they are wanted

throw away the unused milk, or give it to someone else in the family

cold boiled water

BOTTLE-FEEDING IS COMPLICATED

add a level teaspoonful of milk powder for every 30 ml or ounce of water

level

DAWN BRAND FULL CREAM DRIED MILK

FULL CREAM DRIED MILK POWDER

FEED THE CHILD

mix well

add a heaped teaspoonful of sugar for every bottleful

heaped

WHITE SPOON SUGAR

ml or ounces on the bottle

8 - 6, Making a bottle-feed

It takes much time and fuel to sterilize a feeding bottle after *every* feed, and we must not be surprised when mothers do not do it.

WASH AND STERILIZE THE BOTTLE AFTER EVERY FEED

Instead of having one feeding bottle and boiling it five times a day, a mother can have five feeding bottles in a very large pan and boil them only once a day. This is quick and saves fuel, but few mothers will understand why they should buy five feeding bottles.

If a mother is not going to sterilize her feeding bottle every time she uses it, what else can she do? The next best thing she can do is to boil it once a day. But, between every feed, she must wash it with very hot water and a washing powder, rinse it, empty it out, and leave it upside down to drain. The

CHANGE THE HYPOCHLORITE SOLUTION
EVERY DAY

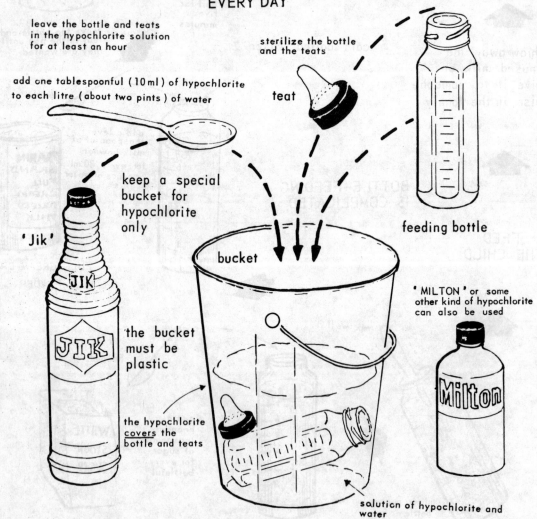

leave the bottle and teats in the hypochlorite solution for at least an hour

add one tablespoonful (10 ml) of hypochlorite to each litre (about two pints) of water

sterilize the bottle and the teats

teat

keep a special bucket for hypochlorite only

feeding bottle

'Jik'

bucket

the bucket must be plastic

'MILTON' or some other kind of hypochlorite can also be used

the hypochlorite covers the bottle and teats

solution of hypochlorite and water

8 - 7. Using hypochlorite to sterilize a feeding bottle

worst thing a mother can do is to leave an unwashed feeding bottle with some milk in it from one feed to the next. In a few hours micro-organisms will grow very well in warm milk. For this reason all milk which is not drunk by the baby at one feed must be given to some other member of the family, or thrown away.

IF A BOTTLE IS NOT TO BE STERILIZED WASH IT AFTER EVERY FEED

If a mother is not going to boil her bottle at all, she must at least empty it, wash it well, if possible with hot water and washing powder, and leave it upside down to dry and drain until she uses it again. A good way of draining a feeding bottle is to leave it upside down on a stick or wire. Micro-organisms do not grow quite so well in a washed, dry, *empty* feeding bottle. **NONE OF THESE THINGS IS NEARLY AS GOOD AS BOILING A FEEDING BOTTLE AND ITS TEAT EVERY TIME THEY ARE USED.** Even if a child is carefully bottle-fed, he will get diarrhoea more often than a breast-fed child.

DON'T LEAVE MILK IN A BOTTLE FROM ONE FEED TO THE NEXT

Mothers with a little more money sometimes keep warm milk in a 'thermos' from one feed to the next. A thermos is a special glass bottle for keeping foods at the same warmth or coldness with which they were put into it. This is one of *the worst possible things to do*, because micro-organisms like growing in warm milk, and the milk in the thermos may be at just the warmth they like best.

8.11 Sterilizing feeding bottles with hypochlorite. There is another way of killing the micro-organisms on feeding bottles besides boiling them. This is to use special liquids called **antiseptics,** which kill micro-organisms on the *outside* of the body. Antiseptics are quite safe if they are used in this way, but they must not be drunk because they are

harmful *inside* the body. The best antiseptic to use for killing micro-organisms on feeding bottles are those which contain a chemical called **hypochlorite,** such as 'Milton' or 'Jik'. Other antiseptics may be dangerous. 'Jik' is the best kind of hypochlorite to use in Zambia, because it is stronger, cheaper, and is also usually easier to get. Use 'Milton' or 'Jik' like this:

1. Put enough water to cover the bottles in a plastic bowl or bucket. Don't use a metal bucket because the hypochlorite will spoil it.
2. Add one *dessertspoonful* (10 ml) of hypochlorite to each litre of water in the bowl or bucket (a litre is about a quart, two pints, or five cupfuls).
3. AFTER EVERY FEED. Wash the bottle and teat well with cold water. Brush out the bottle with a bottle-brush and a detergent. Wash the teat well on the inside and the outside.
4. Put the feeding bottles and their teats into the mixture of hypochlorite and water, so that they are completely under the mixture and the bottles are filled. *Micro-organisms will not be killed on any part of the bottle or teat that is not touched by the mixture!*
5. Leave the bottles and their teats in the mixture for *at least one hour*, or until the next feed.
6. AT THE NEXT FEED. Wash your hands. Take the bottle and the teat out of the mixture. Pour the mixture out of the bottle and make up fresh feed. There is no need to wash away the little hypochlorite left on the inside of the bottle. The little that is left there will not harm the baby, provided the hypochlorite is not too strong.
7. Make new hypochlorite mixture every day.

DON'T FORGET TO STERILIZE THE TEAT AS WELL AS THE BOTTLE

If hypochlorites like 'Jik' and 'Milton' are used in the right way, they are safe. But, if mothers are going to use them, they must buy enough of them each month as well as enough milk.

They must leave the bottles and teats in the hypochlorite mixture for at least an hour, and they must change the hypochlorite mixture *every day*.

All this may seem both difficult and expensive—it shows once again that breast-feeding is best!

CHANGE THE HYPOCHLORITE MIXTURE DAILY

8.12 How much milk to give the baby. Most feeding bottles have ounces and millilitres written down the side. This makes it easy to work out how much milk to give a child.

The rules that we are going to give you only work if a child is fed FIVE times a day. They work from the time a child is born until he weighs 8 kg at about the age of seven months. The rules are these; use whichever is easiest:

Give the baby 30 ml at each feed for each kilogram of his weight.   A 7 kg child thus requires $7 \times$ 30 ml$=210$ ml at each of his five daily feeds.

There are about 30 ml in an ounce; so, if the bottle is marked in ounces, his feed can be worked out like this:

Give your baby the same number of ounces in milk as his weight is in kilograms.   For example, a 6 kg child needs 6 ounces of milk at each of his five feeds.

If you only know your child's weight in pounds and do not want to change it into kilograms, you can use this rule:

Divide your baby's weight in pounds by two and give him this number of ounces of milk.   For example, a 14-pound baby needs $14 \div 2 = 7$ ounces of milk at each of his five feeds.

Because bottles usually hold eight ounces, or about 240 ml, a child of seven months, who weighs eight kilograms, will be getting a bottle full of milk at each feed. He will therefore be getting 5×240 ml $=1,200$ ml of milk during the day. However, by the age of seven months, he should also be taking plenty of solid food, and so from then onwards the amount of milk he drinks can slowly get less, as shown by Table 20 (Section 8.5). He can be given dried skim milk in his porridge instead of full cream liquid milk to drink. A seven-month-

old child can usually drink from a cup quite well; so mothers should be persuaded to stop bottle-feeding at this time if they possibly can. *A child can however only start getting less liquid milk if he is also getting plenty of porridge with added protein.*

If a mother is using a feeding bottle, it is easy for her to measure ml or ounces, because these are marked on the side of the bottle. When she has found the number of ounces her child needs, she must put this amount of cold boiled water in her feeding bottle, and add one *level* teaspoonful of full cream dried milk for every 30 ml (ounce) of water. She will also need some sugar. If a whole bottle of milk is being made, one heaped teaspoonful of sugar must be added. If less milk is being made, less sugar is needed. The milk and water can be mixed in the bottle with a fork. Another way is to measure the water in the bottle, to tip it into a basin, to add the milk powder and to mix it with a fork.

If a baby cries and is hungry before his next feed, he may not be getting enough milk. If this is so, one or more of the spoonfuls of milk should be heaped instead of level. A hungry baby can also be given 30 ml (an ounce) of extra milk at one or more of his feeds.

This way of working out how much milk a baby needs, using pounds and kilograms, can be used with a cup for measuring, but it is not so easy. A cup holds 200 ml, or about 7 ounces. So, by the time a baby is 7 kg, he should be getting a cupful of milk at each of his five daily feeds.

8.13 'The extra bottle'.   Some mothers breast-feed their children well. They give them plenty of porridge with added protein, but they also give them a bottle. Sometimes this bottle has milk in it, but more often it contains only milky tea. What should we tell mothers to do? The best thing to tell them is not to have anything to do with a feeding bottle at any time whatever, because such feeding bottles are seldom properly washed, and if they are left around dirty micro-organisms grow in them and give the child diarrhoea. *When children are given liquid milk or tea, feed them from a cup. If necessary help them with a spoon. Don't feed them* *from a bottle, even if they are being breast-fed at the same time.*

all other foods for a baby, make the fruit juice cleanly!

MOTHER'S MILK IS THE BEST FOOD FOR BABIES

Children, especially small babies, are sometimes given an 'extra bottle' to try to make them fatter. Bottles are a bad way of feeding children, and *if* a mother does want to fatten her child she should give him plenty of porridge with lots of protein food added to it.

8.14   Giving vitamin C.   An artificially fed baby needs a few teaspoonfuls of fruit juice every day to give him enough vitamin C to stop him getting scurvy (Section 4.8). The juice from fizzy drinks, even fizzy orange, usually has little or no vitamin C, so the baby needs *fresh* fruit juice. It is not usually necessary to give breast-fed babies vitamin because there is vitamin C in mother's milk. As with

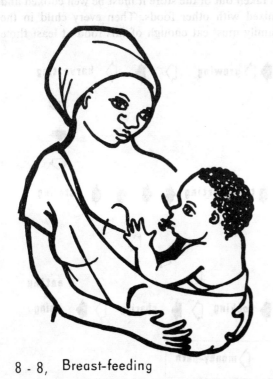

8 - 8,   Breast-feeding

BREAST-FEEDING IS BETTER THAN ARTIFICIAL FEEDING

8.15   Some rules.   Here are some rules to remember:

Don't be afraid to feed your baby; he will not get too much milk.

If your baby is crying and unhappy, feed him.

If you are bottle-feeding, make sure that the hole in the teat is big enough for the milk to get out, but not too big, so that it drowns him!

If your baby is healthy and being properly fed, there is no need to give him boiled water between feeds.

Make all artificial feeds, especially bottle-feeds, as cleanly as possible.

If your child gets diarrhoea, make sure he gets plenty of salt-and-sugar water (Section 7.20).

A feeding bottle is not a plastic breast;
it must be washed;
it must be sterilized;
it must be filled with *enough* milk;
it must be filled with *boiled* water;
          . . . EVERY time it is used!!!

8.16   T H I N G S   T O   D O

(a)   Make a bottle-feed.   If you are one of the readers who may be asked by mothers about bottle-feeding, you must know how to make a bottle-feed and what the difficulties are. Practise making a bottle-feed as it is described here. Try to make a safe bottle-feed in a villager's hut. You will find it almost impossible! Breast-feeding *is* best!

(b)   Make a cup-and-spoon feed.   Make a cup-and-spoon feed and feed a baby. You will find that older babies can drink quite well. Weigh the baby and find out how much milk he should drink in a day.

Chapter Nine

THE FOOD-PATH

9.1 Food-paths. If a child is going to grow, he must eat enough of the right food. This food must come from somewhere. Foods like maize and groundnuts are grown in fields and gardens. Cows are milked and are later killed for eating. Fish have to be caught in rivers and lakes. These foods have then to get to a child's body from the fields and rivers where they grow. We can think of food as going along a path from the fields and gardens where it is grown to the body of the child who eats it. We will call these paths the **food-paths,** and think about all the things that may block them and cause malnutrition. Food-paths are longer for town children, whose mothers have to buy food, than they are for village children whose mothers grow food. We will therefore think about the village food-path first. In Figure 9–1 the village food-path is shown with white arrows and the town food-path

with black arrows. The path that money goes along (the 'money-path') is shown with arrows with lines on them.

The village food-path starts in the gardens where food is grown. If village children are going to eat enough of the right kind of food, plenty of good land must first be dug and good seeds sown at the right time in the right way. People must also be healthy and strong, so that they can work hard in the fields. Then there must be enough rain, but not too much, and no insects must harm the crops (food plants) while they are growing. The crops must then be harvested (gathered in) and stored for eating later in the year. No rats or insects must eat the food while it is being stored. When the food is taken out of the store it must be well cooked and mixed with other foods. Then every child in the family must eat enough of this food at least three

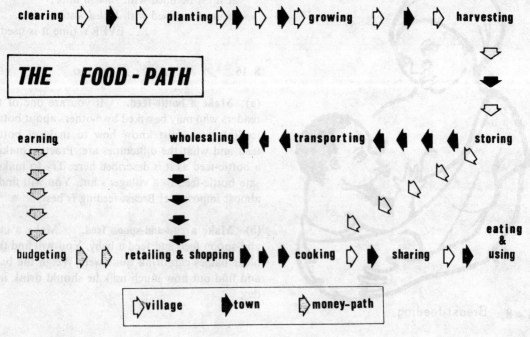

9-1, The food-path

times a day. Last of all, children must not have any diseases, such as measles, diarrhoea or worms, which may stop them eating, or stop their bodies using the food they have eaten. Only if *all* these things happen, will the children of a village be healthy and well nourished.

Town children must also eat enough of the right kinds of food, if they too are to grow and be healthy. The food-path for town children also starts in village gardens. Somewhere villagers have first to grow food, and then to harvest and store it. Next, a wholesaler has to buy this food from the villager and take it to town. A wholesaler is a man who buys and sells in large amounts. The wholesaler then sells the food he has bought to retailers in the shops and markets. A retailer is a person who buys and sells in small amounts. A shopkeeper is a retailer. These retailers then sell food to mothers who buy it for their families.

If a mother is going to be able to buy enough food for her family, her husband must have a job so that he can earn money. He must then give his wife enough of this money, so that she can buy enough food all through the month until the next pay-day. This is a money-path more than a food-path, but it is the same really because money buys food. Food in the markets must be cheap, so that mothers with little money can buy enough for their families. Mothers must buy the right foods and cook them in the right way. Their children must then eat enough of this well-cooked food several times each day to make them grow strong and keep them healthy. Town children must also have no diseases which stop them eating, or stop their bodies using the food they have eaten.

These are not the only food-paths. Fish, for example, follows another food-path from lakes, rivers or the sea, and has usually to be dried before it is taken to the town. Sometimes the food-path in towns is quite short. For example, villagers may grow food in the fields, bring it into town and sell it to mothers themselves. For the very young child the most important food of all is his mother's milk. It has not far to go to get to him! Foods from outside the country, like dried skim milk, have a very long food-path indeed. They have to come across the sea in ships.

ANYTHING THAT BLOCKS A FOOD-PATH CAN CAUSE MALNUTRITION

Anything that blocks a food-path can cause malnutrition. Many of the blocks are the same for the village child and the town child, so we will put them together. The sections below tell you some of the more important things that can block the food-path and cause malnutrition. There are also many others. You can think of these blocks as being like a tree falling across a path and blocking it, or like the bridge over a stream being washed away so the path is blocked.

There is one step on the food-path that we have not said anything about. This is because it is seldom blocked, and thus seldom the cause of malnutrition. This step is **processing.** By processing we mean changing the food in some way, such as grinding maize into flour, drying fish, or making sugar out of sugar cane. Food can be processed in a factory, or in the home. When it is done at home it is really part of cooking. Processing can be put into the food-path between transporting and wholesaling, and you will surely be able to think of some ways in which this step in the path might be blocked.

'Blocks on the food-path' are usually called 'socio-economic factors responsible for malnutrition'. We feel, however, that it is easier to think of the food-path and what blocks it.

BLOCKS ON THE FOOD-PATH

9.2 People may be too sick to work hard.   A farmer and his wife may not be so sick that they have to go to hospital, but they may be a little sick so that they feel tired, do not want to work, and are not able to work hard. Many people are a little sick with diseases like malnutrition, malaria, anaemia, bilharziasis, or other diseases. These diseases are common, and many farmers have some or even all of them. We must not be surprised that they do not want to work. Especially, they may not want to do the important hard work of clearing new bush for planting. A malnourished farmer who does not want to work hard may plant an easily-grown crop like cassava, instead of a better crop like maize, which needs more work.

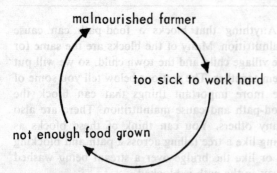

malnourished farmer

too sick to work hard

not enough food grown

9-2, The vicious circle of food production

A malnourished farmer does not want to work hard. He does not grow enough food, so he stays malnourished. This cause of malnutrition therefore goes in a circle. Causes which go in a circle like this are called 'vicious circles'. The vicious circle caused by malnutrition stopping hard work is a serious block at the beginning of the food-path.

9.3   Too many people and not enough land.   In most parts of Africa there is plenty of land. But in parts of Kenya and Malawi there are so many people that there is not enough land to grow food on. In these districts lack of land is therefore a serious block in the food-path. People can move to find land in other places, but they often do not want to do this. They may learn how to grow more food from the same land. People can also have fewer children, say three or four instead of seven or eight. In this way the land does not get filled with people so quickly. Having children only when you want them is called 'family planning'. People in Kenya are learning to do this so that there will be enough land for everyone. There is now no reason why anyone should have a child unless they want to. Read more about family planning in Section 11.22.

9.4   Customs that block the food-path.   Some customs are good for nutrition and some are bad. In many parts of Africa, it is the custom for a mother to go on breast-feeding her child until he

is eighteen months or two years old. This is a good custom because children need their mother's milk during this time. It is also the custom in many tribes for women to do most of the work in the fields. This is not a good custom, because there will be too much work for a woman to do, if the family is to have enough food. In the old days men used to be soldiers fighting other tribes. Now that there is no longer any fighting, many men in the village have little to do. If everyone is to be healthy and well nourished, men must work in the fields, and the old customs must change. Especially, men must clear the bush and help with planting in the important early weeks of the rains. In many places one of the main causes of malnutrition is men not clearing and planting enough land. Many families plant groundnuts, but they plant so little that they only last two or three months. They must grow enough groundnuts to last them all the year. The custom of men not working enough in the fields is one of the most important blocks in the food-path.

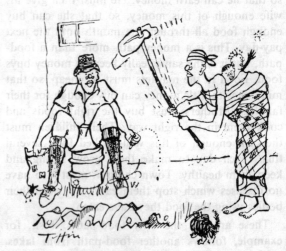

9-3,   Old customs block the food-path

MEN MUST WORK IN THE FIELDS

Some tribes think of cows as money rather than as food. They keep too many bulls, and too many old thin cows that would be better killed and eaten. Other tribes think that eggs should not be given to girl babies, because they will stop them having children or make them steal. These are two more customs that block the food-path.

Some communities think it is very bad for a man to work hard and have a better house and fields than his friends. Sometimes a man who seems richer and more hard-working than his neighbours has his house or his food-stores burnt. This holds the whole community back, because it is difficult for anyone to grow more and better food than anyone else. Some customs were useful and good in the old days but are harmful now.

When villagers do not work as hard as we think they should, we may call them lazy. Perhaps they are lazy, but they may also be malnourished or sick. They may not feel well enough to work hard. Village customs may also make it difficult for them to do some of the kinds of work which we think they should. We should therefore be careful when we talk about laziness blocking the food-path and causing malnutrition. Sickness and custom may also be important.

9.5 Blocks in growing enough food. The best time for planting is early in the rains, and in many villages everyone is very busy for these important few weeks. In these villages one block in the food-path is that there is not enough time for all this busy agricultural work to be done. Time is often shorter than it need be, because people have not done all the work that they could before the rains started. One way to make the work at planting time easier may be to clear and plough the land as soon as the last year's harvest has been gathered. The land will then be much easier to plough when the next year's rains start. Not clearing and ploughing the land just after the harvest can thus block the food-path. Another block is a shortage of tractors, or broken tractors, in the early weeks of the rains when everyone wants them.

In parts of Zambia one of the worst blocks early in the food-path is the *chitimene* kind of farming. Trees are cut down and burnt, and crops planted in land fertilized by the ashes. Crops grow well for some years, after which the land grows poor crops. When this happens families move on to new bush and burn more trees. This is a bad kind of farming, because the land spoilt by burning takes many years to get back to being as good as it was before. It is much better for farmers to stay on the same land, to use fertilizers and farm in a way which does not harm the land.

In the old days villagers had no use for money and used only to grow enough food to feed their families through the year. Now that villagers want money to buy things with, they have to grow crops and sell them. They can do two things to get this money. They can grow more of their food crops and sell the part they do not want to eat. We call these **surplus crops.** They can also grow new crops for sale, such as cotton or tobacco, which cannot be eaten. We call these **cash crops.** The difference between these two kinds of crops is important. In a year when the crops are bad, farmers who grow surplus crops for sale have less food to sell but still have enough for themselves. But the farmers who are growing cash crops like cotton may grow so little cotton that they do not earn enough money to feed themselves through the year. Families who grow cash crops must thus grow plenty of food crops as well, so that if the year is a bad one they have a better chance of having enough to eat until the next harvest.

Farmers may also plant the wrong food crops. They may plant too much cassava and too little maize or millet. They often plant too little maize or groundnuts.

Villagers may plant beans and maize instead of cassava, but they may not plant the best **variety** (kind) of maize or beans. They may have cows, but they may not have the best variety of cow. There are many varieties of maize, beans, cows and goats, and some give much more or better food than others. There are always best varieties of crops and animals for each place. The agricultural department has to find out which these best varieties are and then show people how to grow them. If people want to get the most food from the least work, they must plant the varieties of each crop that the agricultural assistants teach them to. They must also keep the best varieties of animals. All over the world there are people working hard to find and make better varieties of crops, which give more food and are not harmed by insects and plant diseases.

As soon as good new varieties of food plants have been found they must be used.

BETTER CROP VARIETIES ARE ONE OF THE BEST WAYS OF IMPROVING NUTRITION

There are special varieties of maize called 'hybrid maize'. Hybrid maize is made by crossing, or marrying, two carefully chosen varieties of maize. These varieties are the parents, and the hybrid maize is the child. It may produce more than twice as much maize as the ordinary maize plant, especially if it is grown with the right fertilizer and has enough water. One of the best varieties of hybrid maize in Zambia is called SR 52. *New hybrid maize seed must be bought each year*, and farmers should not use the hybrid maize that they have grown as seed. If they do, they will not get a good crop.

There are other kinds of hybrid crops, and farmers in India are now growing much more food by planting hybrid varieties of wheat and rice. One of the best of these is a famous variety of rice called IR 8. Farmers who plant IR 8 rice now get several times more rice than farmers who still plant the old kind of rice.

Another famous crop variety is a kind of maize called Opaque-2. In Section 3.7 you read how ordinary maize has too little of the amino acid called lysine. Opaque-2 maize is different. It has much more lysine than ordinary maize. Because it has more lysine, the protein from Opaque-2 maize is better used for body-building, and has a higher NPU, than the protein of ordinary maize. Opaque-2 maize can be crossed (married) with the ordinary maize of a country to give a maize that grows well in that country, and which has protein that is better for body-building.

New varieties and new ways of farming have made such big changes in India, and have grown so much more food, that they are said to have caused a 'green revolution'. One day Africa must have crop varieties as good as these and start her own 'green revolution'.

Many other things matter besides the variety of a crop that is grown. Fields must be dug in the right way, and seeds planted the right distance apart at the right time. But there are often no seeds to buy, and sometimes there are no tools or the wrong tools. If as much food as possible is to be grown on a piece of land the right fertilizers must be used. As we saw in Section 3.7, a fertilizer is a plant food. One of the foods plants need is nitrogen with which to make the amino acids in their proteins. There is plenty of nitrogen in the air, but plants cannot use it, so nitrogen has to be changed into a kind that the plants can use. Many kinds of fertilizer contain a kind of nitrogen that plants can use. It is the job of the agricultural extension officer to tell people which is the best kind of seed and fertilizer.

Fields are sometimes planted in a way that lets the best soil get washed away into the streams and rivers. This loss of good soil is called **soil erosion.** If the soil is washed away, good crops cannot be grown and the food-path is blocked. Better ways of farming will stop soil erosion.

Diseases may harm the plants as they grow. Fungi may grow on them, and insects may eat them. There are special 'medicines' called **fungicides** that kill fungi, and **insecticides** that kill insects, which farmers can put on their plants to protect them. But many farmers do not know about fungicides and insecticides, they may have too little money to buy them, and the shops may not sell them.

But there are still more blocks to the growing of enough good food. **Pests,** such as mice and insects, may eat the seed in the ground before it has had time to grow. A pest is any harmful animal or insect. If seed is treated with an insecticide before it is planted, the insects at least will not eat it. In some districts birds, rabbits, monkeys and especially wild pigs may spoil the growing crops, and the crops may also be stolen by the enemies of the farmer. Crops may not be weeded at the right time, so that weeds stop the food plants from growing. Much food may be lost when crops are harvested.

Farmers may not be paid for the crops they have sold until it is too late to buy seed and fertilizer for the new season. Sometimes there is nothing in the village shops that the farmer really wants. So he sees no reason why he should work hard and earn money which he cannot spend.

In Zambia, one of the most important blocks to growing enough food is lack of young men in the villages. Too many young men have left the land to go to town, where they cannot find jobs. Many others are in school. Villages are thus left with old people and children, and too few young men to clear the bush for planting. If children are to grow into strong men who are good at hard work in the fields, they must learn to work hard while they are young. Many school children do not learn how to do this hard work, and are less able to work in the fields than their parents who did not go to school.

These then are just some of the ways in which the food-path can be blocked while food is growing.

9.6 Spoilt food stores.   After food has been taken from the fields it has to be stored. Pests, such as rats and insects, may eat the food while it is in store. *About a third of all the food stored in the villages is lost in this way.* This means that of every three sacks of food that are stored, one is eaten by pests and only two are left for the family to eat. This is bad because people need this food. Better food stores have to be built to keep these pests out. Insecticides may have to be put into the stores to kill the insects in them. Agricultural assistants should be able to tell people how to build better food stores, and how to use insecticides. Farmers should ask them what to do so that this block in the food-path can be taken away.

*FOOD IS STORED FOR CHILDREN
NOT PESTS*

9.7 Trouble with transport.   In many rural areas there may be no roads to take food to town, or the roads may be bad. There may be too few lorries, or the drivers may drink in bars and crash their lorries. Lorries may break down, and there may be no lorries or spare parts with which to mend them. Transport is often worse between the villages and the food depots, than it is between the food depots and the town. A depot is a place where the food can be stored and from which it can be sold.

All these difficulties block the food-path for town children, because food has to be transported or carried from villages to towns.

9.8a Blocks in wholesaling and retailing. Wholesalers and retailers may make so much profit that food becomes too expensive for most women to buy. This is serious in the towns of Zambia. In Section 6.3 there is an example of the big profits that are made on the small dried fish that Zambians call *kapenta*.

9.8b Lack of jobs.   Let us now think about the money-path, and how blocks on it can harm nutrition. In Figure 9–1 the money-path is shown with arrows with lines on them. First of all money has to be earned; so this is the first step on the money-path. Then the family must decide how much money is to be spent on food, and how much on other things. Budgeting is thus the next step. Then the money for food must be spent in the best way; so the money-path is shown joining the food-path at the place called 'retailing and shopping'.

In towns the money-path is just as important as the food-path for good nutrition, because people have to have money to buy food. This means that in towns, where people cannot have big gardens in which to grow food, they have to have jobs from which they can earn money. In most African towns there are too few jobs for all the people who want them. Many people have no jobs and are said to be unemployed. **Unemployment** thus blocks the money-path right at the beginning. There are many reasons for unemployment in towns, but, as we shall see in Section 9.17, one of them is that the number of people in a country usually grows so quickly that it is impossible to provide paid jobs quickly enough for everyone to have one.

9.9 Bad budgeting.   Few families have all the money they want, so they must spend their money on the things they need most. Most important of all is enough of the right food. Only when enough of the right food has been bought can the money that is left be spent on such things as radios, bicycles and smart clothes. As we have seen in Section 6.8, planning to spend money wisely is called budgeting. Some families have so little money that it is almost impossible for them to budget well.

In many town families the husband does have a wage each month. It may not be much, but it is often enough to feed his family well on, if it is spent very cleverly. Many families find it difficult to budget carefully enough. They spend most of it as soon as they are paid, and by the middle of the month there is not enough left to buy food. Their children are thus badly fed and become malnourished. Many people do not know that good food is more important for health, especially for their children's health, than smart expensive clothes. Africa is a warm country, and clothes are not necessary for keeping people healthy. Some fathers buy cars without understanding that it will cost more money to run them than they earn. Many people spend more money on beer than on food.

The fathers of some malnourished children earn enough money to feed them well. Malnourished children have sometimes even been brought to a clinic in a Mercedes Benz motor car! These children have become malnourished because the family's money has been badly spent. It has been spent on a car and not on food.

In the rural areas people do not think of money as being used for buying food, because food is grown and does not have to be bought. Thus, when people come to town, they may not think that the most important use of money is to buy food, so we must do all we can to teach them. Thus, we have seen in Section 6.7 that a family needs about K20 each month with which to buy food, and that this does not include fuel. Yet some men, who may earn K50, only give their wives K10 or K15 with which to buy all the food and fuel for their family.

Bad budgeting blocks the money-path, and, if it is to be taken away, families must learn how to budget the money that is earned and spent each month. Careful budgeting is so important that an example is given in Section 6.8.

9.10 Bad shopping.   A family may budget well and put aside enough money for food. But a mother may not buy food in the cheapest way. She may buy food expensively in small amounts,

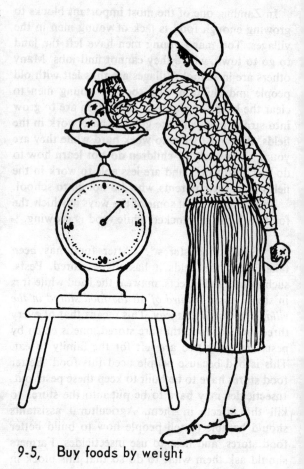

9-5,   Buy foods by weight

instead of buying it by weight in larger amounts. She may buy the expensive foods, such as biscuits, or go to expensive shops instead of to cheaper ones. The expensive shops are often the ones near her home, and a mother may have to walk further to get cheaper food. If she walks to the cheaper shops she will be able to feed her family better. As we have seen in Section 6.3, if a mother buys by weight in larger amounts, she will be able to feed her family better for the same money.

9.11 Alcohol.   When people drink much beer they get drunk. They get drunk because the beer contains something called alcohol. There is even more alcohol in strong drinks, in spirits like gin, or in the drink that they call *kachasu* in Malawi.

Alcohol blocks the food-path in many places and causes a lot of malnutrition. Farmers may be drunk when they should be clearing the bush for planting food. Food, such as millet, may be made into beer when it should be made into a child's porridge. Drunken drivers may smash the lorries that could take food to town. Very many Zambian fathers spend so much money on beer that there is not enough left to buy the food their children need. Some fathers start drinking at 6 a.m. They may lose their jobs and so cannot feed their families. Children may not be fed at all during a long beer-drink. Last of all, children are often

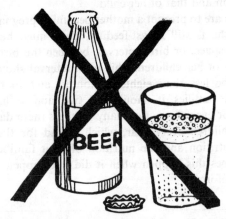

9-6, Alcohol blocks the food-path

given beer when their mothers are drinking. They go to sleep and stop crying for food, even though they are hungry. For all these reasons alcohol is one of the most important causes of malnutrition in many places. It is as if the food-path were washed away in a river of beer!

IN ZAMBIA ALCOHOL IS ONE OF THE MOST IMPORTANT BLOCKS IN THE FOOD PATH

Even so, beer drinking is not altogether bad. People will often work together in the fields if they know that there is going to be beer to drink afterwards. Sometimes they will not even start to work unless they have seen the beer first! Many people say that beer drinking is the only thing they have to do when they are not working, and that it is the best way of making friends and forgetting their troubles. We cannot stop beer drinking even if

we wanted to, although it might help if there were more things to do in the evening. All that we can do is to try to teach people not to drink so much beer so often, and that this is bad for their work, their own nutrition and the nutrition of their families.

9.12 Prestige. Things with prestige are things that people want, because to have them makes other people think you are rich, clever or modern. Big cars give their owners prestige, so do smart suits or a radio. It is also often thought more modern and rich to eat expensive foods like bread or rice, rather than cheaper foods like maize, or to drink bottled beer instead of African beer. Many mothers think it gives them more prestige to bottle-feed their children, instead of breast-feeding them.

Some foods have more prestige than others. Bread often has more prestige than *nshima*, and the larger kinds of dried fish have more prestige than smaller dried fish called *kapenta*. Cassava leaves and the green leaves of the bush, such as the pumpkin leaves the Bemba call *chibwabwa*, have no prestige. Some foods have so little prestige that people may tell you that they don't eat them, when really they do. Mice, snails, caterpillars and flying ants may be like this. These are good foods, and people should go on eating them. In the poem on the inside front cover of this book you read how the mother of the house kept a pocket (bag) of dried white ants to feed her family. This mother did well, however little prestige white ants may have. The prestige of a food does not matter so much as the nutrients in a food, and how cheap it is.

9.13 Bottle-feeding. The most important food-path for a young child is the one from his mother's breast. This is often blocked by bottle-feeding which is badly done. This is such a serious block in the food-path that the whole of Chapter 8 is about bottle-feeding.

9.14 Advertising. Some people make money by selling feeding bottles, tinned milk for bottle-feeding, beer and fizzy drinks. They try to make other people buy these things by putting up posters about them, or talking about them on the radio.

This is called advertising. Much advertising is bad for nutrition, especially the advertising for bottle-feeding. The advertisers of bottle-feeding try to block the most important food-path of all for the young child, even if it is the shortest. They try to block the path that milk takes from a mother to her child.

9.15 Lack of fuel.   Most food has to be cooked. Cooking needs fuel such as wood, charcoal, or paraffin. Wood has often to be carried from far away, and paraffin and charcoal cost scarce money. One of the reasons why many families cook only once a day is that they do not have enough fuel. This is a pity, because young children need porridge at least three times a day. Thus, lack of fuel blocks the food-path and helps to cause malnutrition.

9.16 Broken families.   When a father and mother leave one another (become divorced), their children often become malnourished. When this happens a town mother has nobody to earn money to feed the family, and a village mother has nobody to help her grow food in the fields. Children may also become malnourished when mothers have no home of their own, and have to stay with their relatives. This is probably because they do not get a large enough share of the food that is cooked for everyone, and it may be that the children of visiting relatives are the last people in the house to be fed. Children are often malnourished when their father has no job, or if their mother is not married. The children of families who have just come to town may also suffer from malnutrition. This is because there are not enough jobs for everybody to get one, and especially to get one soon. There may not be enough land for a good garden, and a garden takes some time to grow. It may also be a long way from the house.

*THE CHILD FROM A BROKEN HOME IS
OFTEN MALNOURISHED*

9.17a Children coming too close together.   You will remember that in Chapter 7 we saw how a child needs his mother's milk until he is eighteen months or two years old. Anything which stops

him getting this milk is bad for his nutrition. One of the things that may stop him getting this milk is his mother becoming pregnant again. Although it is quite safe for a pregnant mother to go on breast-feeding her child, she makes less milk, and many mothers do not want to breast-feed. Besides, a mother's own nutrition may be harmed when she has two people to feed besides herself— one at her breast, and another in her womb. Thus it is bad for a mother to become pregnant while she is still breast-feeding. It is bad for her own nutrition and that of her child.

If we are to prevent a mother becoming pregnant while she is still breast-feeding, there must be a proper space, or birth interval, between the births of each of her children. This birth interval should never be less than eighteen months, and in the poorest families it should be two and a half years, or even three. But many mothers these days have children every year, which is bad for their own nutrition and the nutrition of their families. Why does this happen when it did not happen so often before?

*A SHORT BIRTH INTERVAL BLOCKS
THE FOOD-PATH*

In the old days in Zambia, and in many other countries, proper child spacing was thought important. People thought it bad for a woman to have a child every year. After she had had her first baby she was helped to space her children by tying special 'medicine' round her body. Sometimes she was given a string and told to tie a knot in it at the end of every week, starting with the week at the end of her period. She was told to 'jump the third knot', either by going on a visit herself, or by sending her husband out hunting. In these, and other ways, mothers spaced their children in the old days so that there was a proper birth interval. These ways used to work quite well, because the man was also taught what he should do.

But the old ways are changing. Women are not taught these things as they used to be. Besides, men seldom have more than one wife, as they often used to. The result is that children are not so

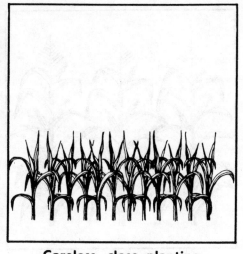
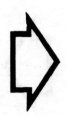
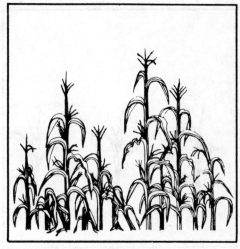

Careless, close planting   **A bad harvest**

well spaced as they once were, which helps to cause malnutrition.

What can we do? Fortunately, many new and much better ways have been found by which parents can have children only when they want to. These good new ways are called **family planning**, and people should be able to get them at every hospital and health centre. They are described in Section 11.22. Family planning means stopping children being conceived (coming alive in the womb) unless the parents wish.

9.17b Too many children. We have just seen that children coming too close together—too

short a birth interval—is bad for nutrition. Too many children in a family can also be bad for the nutrition of that family and of the country.

It is easy to see that children will be malnourished if there are too many of them, and not enough money to buy food. But having too many children is tied to many other blocks in the food-path, besides lack of food for them. Having too many children is closely tied to lack of jobs. As we have just seen, this is a serious block in the food path. Let us say, for example, that a man and his wife have seven children, that two of them die and that five of them grow up to have children of their own. This means that, whereas there are two parents

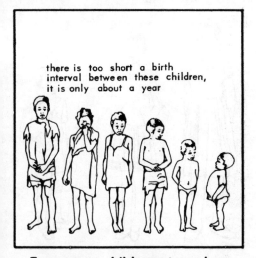
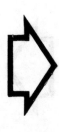
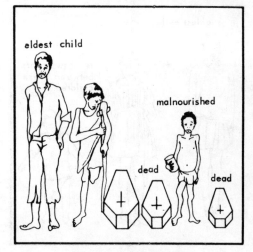

Too many children, too close   **A wrecked family**

9 - 8, Plan your family

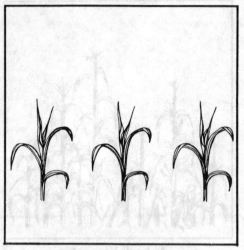 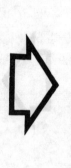 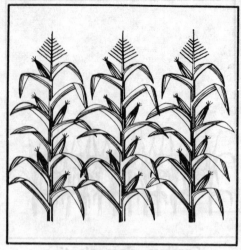

Careful planting   **A rich harvest**

now, there are going to be five living children, or more than twice as many children as there are parents. When these children marry and each of them has five living children in their turn, there will be more than six times as many grandchildren as there were grandparents. When most parents have as many children and grandchildren as this, the number of people in a country grows very fast. This is happening in many countries of Africa, which now double the number of their people about every 25 years. Thus, if a country has four million people now, it will have eight million in 25 years' time.

When a country grows as fast as this, it is difficult to build schools, hospitals and clinics fast enough, or to build enough factories and offices to give people paid jobs. For every job that is made in an office or factory, or on a good farm with tractors and machines, at least K5,000 has to be spent to give the worker a place in which to work and the tools and machines he needs. Most governments do not have enough money to provide these kinds of jobs fast enough. This means that many people cannot find paid jobs. They can, of course, stay in the rural areas or go back to work there, but many of them do not want to do this. So towns grow fast, and there are too few schools, jobs, clinics and houses. People have to have somewhere to live, so they build houses for them-

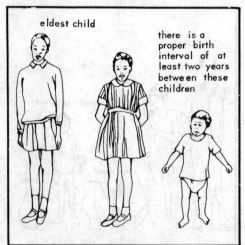 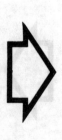 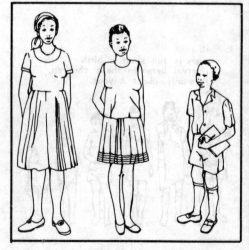

eldest child

there is a proper birth interval of at least two years between these children

Spaced children   **A happy family**

9 - 8, Plan your family (continued)

selves in the shanty-towns. They have to have something to eat, even if they have no job, so they eat the food of their relatives, or sometimes become thieves. The food-path for their relatives is blocked, and if food is stolen from the fields, people may not trouble to plant it.

Many parts of Africa have much land and few people, so it is often thought good for the number of people to grow fast and quickly fill up the empty bush. This might be right if people stayed in the bush, and if they did not come to the shanty-towns and want paid jobs. It might also be right if they did not want schools, roads, hospitals and clinics. But everyone wants these things. It is therefore important that the number of people in a country should grow more slowly, so that each person can have the job, school and clinic that he needs. Family planning helps the numbers of people in a country to grow more slowly, because it allows there to be a longer time between one child and the next, and families can be smaller.

The number of people in a country must stop growing some time because in the end there would be so many people that there would not be enough room for each of them to sit down! The number of people must stop growing long before this, and there must be a right, or best, number of people for a country. This is the number that will give each person the best life. It is difficult to know what this number is, *and family planning does not stop it being any less than it should be.* Family planning does, however, make it possible for the best number of people in a country to be reached *more slowly than at present.* Let us put it in another way. It is not the total number of people in a country that stops them having a good life. This can, in time, be large. *What does matter is that the rate (speed) of growth must not be too fast.*

If only the number of people in a country could grow more slowly, each person could have a better life. He would have more chance of a place in school, a paid job, or a bed in hospital when he was ill. Several blocks in the food-path would be removed, and his nutrition would be better. This is one reason why family planning is *so* important, and why every clinic should be able to tell mothers and fathers about it. In the old days it used to be

necessary for families to have many children, because so many of them died. But already more are living, and as we prevent malnutrition even more will live. If each of those who live is to have a better life, and especially a place in school and a job, fewer children must be born and the number of people in a country must grow more slowly.

9.18 Unfair shares of food.   A mother may grow or buy enough food and she may cook it well. But her younger children may still become malnourished because they do not get their share of the family's food. A young child needs a lot of food for his size; he eats so slowly that the rest of the family, especially any 'relatives' or 'lodgers', may have eaten everything before he has had enough. In many families it is the father who gets the biggest share of the food, especially the protein. As we have seen, meals like this may be a competition to see who can eat the fastest. The youngest child always loses this competition and thus does not get enough to eat.

This is an important block in the food-path, even in families who buy and cook plenty of food. You read how young children should have a plate to themselves, how their food should be mixed, and how they should be helped to feed themselves with a spoon. By doing these things one of the last blocks in the food-path can be taken away.

9.19 Mothers not knowing the best way to feed their young children.   Many mothers do not know the best way to feed their children. They may not give their children porridge until they are seven or eight months old, and do not know that children should start eating porridge at the age of four months. They may not add any protein food, such as groundnuts, to the porridge. They may only feed them once or twice a day, and do not know how important it is to feed them three or four times a day. There are several reasons why mothers do these things. One of them is that they do what is their custom, and do not know that there is any better way of feeding children. This block in the food-path can be removed by teaching mothers to feed their children better.

9.20   Diseases which waste food and stop the body using it.   A child may be ill with measles, whooping cough, diarrhoea, worms or other diseases. His illnesses may make him not want to eat, and because he does not eat he becomes malnourished. Measles is a good example, because it makes a child's mouth so sore that it is painful for him to eat. If a child has diarrhoea, the food that he has eaten may go out of his body again in his stools. If he has worms, they may eat some of the food he has eaten and stop him getting it. Diseases like these are therefore the very last of all the blocks in the food-path, and they have to be removed. Children can be given special medicines called vaccines to stop them getting measles. Children do not get worms or diarrhoea if they live in a clean place, where people use pit latrines, and are given clean food and clean water.

MORE ABOUT THE BLOCKS ON THE FOOD-PATH

9.21   Tied together like a spider's web.   *Many of the blocks in the food-path are tied to one another.* Bottle-feeding and the wish to have prestige are closely tied together. Custom is tied to many blocks in the food-path, such as beer drinking, the way the fields are planted, and how children are fed. Lack of knowledge is tied to bad budgeting as well as to the wrong ways of feeding children. Diseases both stop people working hard and stop children eating. From these examples you can see that blocks in the food-path are tied to one another in many ways. It is as if they were tied together like the threads of a spider's web.

9.22   Many blocks at the same time.   *The food-path is usually blocked in several places at once.* Sometimes one block is the main cause of malnutrition, sometimes it is another. In one place one year insects may destroy the crops, block the food-path and cause malnutrition. In another place, or in another year, heavy rains at the wrong time spoil the crops. Sometimes drought (lack of rain) blocks the food-path. Occasionally, war blocks the food-path very seriously indeed. Usually, there are several blocks at the same time. In Lusaka in

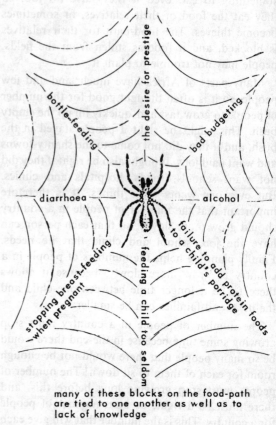

many of these blocks on the food-path are tied to one another as well as to lack of knowledge

9 - 9,   Tied together like a spider's web

1970, for example, malnutrition was partly due to too little of the right foods being grown, partly due to the big profits made by wholesalers and retailers, and partly due to mothers not knowing the best ways of feeding their children. Fathers without jobs, too much beer drinking, and bad bottle-feeding are further blocks on the food-path, which also help to cause malnutrition. Towards the end of 1970 the very bad harvest in the previous year became a very serious block in the food-path. The harvest was one of the worst there had ever been, partly because of lack of rain, and partly because many of the big maize farmers had left the country. Much maize had to be bought from other countries, but there was still a great shortage in the rural areas. Each time and each place thus has its own special mixture of blocks.

MOST MALNUTRITION IS THE RESULT OF SEVERAL BLOCKS IN THE FOOD-PATH

9.23 Many things block the food-path for some children. Just as malnutrition in the community may be caused by many blocks in the food-path working together, so also many things may combine to block the food-path of a particular child. Here, for example, is the true story of how one child in Lusaka came to be very malnourished. He was found at home because his family did not think him ill enough to take him to a clinic.

David was exactly two years old. He weighed 8.3 kg and had an arm circumference of 12.5 cm (a well-nourished child of this age weighs 12.5 kg, and has an arm circumference of about 16 cm). He did not look too malnourished until he stood next to a well-nourished child of the same age, when he was seen to be much shorter than he should be. His arms were thin, his head looked too big for the size of his body, and his stomach was swollen. Some of the hairs on his head were pale. His skin was a little pale, and his legs were thin, but not swollen. He looked sad and spent most of the time sitting quietly in someone's lap, and not playing.

His mother was away out of town looking after her mother who was sick in the village; so he was being looked after by his great-grandmother, a very old lady who was nearly blind. David's great-grandmother did not think he was ill, but she was worried because he was not eating well, and she tried to feed him extra bits of bread and *nshima* between meals.

David had one elder brother, Joseph, who seemed quite well nourished, and a younger sister, Joyce, aged three months, who had gone to the village with her mother. As soon as David's mother had become pregnant with Joyce, she had stopped breast-feeding him. She had tried to bottle-feed him, but his great-grandmother said that he had only been bottle-fed for three days.

David's father had left his mother, who was trying to get a divorce. The family were living with David's uncle, a retail vegetable seller, who was very often drunk. He gave the family K3 each month for maize meal, but almost no other money. When the family were visited, the uncle was away, and the great-grandmother had no money. They lived in a small two-roomed mud house without windows in a shanty-town. The family had two pots, a small table, two chairs, a broom, an empty fizzy drink bottle and almost nothing else. There was no fuel in the house. The hot season was beginning and the wells in the shanty-town were starting to run dry, so water had to be carried for over a mile.

Great-grandmother said she gave David bread and tea in the morning, and porridge twice a day. Sometimes they had a relish of green leaves, and although he sometimes had fizzy drinks, he never had relish of meat, milk, eggs, fish, beans or groundnuts.

David had never been to the under-fives clinic, even though it was only two kilometres away, and a doctor had told his mother to take him there. David's mother had said she thought it was too far to walk.

We see from this that David was very much underweight for his age. Although his hair was that of kwashiorkor, and he was sad and did not run about, his skin was healthy and he had no swelling of his legs. He was not thin enough to be a real case of marasmus. He was thus a very underweight child who was showing the beginnings of kwashiorkor, and who might get it properly at any time, especially if he got measles. Many things were blocking his food-path. His parents were divorced, the family were staying with relatives, the worker of the family had not got a good job, and often got drunk with money that should have been spent on food. His mother was away in the village and he was being looked after by an old blind, great-grandmother, who could not feed him well. His mother had stopped breast-feeding him when he was only a year old, because she had become pregnant again. He was not fed often enough, no protein was added to his porridge, he did not have a plate of his own, and he was not helped to feed himself with a spoon. There were thus very many blocks on his food-path.

The most dangerous time for malnutrition in many communities is during a child's second year. That is between his first and second birthdays. You can see from the story of this child how many things can block his food-path at this age. Breast-feeding is ending, he is not big enough to eat like the older people in the family, and yet he needs much protein and many joules for his size.

If you are a health worker, you will see many malnourished children. Whenever you see a child with kwashiorkor, or marasmus, or even an underweight child, try to find out *why* he is malnourished —what are the blocks on *his* food-path? The diagnosis of a malnourished child is not complete until the blocks on his food-path have been looked for and listed.

WHENEVER YOU SEE A MALNOURISHED CHILD LOOK FOR THE BLOCKS ON HIS FOOD-PATH

9.24 Health education can remove many blocks. We have now made a long list of blocks on the food-path. When we look at them we see that many of them are due to *people doing things in the wrong way for good health*. Another way of saying this is that people *behave in the wrong way for good health*.

We must be careful about using the word 'wrong'. It has different meanings, and they are important. Some of the things that we say are wrong are those that most people say ought not to be done, like stealing. Most of the blocks in the food-path are not like this. People are doing what they think of as the 'right' thing. They may be doing things that most people do in their tribe and country, such as feeding children plain porridge. Also, when women stop breast-feeding when they get pregnant, they may be doing the right thing for their custom. We can say it is wrong because we have found that it is bad for the health of children. We should not therefore blame women for doing these things, even though we try to teach them differently.

Other blocks are due to people doing new things that everyone else is doing, such as drinking bottled beer or feeding children from bottles. Someone may have told them that these things are good, and it even says on the outside of many milk tins how good the milk is for bottle-feeding babies!

Many of the blocks in the food-path are examples of behaving in the wrong way for the health of the family, even though many of the ways seem 'right' to the people who do them. These blocks can be removed, if we can persuade people to change their behaviour, and to do the right thing for their own health and that of their families. This is called **nutrition education,** and it is the most important way of fighting malnutrition.

HEALTH EDUCATION IS USUALLY THE BEST WAY OF IMPROVING NUTRITION

Nutrition education is only part of the much bigger subject of **health education,** which tries to prevent diseases of many kinds by persuading people to change their behaviour. Health education also tries, for example, to prevent death on the roads by getting people to change their behaviour by fastening their safety belts, and not driving while they are drunk. Agricultural and nutrition education often try to do the same things. For example, when we teach a farmer how to grow better groundnuts and eat more of them, we are teaching him both better agriculture and better health at the same time. Health education, especially nutrition education, is of such great importance that it is why much of this book, especially the next chapter, has been written.

We have now thought about the many things that block the food-path in the community, and how several of them can join together to cause malnutrition in a particular child. We have also seen that many blocks in the food-path can be removed by nutrition education. Now we can put together much of what we have learnt to make the community diagnosis.

THE COMMUNITY DIAGNOSIS

9.25 How much malnutrition is there? What are the blocks in the food-path?   In Section 1.5 you learnt how we could find out *how much malnutrition there is in a community*. One way to find this out is to weigh many children under five years old, and to see how many of them come below the lower line on the road-to-health chart. Another way is to find out how many children between the ages of one and five years have an arm circumference of less than 14 cm. These are only very simple ways of measuring the malnutrition in a community, but they are useful ones.

If we find that a community has many malnourished children, the next thing to find out is *why they are malnourished*. When a sick person comes to see a doctor, the doctor talks to the patient, looks at him, and then does various tests. He first tries to find out how sick the patient is, and then why he is sick. This is called making a diagnosis. When we find how much malnutrition there is in a community, and then why there is malnutrition, we can say we are making the **community diagnosis of malnutrition.**

The amount of malnutrition in one district differs from that in another, and it may change from one year to another. In the same way the blocks in the food-path will differ from district to district, and from year to year. *The community diagnosis of malnutrition will thus be different at different times and in different places.* For example, it will be different in Dar es Salaam in Tanzania, in Serowe in Botswana, and in the Namitambo district of Malawi. In all these places it is likely to differ in 1977 from what it was in 1972.

It is quite easy to find out how much malnutrition there is in a community. It is also not difficult to give a list of the things which are causing it (the blocks in the food-path, as we have called them), and to say how bad we think each one is. It is however very difficult to *measure* exactly how serious each block is, and we shall not try to do it here. Even so, we can make a very useful community diagnosis of malnutrition by finding out how much malnutrition there is, and then thinking about important blocks in the food-path for the district in which we live.

You can now start to make the community diagnosis of malnutrition in the district in which you live. If you think carefully, you will probably find that you already know many of the things that you need to know. You will know if lack of rain is a problem in your district, or if the roads are bad. You can get help in making other parts of the community diagnosis by asking special questions and looking for the answers.

Many of the questions needed for making the community diagnosis of malnutrition can only be found by visiting families in their homes. Some questions can only be answered by a doctor or medical assistant, or by visiting hospitals and health centres. Other questions can be answered by the agricultural department. You can find out how much malnutrition there is in a community by doing a nutrition survey as it is described in Section 1.6.

9.26 Questioning the family.   Before you do this, you must choose which families to visit. A community is made of many families, and each one will be different. Some may be very poor, and some not so poor. In some all the children will have died, and in others they will all be alive. If you just go from any house to any other house, you may choose the richest houses, or those with the most children playing outside them. Because you notice these houses more easily, you will not choose the houses fairly. The best thing to do is to visit every house, and if this is not possible then to *give each house an equal chance of being chosen.* The best ways of doing this are rather difficult, but quite a good way is to visit, say, every fifth or every tenth house in the village.

Start by visiting the chief or headman of the village, and telling him who you are and what you want to do. When he understands why you have come, he will probably let you visit the families in his village. The next thing to do is to *observe*, which is only another way of saying 'look carefully'. Look around and notice all you can about what anyone is doing that may have anything to do with the food-paths. Are the gardens good or bad? What is in the food stores? Are people drinking or working? What do you see when you get inside a house? How much food is there? What cooking pots are used? If any of the family are eating, who is eating, and how are they eating? If you look carefully you will soon learn a lot about the food-paths and what is happening to them. Remember, when you see something happening you *know* it is happening. When you ask someone a question, the answer may or may not be true.

After looking, the next thing to do is to talk to people and ask questions. Asking questions in this way is called 'holding an interview'. There are very many things that you may want to know, and later on in this section you will read many questions that can be asked. You cannot ask everybody all the questions at one time. How many questions you can ask will depend on how much time you can spend, and you will probably have to choose to ask only a few of the more important questions. It may perhaps be possible to ask some of the other questions later on at another visit, or to ask different families different questions. Make a list of the questions that you want to ask, write down the answers the people give, and make notes on what you see. When you are asking questions try to make a conversation out of them instead of just a list of questions. This will be more interesting for the families you visit, and you may get better answers.

It is not easy to get true answers; so if you are not sure an answer is right, try asking it later in a different way. Perhaps, for example, you do not think that a mother is right when she says she feeds her child three times a day. Later on, ask her what times of day she feeds her child. If she does not give three different times, the answer to one of these questions must be wrong. Mothers may try to please you by telling you what they think you want to hear instead of what they really do. They may also not be able to give the right answers about the quantities of the things that they buy and use.

People do not like answering some questions. It may be difficult, for example, to get the right answers from them about how much money they have to spend, or about the children who have died. You have to be very careful when you ask these questions. It may be better to ask a mother how many children she has had, and then how many are still alive. If a woman does not want to answer questions, do not force her to give an answer, as she may just guess so as to get rid of you. Most women are pleased to talk to people who are interested in them and their children.

The questions in the list below tell us the kind of things that we need to know about the food-paths within a family. It will not be possible to use them exactly as they are, and you will have to change them to make them easier to use. You will, for example, have to ask separately about each child in the family.

Introducing yourself to the family. First of all tell the people in the house who you are, and why you have come. Tell them you are interested in the feeding of children, and would like to ask them a few questions. Make people feel that you have come to learn about their difficulties and not to criticize. Try to see that everyone sits down during the interview.

Take the name of the head of the house and the address of the house if it has one. Ask who lives in the house, how they are related, and what jobs people do.

Some general questions about food. Where does the family get its food from? How much is bought, grown, picked from the bush or fished from rivers? What sorts of food are eaten and how often? What kind of meals do the family eat during the day? Do people eat together or separately? How many people in the house are eating from the same pot? How much is cooked for them all? How does the food they get differ at different times of the month, and at different times of the year? What food have the family eaten in the last twenty-four hours? Many people can remember this far back. Few can remember any further. What visitors or relatives are living in the house? What do they eat and how are they given it? How much alcohol is drunk? When is it drunk, and by whom?

The children. What are the ages of the children? How many children has the mother had? How many are alive? How old were those who died? What diseases caused them to die? When was each child given his first porridge? Is any protein food added to this porridge? Is milk ever given to children? Are any children bottle-fed? How is the feeding bottle washed and sterilized? What is put into the feeding bottle? Have the children got road-to-health charts? Are they on the road to health, or below it? How much do the younger children weigh? What is the arm circumference of the children between the ages of one and five? Weighing children and measuring their arm circumference are not usually part of an interview, but they are useful things to do when you are interested in the nutrition of a family.

How do the family eat their evening meal? What meals do the children have each day? How often are they fed? What do they eat? Do the parents and children eat together? If the family does not eat together, how much of each food is put on the husband's plate, and how much is left for the rest of the family? Do the younger children have a plate to themselves? Who helps to feed the younger children? Do they use spoons, or do they try to eat relish with their fingers? Are the porridge and relish mixed together for them? These questions are important, so try hard to find out how much food a young child gets each day, and how he is fed. One way to find this out is to ask a mother what she fed her young child on yesterday. *Best of all, try to see young children eating.* You will then see what happens for yourself.

How far do children have to walk to school? Do they have breakfast before they go? Do they get any food in the middle of the day?

LEARN FROM FAMILIES BEFORE YOU TRY TO TEACH THEM

What are the local names for kwashiorkor and marasmus? If there are local names, what does the mother think caused them?

Some important customs. Are children sent away to stay with relatives, such as a grandmother? How do these relatives feed them? What do people believe about breast-feeding and the time a child should be taken from his mother's breast?

Are there any foods that a pregnant mother should or should not eat? Are there any foods that children should not eat? Are women free to try new methods of looking after children, or do they have to ask their husbands or some other member of the family before making any changes?

What new ways of eating and cooking has a mother learned in the last year? Where has she learned them? To whom does she go for help and knowledge when she needs it?

Cooking, fuel and water. How does the family cook? What local recipes are there? A recipe is a way of cooking something to eat. What cooking pots are used? Is there a pestle and mortar or a sieve in the house? What fuel is used? How is it bought? What does it cost? Where does the water come from? Who carries it?

Mainly for people in towns—the buyers of food. How much money does the husband earn? Many husbands do not tell their wives this, and you may have to try to see the husband himself. How much money does the husband give his wife to buy food? Many women find it difficult to answer these questions, so it may be better to put them late in the interview, when she knows you a little better, and is more used to answering questions. You may not get answers to these questions, and may have to guess from the husband's job how much he earns, or guess from the look of the house whether they are rich or poor.

Who buys each kind of food? You have already asked how many children there are in the family. Now you will be able to work out how much money is spent on food for each person. How does this compare with what you found in Sections 6.7 and 6.8? Does the money last all the month, or does it run out in the third or fourth week? Do families get 'credits' or 'balances'? Do they pay extra for these? People are often very shy about answering this.

Are large or small quantities of food bought each time? Does the mother understand buying by weight and volume? Does she know what is meant by grams and kilograms, or pounds and ounces, or litres and pints?

If the family is in a town, do relatives bring in any food from the country? Does the wife have a garden? What do they grow in it?

Mainly for villagers—the growers of food. Have the family got a garden? How big is it? What foods do they grow? How much was grown— last year for instance? Who works on the garden and at which times of the year? How long do they work for? Which members of the family do the various jobs in the garden? Who clears new land for planting? Have the crops had any diseases? If they grow cassava, how big are their cassava gardens? Are they digging up their cassava when the gardens are one or two years old, or are they able to leave it until the roots have got bigger when the garden is three or four years old?

What foods are got from the bush?

Have the family any cattle, pigs, goats, pigeons or hens? When are they killed? Who eats them? How many eggs do the chickens lay? What happens to these eggs? Are the cattle and goats milked? Have the animals had any diseases?

What foods are sold? How much food is sold and how much is kept for eating?

How are foods stored? Do rats or insects eat any of the foods while they are stored?

What do the family think they need? These are sometimes called the family's 'felt needs', and it is important to ask for them. You may find that the children of the family are malnourished, and yet a mother may not say that she wants more food for her children, because it is not one of her 'felt needs'.

Giving the family a chance to ask questions. When you have asked the questions you wanted to, it is only fair to give the people you have been talking to a chance to ask you some questions. Many mothers are very keen to know how they can feed their children better. You may be able to tell them from what you have read in this book.

Last of all, when you leave, do not forget to thank the family and say that you look forward to seeing them again. More is said about visiting families in Section 9.30b.

THANK THE PEOPLE WHO ANSWER YOUR QUESTIONS

9.27 Questioning the agricultural department. Many of the blocks in the food-path concern the agricultural department; so see if they can answer

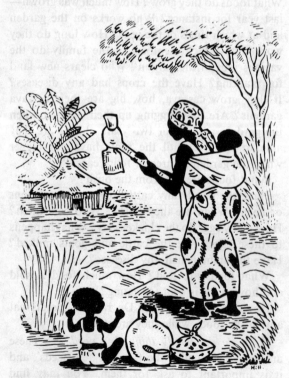

9 - 10, Have the family got a garden?

these questions. These are only some of the questions that need to be asked and answered. From what you have already read, you will easily be able to think of many more. An agricultural assistant, or agricultural officer, may be able to give you the answers to them.

Is enough land being cultivated?
Are people growing the right crops?
Are people growing the best varieties of crops?
Are fertilizers being used in the right way?
Are insecticides being used in the right way?
Are the fields and gardens being dug and planted as they should be?

9.28 Questioning the medical department. A doctor, a nurse or a medical assistant may be able to tell you the answers to some or all of these questions. You may already have found the answers to some of them in Sections 1.5 and 1.6.

About how many children died partly or wholly as a result of malnutrition last year?

How common is kwashiorkor in the area?

How many cases were seen in the hospital or health centre last year?

How common is marasmus in the area?

How many cases were seen in the hospital or health centre last year?

How common is marasmic kwashiorkor?

How many cases were seen in the hospital or health centre last year?

Remember that children may die without going to the hospital, and that many underweight children do not go to under-fives clinics. You may be able to find out more than the hospital knows by visiting people at home and weighing children.

How many underweight children are there? By this we mean how many children are there below the lower line on the road-to-health chart. How many one- to five-year-old children are there with an arm circumference of less than 14 cm? If you have not already done so, can you find this out? See Sections 1.5 and 1.6.

What diseases are there in the district that make malnutrition worse or are made worse by malnutrition? See Section 2.3.

9.29 Making the community diagnosis of malnutrition. We have already seen that it is not too difficult to measure how much malnutrition there is in a community, but that it may be very difficult to measure how serious each of the blocks in the food-path is. You will have been able to measure some things, such as the percentage of underweight children in a village. If you have visited many families (say more than 20) you will be able to count how many of them do such things as using feeding bottles, or how many of them run out of groundnuts before next year's harvest, or how many of them eat cassava only instead of maize. Always try to measure things when you can. But there will be many things that you cannot measure, such as how difficult transport is, or how bad the roads are. All you will be able to say is roughly how important they seem to be, and whether one is more important than another. Put a '+' in pencil opposite the blocks which you think are important in the place where you work. If necessary, put in more than one '+', like this:

Block of no importance   0
Block may or may not be important,
  don't know   ±
Block is there but of little importance   +
Block quite important   ++
Block very important   +++
Block so important that it is the
  only one which really matters   ++++

TABLE 21
The Community Diagnosis of Malnutrition

Place.. Date ....

THERE IS THIS MUCH MALNUTRITION IN THE COMMUNITY
........................% of children in the district are below the road to health.
........................% of one- to five-year-old children have an arm circumference of less than 14 cm.
.... children died of malnutrition in the hospital last year.
Kwashiorkor is not seen/uncommon/quite common/very common. There were .... cases of kwashiorkor in the hospital or health centre last year.
Marasmus is not seen/uncommon/quite common/very common. There were .... cases of marasmus in the hospital or health centre last year.
Marasmic kwashiorkor is not seen/uncommon/quite common /very common. There were .... cases of marasmic kwashiorkor in the hospital or health centre last year.
  You may not be able to get figures of the different kinds of malnutrition, and it may be necessary to put them all together as 'malnourished children'.

THESE BLOCKS IN THE FOOD-PATH CAUSE MALNUTRITION

Block in the food-path	The importance of the block	Removal possible by health education	Removal by health education easy or difficult
People too sick to work hard			
Too many people and not enough land			
Men not working enough in the fields			
Not enough land cleared for planting			
Soil erosion			
The wrong crops grown			
The wrong varieties of crops grown			
Fields dug and planted in the wrong way			
Fertilizer not used			
Insecticide not used			
Not enough men in the villages to work			
Drought			
Plant and animal diseases			
Other kinds of farming which could be done better			
Insects spoiling the food stores			
Rats and mice spoiling the food stores			
Not enough roads			
Not enough transport			
Not enough markets			
Too large profits by wholesalers and retailers			
Bad budgeting			
Wasteful shopping			
Bottle-feeding			
Advertising the wrong food and drink			
Lack of fuel			
Broken families			

Families too large for one wage earner to feed

....

Birth interval commonly too short

....

Not enough jobs

....

Unfair shares of food

....

Mothers not knowing the best ways of feeding their young children

....

Customs block the food-path in these ways

....

....

....

Alcohol blocks the food-path in these ways

....

....

These diseases are seen that make malnutrition worse

....

....

The food-path is blocked in these other ways

....

....

....

It may help you to complete the community diagnosis of malnutrition in your district if you make a list of what you think are the most important blocks in the food-path.

The ten most important blocks in the food-path in the .... district are as follows:

1. ....

2. ....

3. ....

4. ....

5. ....

6. ....

7. ....

8. ....

9. ....

10. ....

In this chapter we have been studying why there is malnutrition in a community. What we have really been studying is what is called the **ecology** of malnutrition. The ecology of something is the study of how it fits into, and is related to, the rest of what goes on in a community.

After doctors have diagnosed patients, they try to cure them. Now that we have made the community diagnosis for our district, we can think first of how the family and then of how the community can cure themselves. This is what the last two chapters are about.

9.30   THINGS TO DO

(a) How many blocks can you find in the food-path? If you visit families carefully and go and see them often, you will soon get stories like that of David in Section 9.23. These can either be read out in class or handed round on a duplicated sheet, and the class asked to list all the blocks on the food-path that they can find. They can then discuss what they might do about them. Here is a story that will do as an example—but it is much better to find your own.

Hariet was the first child of the second wife of a night-watchman living in a Lusaka shanty-town and earning K48 a month. When she was first seen she was 17 months old, weighed 7.9 kg and had an arm circumference of 12.8 cm.

Earlier on Hariet's father had lived in the village, where he had had two wives, the first of whom he had divorced after three of her children had died before they were a year old. After two years in town, he had sent for his second wife and Hariet, who was then 16 months old.

Hariet had never been a healthy child. She had had measles at the age of 10 months and had had diarrhoea most of the time ever since. First, a *nganga* had tried to cure her by making cuts on her chest, but this had not helped. (A *nganga* is often called 'a traditional practitioner'.) When she arrived in town her father had next taken her to a private doctor, who had given her injections as long as there was any money to pay for them, but these also had not cured her. She then went to the clinic, but the medicine that they gave her did not help either. Several people gave her mother advice. At the hospital near her home in the village, they had said that breast-feeding should stop, and Hariet had been given some dried skim milk. However, Hariet's mother neither gave her this milk nor did she stop breast-feeding, because she did not trust the hospital. So Hariet had continued breast-feeding and was said to be very hungry. She had her own plate of *nshima* and relish but no extra milk. Even though her father earried a good wage, her mother was only given about K15 to buy food, and the family had almost no money by the middle of the month, and for the last two weeks of it their relish was usually cabbage.

Meanwhile Hariet got worse; she became thinner, and, whereas she had been walking, she now stopped crawling and lay still. Her father decided that because the private doctor, the clinic and the hospital had failed, her mother must have 'witches in her breasts' and that her milk must be bad. He was determined that Hariet should stop breast-feeding and would feed from a bottle instead. So she was given a bottle, even though she could easily drink from a cup, and in fact usually drank unboiled well-water like this anyway. When the house was visited this bottle was seen to be full of dried lumps of milk and covered with flies. She was only given it once a day, and it usually contained only a single spoonful of milk powder. When the family were visited a week later Hariet had lost a whole kilogram, and her diarrhoea had come back. Meanwhile the clinic had given her more 'diarrhoea mixture', but this had not helped, nor had some more 2-kwacha injections given her by the private doctor. Her mother had given her some herbs (plants), but even these had made no difference.

Two weeks later Hariet had lost another half kilogram, and her arm circumference was now only 10.8 cm. She was obviously marasmic, and she still had diarrhoea. Her mother was therefore asked to buy some dried skim milk, and to add it to her porridge three times a day. When her mother said that she had no money and that her husband would not give her any, they were shown that it was cheaper than expensive injections. Fortunately they were told this on pay day, so her father was able to buy a kilo of dried skim milk and several times bought Hariet fresh milk.

Two weeks later Hariet was much better; she was gaining weight, her diarrhoea had stopped, she was crawling about once more, and was beginning to walk again. However, the milk soon finished, so did her father's money. Thus Hariet went back to eating porridge and cabbage, and her weight stayed the same. When she was visited a few months later she was gaining weight slowly on her old diet, without any extra milk. It seemed that the few weeks of extra protein food that she had been given had cured her diarrhoea, so that she could now absorb food properly and gain weight slowly *on her old diet.*

Besides showing many blocks in the food-path, this story also shows how important food can be in treating chronic diarrhoea in underweight children—see Section 7.20.

(b)   Visiting a community.   In Section 9.26 we saw that we could learn much about the nutrition of the people we wanted to help by visiting them in their homes. The home is so much the best place to learn many of the things we need to know that *everyone learning about nutrition must visit families in their homes.* Teachers sometimes think that this is difficult to arrange, and that families will not be pleased to see their students. This is not so. Arrangements are usually easy, and most families are pleased to talk to visitors, if they follow the rules in Section 9.26, and if the headman is told about the visit first.

Visits can be arranged in various ways. Sometimes students can walk from their school to the homes they want to visit. They can also go in a bus, or cycle, or borrow a hospital ambulance, or lorry. The whole class can go at once, divide themselves into pairs, spread themselves out around a village or township, and introduce themselves to the families they find. Two or three families can usually be visited in an afternoon. depending on how many questions are asked, Questions can be asked about everything to do with nutrition, or different pairs of students can ask about different parts of it, such as about children, customs, cooking, fuel and water, or about buying food and growing it. Ask students to list the questions they are going to ask before they start their visit.

Students can also visit families in their own time. They may perhaps decide to visit between them all the families in part of a village or township, and to write a joint report. The homes to be visited can also be chosen in various ways. Malnourished children can be found in a hospital, or under-fives clinic, and their homes visited. The homes of well- and badly-nourished children might be compared. If there are enough weighing scales, the children who are visited can be weighed—see Section 12.3. The arm circumference of all one- to five-year-old children should always be measured—see Section 1.6b.

Home visiting does not end with the visit. If a whole class of students have been visiting families in a village, they should gather with their teacher and talk about what they have found before they have forgotten it. One subject should be discussed at a time, and the students asked what they have found in their families. If income, for example, is being discussed, various income groups can be written on the board, say less than K30 monthly, K31–40, K41–50, and so on, and a tally made of family income, in the same way that a tally was made of arm circumference in Figure 1–23. Students should be asked to write down what the class as a whole has found. They can also be asked to write essays on their visits.

Nurses who have to do a dissertation might find nutrition home visiting of this kind very useful, and if several of them do the same thing in different places, they will be able to compare what they find, and learn even more.

If possible families should be visited more than once. Are families doing any of the things that they were told about on their first visit? Learning about nutrition is not something that can be finished after one visit. It must go on all through the life of anyone who has anything to do with nutrition.

(c) Visiting a malnourished child. Visit the family of a malnourished child to find the various blocks in the food-path that have caused him to be malnourished. Each member of the class should try to write his own 'David story' or 'Hariet story' for at least one child in the way that these are described in Section 9.23.

(d) Making the community diagnosis. Make the community diagnosis of malnutrition as it is described in Section 9.29.

(e) An essay on food customs. Write an essay describing the food customs in your own family.

(f) A farming diary. Make a diary of the work that is done to grow food during each month of the year. Describe the jobs which are men's work, women's work and children's work.

(g) An exercise for a civics class. A good exercise for a civics class is to describe the blocks in the food-path, and then to discuss whose job it is to remove them. They should think about which government departments are concerned, which person in them is responsible for removing a particular block, and how he might do it. After thinking about what the government might do, the class should discuss what other people and organizations in the community could do.

(h) A nutrition play. Make and act a nutrition play to show some of the blocks in the food-path, and how they can be removed. Many classes greatly enjoy these plays—one of the best liked parts is that of the baby! Here is a play that one class acted.

> A father did not share his money with the family. He gave his children no school uniform and no money for food. He went to the bar, got drunk and was robbed. Meanwhile his wife was being taught by a nutrition worker how to care for her very small hungry child. The nutrition worker had learnt how to do this on a course like the one described in Section 11.2c. When the father understood the importance of what the nutrition worker had to say he promised not to waste his money again.

(i) Thinking about advertising. Let each student bring in an advertisement and discuss it in front of the class. What does the advertisement claim? Why do people buy the product? Do people need it? If it is a food, what do people feel is contained in it?

(j) Nutrition from the newspapers. During a nutrition course one of the students should collect from the newspapers all the cuttings that have anything to do with nutrition and report them to the class.

A missing block in the food-path—lack of love. One of our readers (Dr R. C. Braun) has pointed out that we have forgotten an important block in the food-path—lack of love (emotional deprivation). If a child is not loved, he is unhappy. If he is unhappy he does not eat, and if he does not eat he does not grow. If he is very unhappy he may eat so little that he dies. So, when we are looking for blocks in a child's food-path, we must not forget to ask if he is loved and wanted. Here is an example. A man had two wives who did not like one another. One wife died after giving birth to a baby boy, so he was given to the other wife who already had a six-month-old child of her own. The other wife seemed to be caring for the new baby and put him to her breasts first. But she did not love or want him, so he died.

Chapter Ten

HELPING FAMILIES TO
HELP THEMSELVES

10.1 The educational diagnosis. In the last chapter you made the community diagnosis of malnutrition for your district. You tried to measure *how much* malnutrition there was, and *why* there was malnutrition. You listed the 'whys' of malnutrition as blocks in the path that food takes from the fields where it is grown to the body of the child who needs it. You probably found many blocks, some of which were very important and some not so important. Our job now is to see how we can remove these blocks.

In Section 9.24 we saw that many of the blocks were due to people not doing things in the best way —they were due to people behaving in the wrong way for the good of their health. We saw also that these blocks might be removed, if only we could teach people to change their behaviour in a way that would make their own health and that of their families better. Trying to get people to change their behaviour in this way is called health education, which includes nutrition education. A list of the knowledge people lack, which prevents them improving their nutrition by changing their behaviour, is called the **educational diagnosis** of malnutrition. It is a list of the blocks on the food-path which could be removed by changing people's behaviour, and a measure of how serious each block is.

Turn back to Section 9.29 where you made your community diagnosis. On the right hand of your list of blocks you will see a column marked 'Removal possible by health education'. Go through each block and put a '+' opposite it if you think that health education might help to remove it. Put a '0' if you think that health education cannot help. Health education cannot, for example, remove the block caused by drought, but it might take away that caused by bad budgeting. You will probably find that health education

can play some part in the removal of most blocks. For example, mothers may not know that it is possible for them to have no more children than they want and can feed, and may need to be educated about family planning.

Some blocks are much more easily removed by health education than others. So, think carefully about the community you are studying, and fill in the third column in the community diagnosis in Section 9.29. Put 'easy' or 'difficult', or perhaps 'very difficult', against each of the blocks that might be removed by health education. You will need these ideas when you come to make your health education plan later in this chapter.

TEACHING IS USUALLY THE BEST WAY OF PREVENTING MALNUTRITION

Everyone must teach whenever they possibly can. Health education is of the greatest importance, and everyone who can must help. Medical assistants, dressers, nurses, midwives and sweepers must teach the patients who come to their clinics and health centres. Sweepers may not be able to read this book, so medical assistants may first have to teach them. School teachers must teach their pupils. Community development and homecraft workers must teach the mothers who come to women's clubs. Agricultural workers must teach farmers both how to grow more food, and how to feed their children. Priests must teach the people who come to their churches.

Teaching is also very important in hospitals. This is just one good reason why the mother of a malnourished child must come into hospital with him. She must be taught by the hospital staff as a very important part of their treatment of the child. *The mother of every malnourished child must leave* hospital knowing how she should feed him. Many children are cured of their malnutrition in hospital, but become malnourished again and die when they go home, because their mothers have not been taught how to feed them well enough to prevent malnutrition happening again.

Individual and group teaching. We can either teach one person at once, which is called *individual teaching*, or several people together in *group teaching*. There is such a great need for health education that we should not lose any opportunity for teaching, and particularly for individual teaching. Thus any health worker who sees an individual patient should always try to teach him something to improve his own health, or that of his family, as well as treating his disease. Many teaching opportunities, or 'teachable moments', are lost, both for individuals and groups, and we should try to make the most of them.

Most teachers will have to teach in slightly different ways, and there is room for one example only here. The example of group teaching that we shall take is a class of mothers being taught by a medical assistant or a nurse at a health centre.

'*Practise what you preach.*' Before we can begin teaching other people, we must be quite sure that we ourselves are doing all the things that we are teaching. People often do things they see other people doing, especially if they respect them. They will also quickly see if their teacher does not himself do the things that he teaches. If we want other people to breast-feed their children, to give them three protein meals a day, and to boil their water, we must first do these things ourselves.

ONLY TEACH WHAT YOU ARE PREPARED TO DO YOURSELF

CHANGING BEHAVIOUR THROUGH TEACHING

10.2 Knowing and doing. Before we begin to teach we must think a little more about what we are trying to do. We teach so that we can change what people do in ways that will make their health better. If a mother does not add protein foods to

her child's porridge, we try to change her behaviour so that she does add them. If she feeds her child only once a day, we try to make her feed him three or four times. We know that if she does these things her child will grow. We also try to persuade fathers to give their wives more money for food, and farmers to grow more protein foods. In all these ways we are trying to make people do something different. *It does not matter very much if a mother knows about protein foods. What does matter is whether she adds groundnuts or dried skim milk to her child's porridge.* However she will need to know something about why she should be doing this, and some 'knowing why' usually has to come first, before doing. People seldom do things just because they are told to, without knowing why. First they must know *why* they should do something, and then they *may* do it.

THE MOST IMPORTANT PERSON IN A CLINIC IS THE PERSON WHO TEACHES

It is sometimes thought that teaching people is like filling up an empty bottle, and that all we have to do is to 'fill people up with knowledge'. But it is not as easy as this. 'The bottle is already full'—people know many things, but they often do not know the most useful things. For example, a mother may know a lot about how to feed children by the customs of her own tribe or village. We may have to persuade her that some of her ideas are not the best ones, and, if necessary, that some of them are wrong. What we have to do is more like changing what is already inside a full bottle. This is more difficult, and we have to try to change people's ideas by talking to them very patiently.

It is sometimes wise not to try to change important ideas or beliefs—*we may do better by adding to them.* For example, a mother may think that her child has kwashiorkor because of witchcraft, because her husband has been with another woman, or because she became pregnant while she was still breast-feeding him. She may not believe us when we say this is wrong, and that he is ill because she has not been feeding him properly. Her reason may be an important belief to her, and it may be very difficult for her to change. We might, however, begin to change her *behaviour*, if we worked together with her beliefs and said, 'A good way to fight the witchcraft is to add some special medicine to the child's porridge—dried skim milk is a very special medicine. Add one large spoonful of it to his porridge, and feed him four times a day'. If she finds her child getting better, she may begin to think that you know a lot of witchcraft! She may also do the other things you teach her, and even tell other people.

TEACHING IS THE MOST IMPORTANT PART OF AN UNDER-FIVES CLINIC

Now let us say that we have taught a mother something, and we are sure that she understands it. How can we make sure that she *does* it? This is not easy, but there is one thing that we can do. *We can try to find something that she wants very much, and then show her that she can have it, if she does what we have taught her.* Say we find that she wants her child to do well in school, and that we want her to give him breakfast before he goes to school. We can say to her that her child will do better at his lessons if she gives him breakfast before he goes to school. Because she wants him to do well at school, she may give him breakfast before he goes. Sometimes there may be nothing that a mother seems to want. When this happens we have to try to make her want something, and to show her that her wants are serious. We have to show her, for example, how important it is for her child to do well at school.

Our job is thus to try to make people *do* things. Knowing what to do, and understanding why it is better, is only the beginning. *Doing is what matters.* If we want to make people do things, we can see if we have succeeded by looking to see if they are doing what we told them. Perhaps we are teaching mothers to add protein foods to their children's porridge. Are they doing it? We can find this out by visiting their homes and seeing if they do so. We can also weigh their children and see if they are gaining weight. Finding out if health education is working is called **evaluating** health education. It is

important. What is the use of teaching something, if we do not try to find out if what we are teaching is being done?

LEARN TO THINK LIKE THE PEOPLE YOU ARE TRYING TO HELP

Many mothers need health education, and yet few can come to our classes. What can we do for the others? The answer is really very simple—each of the mothers that we teach must teach her friends. Health education has thus only really succeeded if the people we teach change their behaviour, *and go and teach other people to do the same.* We must try to make each mother a teacher.

Mothers can become teachers in two ways. Let us take the use of dried skim milk as an example. A mother might make a special effort to try to make her friends use this milk, in much the same way that she has been taught in the clinic. On the other hand, she might just let her friends see what she does, and perhaps they will follow her example. Both ways are important, and we should try to see that mothers do both of them.

MAKE MOTHERS INTO TEACHERS

It is not easy to make people change their behaviour, and it is useful to think of there being seven steps in health education.

THE SEVEN STEPS TO HEALTH EDUCATION

10.3   First step: learning about the people we teach, and making the community diagnosis.   We cannot remove the blocks in the food-path of a community unless we first know what these blocks are, and which of them might be removed by health education. We must thus start by making the community diagnosis, as it is described in Section 9.29.

Making the community diagnosis is a good beginning. But once we have made it we must not stop there. We must go on learning as much as we can about the families we are teaching. We need to know about how and *why* they do things. We must know about the way they live, and cook, and feed their children. Only when we know this can we teach them what they might be able to do. Other people in other places will be different, so we need the answers to as many as possible of the questions in Section 9.26 *for the families we are teaching*.

It is seldom possible to ask one person all these questions, but by asking several people we can find out what most of them do. Much can be learnt by talking to mothers at clinics. More can be learnt by visiting them at home. It is not possible to visit every mother, but we should try to visit the homes of some mothers, especially those whose children are sick.

Most families will probably be nearly the same. They will have nearly the same cooking pots, eat nearly the same foods, and feed their children in much the same way. But no two people are exactly the same, and each mother is likely to have her own special problems. So it is important to try to talk to each mother by herself at some time, as as well as talking to her in a group with the others, so that you can find out her individual problems, and perhaps give her some individual teaching. Perhaps she is her husband's oldest wife, and her children are malnourished because he does not clear the ground for her garden, as he does for his younger wives.

Many people are afraid to talk about their problems in front of others. So you should try to take a mother by herself, and talk quietly to her where other people cannot hear. This may be difficult in a busy clinic, but she may find it easier to tell you the truth. Try to make her feel that you are really interested in her problem, and that you really want to help her.

SOME MOTHERS HAVE SPECIAL NUTRITION PROBLEMS OF THEIR OWN

10.4 Second step: making a nutrition education plan.   Once we have found out as much as we can about the people we are teaching, the next thing

to do is to see which of the blocks in their food-path might be removed by changed behaviour.

We started to do this at the beginning of the chapter when we made the educational diagnosis of malnutrition. We saw that some blocks in the food-path are more important than others, *and also that some might be easier to remove than others*. For example, in Lusaka one of the most important blocks is mothers not feeding their children often enough. It is also probably one of the easiest to remove. Most mothers have enough maize meal most of the month, and they could do this quite easily. It should thus be easier for them to remove this block than it would be, for example, for them to remove the block caused by bad budgeting. Bad budgeting is an important block, but it is harder to remove, because it is tied to the way families share money, to beer drinking, to lack of education, and to how women can make decisions in a family. These can in their turn only be removed very slowly, so bad budgeting is likely to be a difficult block to remove.

In thinking about health education we should thus look both for the important blocks, *and for the easier blocks to remove*.

TRY TO ATTACK BLOCKS WHICH ARE BOTH IMPORTANT AND EASILY REMOVED

There are so many blocks to be removed, and so much for mothers to learn, that teaching time must be used in the best possible way. To do this we need a **health education plan.**

A health education plan for a health centre is a list of the behaviour changes that are needed, so that we can teach families to make these changes. Because this is a book on nutrition, the health education plan that we shall describe is about nutrition only. But other behaviour changes are also important, especially those about such things as the proper use of latrines. Each of our lessons needs to be about *one* of the behaviour changes that we want our families to make. Each lesson also needs a short name, so that we can easily record it on a child's road-to-health chart, as described in Step six. (Section 10.7b.)

Here, for example, is a nutrition education plan that a clinic in Lusaka might use.

A Nutrition Education Plan for a Lusaka Clinic in 1971

Behaviour change wanted	*Short name to record the lesson on the road-to-health chart*
1. Three or four meals to be given daily, instead of only one or two.	Feed often a), b), c)
2. The addition of dried skim milk to porridge, as this happens to be a good protein buy—see Section 6.4.	Dried skim milk
3. Children must be given their first porridge at four months, and not at eight or ten months as at present.	Porridge at four months
4. Powdered groundnuts must be added to a child's porridge.	Groundnuts
5. Mothers should continue to breast-feed wherever possible.	Breast-feeding
6. Mothers must understand what the road-to-health chart is for, keep it safely, and bring it with them each time they come to a hospital or clinic.	Road-to-health chart
7. Mothers must come for immunizations and be able to explain what they are for.	Immunizations
8. Families not to spend money on fizzy drinks for children, but should buy milk instead.	Fizzy drinks
9. When children have diarrhoea, they should be given salt-and-sugar water, as described in Section 7.20.	Diarrhoea
10. School children should be given breakfast and lunch.	School meals

In this plan we have shown one lesson for each behaviour change we want. But some behaviour changes are so important that they need several lessons, each one trying to make the behaviour change in a different way, with different examples and different visual aids. This is why we have put (a), (b), and (c) after the first lesson. For example, in Lusaka when this nutrition education plan was made, there needed to be three lessons on why children need to be fed often. Each health centre must thus be able to give many lessons, and it might take a mother several months of coming regularly to hear all of them.

The nutrition education plan, as you see it above, is a list of lessons only, and is not yet complete. When the staff of a health centre have discussed and agreed to the behaviour changes that the families in their district need, they must next discuss what is to go into each lesson, and write it down for all to see. They should also list the visual aids that are needed, the people's 'wants' that can be used (fourth step), the things that mothers can practise during the class, and the questions that can be asked to evaluate the health education that has been given. If you want an example of how to write out a lesson, look at the very end of this chapter—Section 10.13f.

If you have difficulty in writing out a complete lesson about just one behaviour change, you may be helped in filling it out with what you find in Section 10.11 on 'What to teach'. This lists many things, such as the usefulness of recognizing the healthy child, which may not need complete lessons in themselves, but which can usefully be brought into other lessons. Thus the main part of the talk might be on the healthy child, after which mothers might be told that one way to make their children healthy is to add dried skim milk to their porridge.

A nutrition education plan is only complete when every lesson has been written out, complete with its list of visual aids and the questions that will help in evaluation.

A NUTRITION EDUCATION PLAN MUST BE WRITTEN DOWN

Now that we have decided what changes in behaviour we need, and have made our nutrition education plan, and written it down, we can think more about how we can get our families to change their behaviour. The next thing to do is to make friends with the families we teach.

10.5 Third step: making friends with the people we teach. People will learn from you more easily if they think of you as a friend. So, say 'Good morning' to mothers before you start. Be friendly, polite and respectful towards mothers. Do not be proud, or get annoyed. Never, never tell a mother she is stupid. Don't make a mother a bad example in front of her friends, so that she feels unhappy in front of them. If, however, she has done well, be quick to praise her. Don't judge her—help her. Be her servant, not her master.

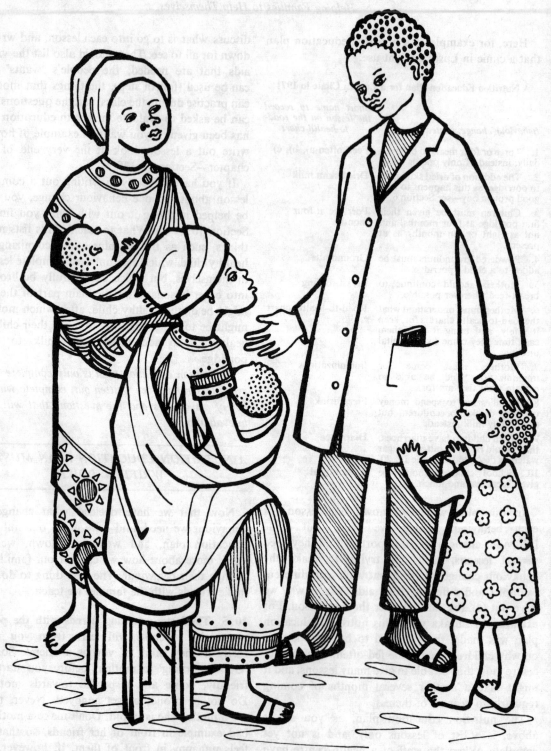

10-1, Be friendly, polite and respectful towards mothers

Say 'Good-bye' to your class when it is finished, and say that you hope you will see them again.

10.6 Fourth step: finding people's wants, and making sure that they are serious. Try to find a mother's wants. Does she want her children to be healthy, able to work hard, and get a good job? If her child is sick, she will want him to get well again. Does she want him to do well at school? If, for example, she knows that because he is underweight he will not do so well at school, she may perhaps feed him better.

Mothers must also see that their wants are serious. They must be told that their underweight children may get a disease from which they may die. A mother must be made to see how serious it is that her child does not grow up as healthy, clever or hard working, as he could be. If you tell mothers that a child who is not clever will not be able to earn so much money, and will not be able to help them, they are likely to think that this is serious.

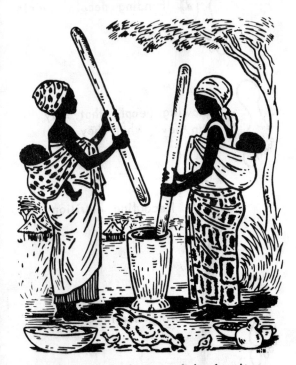

10-2, Visit the homes of the families you teach

Finding these wants is an important part of health education, so try to write them down as part of your health education plan.

10.7a Fifth step: showing people that there is a way out of their problem, and that they can have what they want. Help mothers to see that there is a way out of their problem by changing their behaviour. If mothers have a problem in that their child is not growing up strong and clever, make them see that the way to stop this is to give him more protein foods, and to feed him often. *The way out of the problem must be possible.* Never suggest things to a mother that are impossible for her. This is why it is so important to find out, in the first teaching step, what is possible. Never tell a mother to give her children meat every day when she has no money, or to come to a clinic every day when she has to walk twenty miles. Never talk about fridges, or electric stoves, or pressure cookers, because most mothers do not have these things. Most of this book is about what is possible for people.

DON'T TEACH PEOPLE THINGS THAT ARE IMPOSSIBLE FOR THEM TO DO

10.7b Sixth step: recording health education. When mothers come to a clinic several times it is useful to be able to find out what they have been taught on earlier visits. Can they remember what they have been taught a month or six months later? If they cannot remember anything, something must be wrong with the teaching. The only way to find out what a mother has been taught is to record it.

In the second step we made an educational diagnosis and divided the health education that families need into several lessons, each of them with a number. Write the name of the lesson, if it is a short one, or its number, on the top of the road-to-health chart opposite the month in which the lesson has been given. Try to do this after every health education talk you give. If these records are to be useful, the content of each lesson on a particular subject (the message in the lesson) must be the same each time it is given. For example, the things that are said about feeding school children should be the same in each talk, although the way in which it is given might be made better each time.

10.8 Seventh step: evaluating health education. This, as we have seen, means finding out if our health education is working. Are people doing the things they have been taught? One way is to visit them in their homes, and ask them the questions that you listed when you wrote down the lessons in your health education plan. If mothers have road-to-health charts, and you have recorded on them which lessons they have been taught, you will know which questions you should ask them.

A much better way to evaluate health education is to visit people's homes, and see what they are doing. Perhaps there is a maize mill in the village, and you have been teaching families to grind maize and beans together into a meal. Are they doing it? What do the children you visit weigh? Are they on the road to health?

If your health education is succeeding, and families are doing what you tell them, this is good. Your efforts are working, and you will surely be pleased. But what if they are not? Think carefully about what you are doing. Perhaps you should change the way in which you teach people? But do not get too impatient—people take a long time to change what they do!

IS YOUR HEALTH EDUCATION WORKING?
GO AND SEE!

HOW TO TEACH A GROUP

10.9 Putting the seven steps into practice. The seven steps can be used in individual teaching, as well as in group teaching. But what follows here is about group teaching only, and how it should be done. We shall go on taking health education in a health centre as an example. There are many things to think about in successful group teaching of this kind, so we will make them into a list.

Who?   Health education is the most important and the most difficult part of an under-fives clinic.

1 Learning about the people we teach

2 A nutrition education plan

3 Making friends with the people we teach

4 Finding people's wants

5 Showing people that they can have what they want

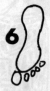
6 Recording nutrition education

7 Evaluating health education

10 - 3, The seven steps to nutrition education

It is thus usually best done by the most senior person who can speak the local language. Sometimes, in a very busy clinic, it may be best to have a special person whose main job it is to do health education. Whatever happens the person in charge of a clinic must see that *good* health education is given in his clinic!

Where? This is very important. The people you are teaching must be able to hear you, they must be able to sit down, and the place where you are teaching must not be too hot, crowded, uncomfortable or noisy. It should also be out of the wind and easy for people to come and go without upsetting the class too much. A small, hot, noisy room is the worst place in which to teach. Outside the clinic in a special shelter, or under a tree is likely to be much better. It will also be easier to use the kind of stove that the mothers have if you are outside. When a clinic is being planned, see that a simple, shaded shelter, with seats and a concrete table, is built as well.

How many mothers? Everyone must be able to hear you, so don't try to talk to too many mothers at once. Twenty mothers at a time is as much as most people can manage.

When? This again is important. In most clinics a health education talk is best given first, before children are weighed, seen and immunized. If talks are given at the end of a clinic, mothers may not wait for their lesson.

How often? A health education talk should be given at every under-fives clinic, and also at every clinic to which mothers bring their children. One talk a week is not good enough, and at a busy clinic several talks should be given during a morning or afternoon.

What with? Health education tries to change what people *do*. This is much more likely to happen if they can see and practise in a clinic what they should later do in their homes. The Chinese have a saying which is very true for health education. It is this:

What we hear — we forget.
What we see — we remember.
What we do — we know.

So don't be content with only talking. If you want mothers to pound groundnuts and add them to their children's porridge, show them how this can be done as part of your talk. Then let one or two of them pound groundnuts themselves and make a child's porridge, with the rest of the class watching. If mothers are going to be able to do things like this, you must get everything you need ready before the class starts. The things for this kind of teaching are best gathered together in a nutrition teaching outfit, as described in the next section.

'IF I DO IT I KNOW'—LET MOTHERS PRACTISE WHAT YOU TEACH THEM

The best helps or aids to teaching are the real things themselves that people can see and touch and use. They are often called **visual aids.** Visual means seeing, and many of them are helps in seeing. Thus, if you want to get mothers to give salt-and-sugar water to their children with diarrhoea, get salt, sugar, water, cups and spoons and make these your visual aids. If you want them to buy something at a shop, such as dried skim milk, show them the packet that they must ask for and visit the local shops to make sure that they sell it. Pictures are not so good as the real thing, but whatever visual aids you use, be sure to get them ready before the class starts.

GET YOUR VISUAL AIDS TOGETHER BEFORE THE CLASS STARTS

The first two steps. There is much to do before you can begin to talk. You should have made the community diagnosis (first step) and the educational diagnosis with its nutrition education plan (second step). You should also have written out your lessons with their lists of questions for evaluating how successful you have been. The class should be comfortable and easily able to hear you, and all your visual aids should be ready. Try hard to get mothers to give you the answers.

The third step. The talking part of teaching only starts with the third step—making friends with the people you are teaching. Tell them who you are, if they may not know, and how pleased you are to see them. *Tell them the name of the lesson.*

The fourth and fifth steps. Try to work these two steps into your talk. You will remember that they were finding out people's wants, and showing them that they can have what they want if they do what you are teaching them. A good way to begin is to ask questions. Do the mothers in the class want healthy children? If they do, and your lesson is on good budgeting, ask them how much money they have and how much they spend on food. Tell them that they can have healthy children if they budget wisely, and then show them how they can budget in the best way.

Try to make your talk partly a conversation with the mothers. Don't talk for more than three minutes before asking more questions, even though your whole lesson may last 20 minutes. Try to discuss what you are teaching about from several points of view—that is in several different ways. Try hard to get mothers to give you the anwers.

After you have been talking for a few minutes, ask questions, listen to what mothers say, make a joke or show them something, and then talk again. Use easy words and make sure the class understands, them. Be sure to give people a chance to ask you questions.

Teach one thing at a time. If you have had difficulty with your educational diagnosis, and are not sure what to teach, teach one of the 'ten good rules' that you will find at the end of this chapter. In most districts these will be the behaviour changes that you will really want to happen. Most other things come a long way second. If only every mother would follow these rules there would be no malnutrition in most districts.

TEACH ONLY ONE BEHAVIOUR CHANGE AT A TIME

Go through your lessons one after the other during a few weeks or months, and then go through them again, changing them as you think best.

Change your teaching with the seasons. If it is the planting season, encourage families to clear more land and plant more protein crops. If you can only teach once in a place make sure that you teach what is most important.

Sixth step. As the class ends and you are about to say good-bye, don't forget to record the name or number of the lesson you have just given on the mothers' road-to-health charts.

Seventh step. As we have seen, the best way to evaluate health education is to visit mothers at home. But if you have recorded the lessons that you have previously given mothers on their road-to-health charts, you will be able to ask them the test questions that you listed when you wrote out your lessons.

Another way of evaluating your health education is to ask a mother to tell the class what she was taught when she last came to the clinic. Let her teach the class for a few minutes. Many mothers like doing this and the class will laugh a lot!

10.10 More about visual aids. If you are going to teach properly, you must have ready all the things you need before the class starts. You will find it useful to keep all the things you need together as a *nutrition teaching outfit*. The outfit in Figure 10-4 contains everything that is needed for making a child's porridge and adding pounded protein foods to it. Outfits for other kinds of nutrition teaching could easily be made.

There is a box (1) in which things are packed, a bottle of clean water (2), a charcoal stove (3), some charcoal, a piece of candle to get the charcoal lit (4), matches (5), a local kind of wooden spoon (7), a knife and board to chop on (8), a sieve (9), a small clean pestle and mortar (10), and several small tins or jars to keep pounded protein foods in (11). There is an egg (12), and a cloth to dry things with (13). The porridge in the pot has been made from the maize in the bag (14). The three cups of porridge have had either roasted pounded ground-nuts (15), or an egg (16), or dried skim milk (17) stirred into them. If flies are a problem, take some plastic plates to put over the food.

NOBODY CAN TEACH NUTRITION WITHOUT THE RIGHT FOODS AND EQUIPMENT

When you are using this outfit, make plain porridge and pour it into the cups. Add a large

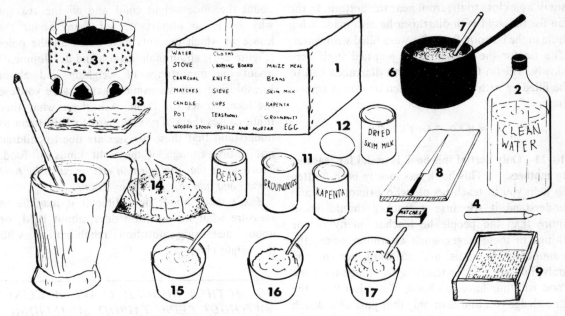

10 - 4, A nutrition teaching outfit

spoonful of one of the protein foods to each of the cups. Show them only one new food at each lesson. Another time, make the pounded protein foods with mothers watching, so that they can learn how to do it.

EVERY HEALTH CENTRE NEEDS A NUTRITION TEACHING OUTFIT

Keep your outfit in a box and make a list of the things that it should contain, so that you do not forget them. If you keep an outfit like this always ready, you will find that it will save you much trouble. It packs away quite small, but even so you will probably not be able to carry it on a bicycle. If you are cycling to another clinic, you may have to take some things one week, and other things on another visit.

Teaching charts and pamphlets. A poster is a big picture that stays on the wall and is supposed to teach people something. They seldom do, because people soon stop looking at them. If you have any posters of this kind, use them as teaching charts. Put them up only when you are going to teach, explain them to your class and see what they

think about them. People who are not used to seeing pictures may find them difficult to understand. Colour them, and if they are not in the local language, stick new names on them which are in the local language. When you have finished teaching with a poster or teaching chart, take it down and put it away until you want to use it again.

If you have pamphlets (pieces of printed paper), give them only to people you are teaching. Explain what the pamphlets mean, and make sure they are in the local language. They will help your class to remember what they have been taught. Even if a mother cannot read herself, someone else in the family (her husband or a schoolboy) probably can.

Another very useful teaching aid is the **flannelgraph.** This is a special kind of picture made out of flannel and is described in the 'things to do' section at the end of this chapter.

Try to collect teaching aids and do your best to make your own. Mr. Liwakala, a medical assistant, made a very good one to show how important it is to give a child with diarrhoea plenty of salt-and-sugar water to drink. He took two tins as 'models' of two children, one a healthy child, and the other a child with diarrhoea. In each of them he made a small hole close to the front near the bottom. In the tin for the child with diarrhoea he also made a big hole in the bottom. Both tins were filled with water. The tin for the normal child emptied itself very slowly. The tin for the child with diarrhoea had to be filled up with water very often to stop it emptying!

WHAT TO TEACH

10.11   Only part of this book is useful for teaching to mothers.   This book has mostly been written to help you to teach people who cannot read and understand it. Because a teacher should know more than the people he teaches, many of the things in these pages, such as amino acids, the community diagnosis, and aflatoxin, are for you only, and are not for teaching to village mothers. You will thus have to choose and select from the knowledge you find here only that part of it which will be useful for the people you teach. Deciding which behaviour changes you want, and making your health education plan, will help you to choose. But, even so, you may still need the help of this section which lists the things you may need to teach. Many of them are quite small and can be used to fill out the lessons you are writing about some important behaviour change. Once again we have been thinking of a group of village mothers at a clinic, and when you teach other groups the list may need changing.

Chapter 1: Growth.   Teach about the road-to-health chart, how it should be kept with great care and brought with a child every time he comes to a clinic or hospital; teach about growth, and where a healthy child should be on the road-to-health chart; about immunizations and what diseases they protect children from, and about what an under-fives clinic tries to do. Ask mothers what they mean by a healthy child. Show them the things that tell us if a child is healthy and which are listed at the end of Section 1.2. Talk to them about the words in their language for 'healthy', 'fat', 'well nourished', and 'badly nourished'.

Don't teach them about children's weights at particular ages, about nutrition surveys, or about arm circumference.

Chapter 2: When growth fails.   Teach mothers about the underweight child and all the reasons why he is so important; tell them about the house in which the ants have eaten all the poles (Figure 2–3); about malnutrition and development; about the importance of weighing and about kwashiorkor and marasmus, making sure you use the local names for them. Ask them what they think causes them. Try very hard to help them to understand that these diseases are due to children not getting enough of the right kinds of food. *Teach them that malnutrition can be cured by food alone, and not by giving injections.*

Don't teach about how difficult it may be to measure what malnutrition does, about PJM, or about measuring nutrition rehabilitation with the weight chart.

NO MOTHER SHOULD LEAVE A CLINIC WITHOUT BEING TAUGHT SOMETHING

Chapter 3: Nutrients and proteins.   Teach mothers about body-building foods, energy foods and protective foods. Some people think that mothers should be taught about 'protein', and that it would be good if the word 'protein' was used by villagers. This is happening in Uganda where the word 'protein' is getting into the Luganda language. Try to get them to use the word 'protein' and to tell you which are the protein-containing foods. Tell mothers that proteins are a brain food which will make their children clever. Teach them how protein is used for repair and growth, and use the idea of 'feet and shoes' as in Figure 3–2. Tell them how useful it is to mix foods.

Don't tell them about nutrients, carbohydrates, fats, vitamins and minerals, percentages, amino acids, atoms, cells, the 'letters', NPU or reference proteins.

Chapter 4: Energy foods, etc.   Teach about energy foods and protective foods, non-foods, fizzy drinks, safe water, and perhaps about the food groups, although these are not very important. It may also be useful to teach about iron and anaemia.

Don't teach about joules, staples, vitamins and minerals, nicotinic acid, folic acid, iodine, calcium or fluorine.

Chapter 5: More about food. If you have taught about food groups, teach about balanced meals, but not otherwise. If milk is a good thing to buy in your district, teach about which are the best kinds to buy, and show them the tins or packets they should ask for.

Don't teach about aflatoxin or cyanide.

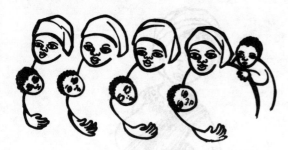

10 - 5, No mother must ever leave a clinic without being taught something

Chapter 6: The need for food and its cost. Teach mothers which kinds of people need extra body-building or protein foods, and which kinds of people need extra energy foods. Tell them about the cost of food, and about budgeting and selling food.

Don't teach them about protein needs in grams, or joule needs, or about protein and joule 'best buy' lists.

Chapter 7: Feeding the family. Teach almost the whole of this chapter, choosing the parts which are most suitable for your district, and changing them if necessary. Remember most especially to teach them to give their children salt-and-sugar water when they have diarrhoea.

Don't teach them about 'bulk', lactose, the vicious circle of malnutrition and infection, or about dehydration—explain what happens using ordinary words.

Chapter 8: Bottle-feeding. Don't teach any of this chapter, except how bad bottle-feeding can be, unless mothers have started bottle-feeding—then they need it all. Try to teach each bottle-feeding mother by herself.

Chapter 9: The food-path. This is probably not suitable for mothers, although it is very good for other groups, such as those in schools, agriculture and government.

Chapters 10 and 11: Helping the family and helping the community. These chapters are to help you to help families and the community and contain nothing suitable for teaching a group of mothers.

DON'T TEACH PEOPLE WHAT THEY ALREADY DO

Explain to mothers that you are telling them things that may be new to them, and that you know that lots of other people in the village, especially older women and grandmothers, will not believe them. Tell them that you are teaching them these things because you know they are important, and will help their children. Explain that you understand how difficult it is for them to bring new ideas to a village where many people believe something different.

If you are still in doubt about what you should teach, you will not go far wrong if you teach these 'ten good rules'.

1. **Breast-feeding is best.**
2. **Bottle-feeding is dangerous.**
3. **A child must start eating porridge when he is four months old and be eating porridge with added protein by the time he is six months old.**
4. **Children need at least three meals with body-building foods every day.**
5. **Children need some protective foods every day.**
6. **School children need food before going to school and also something to eat while they are at school in the middle of the day.**
7. **Children with diarrhoea need a lot to drink, and all sick children must be fed, even though they may not want to eat.**
8. **Maize or millet are much better foods for children than cassava, potatoes or plantains.**
9. **Plain porridge is not good enough—some protein must be added. A good food is a mixed food.**
10. **Pregnant women and breast-feeding mothers need extra food of all sorts, especially protein and protective foods.**

If every mother did these things, children would be much more healthy than they are now. Most of these things are on the back cover of this book. Teach everything that you read there.

10.12   Two special kinds of mothers—and fathers. This book has been written for the poorest and hungriest families, but before we end this chapter two other kinds of mother must be mentioned, and something said about fathers.

How has the successful mother done it?   When we weigh children and put their weights on road-to-health charts we will probably find that many children are below the road to health. Some children will be on the road to health and some may even be above it. Some of these healthy children will be from very poor homes, yet somehow their mothers have been able to feed them well—how have they done it? How do these children from very poor homes come to be on the road to health?

There are several possibilities. One is that these children are lucky. They have one block in their food-path—they come from very poor homes. But they may have avoided many other blocks. Their parents may not drink, or be divorced. They may be fed often, even if it is only with maize porridge. As we have seen, malnutrition is usually caused by there being many blocks on a child's food-path, and these children may be lucky in having escaped many of the other blocks, even though they are poor.

Another possibility is that children differ from one another in the ways in which their bodies use food to grow with. If given the same food, one child may grow more than another, and it may be that these healthy children are better at using, and growing with, the little food that they are given. But this is probably only part of the answer.

It is also possible that the healthy child's mother may have been doing the things that you have read about in this book, like adding protein foods to his porridge. She may also have found ways of feeding him that are specially good for the place where she lives. She may have found some ways of feeding her child that other mothers might find useful. *Can we learn from the mothers who have* *succeeded in feeding their children well?* Can we teach other mothers to do the same things? What one mother can do to get round the blocks on the food-path, another mother can also do. We must learn from the more successful mothers as we teach the less successful ones.

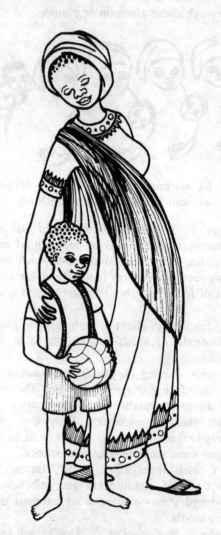

10 - 6, Teach mothers that they themselves need extra food when they are pregnant

The richer mother.   Some of our mothers will be much richer than the others. They will be able to buy more animal-protein foods, especially milk, meat and eggs. Because they can get these foods they need not breast-feed their children for the full eighteen months or two years that is best for poorer mothers. They need only feed their children for nine months or a year, but it is better if they continue longer. Other mothers will follow their example, so it should be the right one. By the time a child is a year old he can get all the protein he needs from the animal-protein foods that can be added to his porridge—if his mother is rich enough to buy them. It is the children of poorer mothers who need the animal protein of their mother's milk until they are two years old.

If you have richer mothers and poorer ones in the same class, don't separate them into two. Instead, teach both together, and tell the more fortunate mothers the extra things that they are able to do.

Don't forget father. Many men want to know how children should be fed, and do not understand how much money their wives need to buy food for the family. It is also important for them to know how a woman should eat when she is pregnant or breast-feeding. So try to teach them whenever you can. Some fathers will come to an 'open day' or 'husband's day' at a women's club, especially if some important man is to come and speak.

10.13   THINGS TO DO

(a) Teaching. If you are at school, visit an under-fives clinic and try to practise what you have learnt in this chapter.

If you are a medical assistant or a dresser, make sure you teach at every under-fives clinic you hold. Teach the cleaners at your health centre what you have learnt. They may be able to help you teach. See if you can do some teaching at women's clubs. Can you talk to farmers who are being taught by the agricultural assistant? Can you teach in the schools? Can the boys and girls from the secondary school come and help you? Can the agricultural assistant come and teach the mothers at your clinic how they can grow more protein foods? Can you talk at the meetings of the Parent Teacher Association, to youth groups, church groups, community development clubs, or at meetings of the political party? Can plans be made so that all these people are teaching the same thing at the same time?

EVERYONE MUST TEACH BETTER NUTRITION WHENEVER HE POSSIBLY CAN

(b) A play. If you are using this book in class, act a play to show some of the important things in nutrition teaching. One member of the class can be the teacher, and the rest a group of mothers. They can then ask their teacher all the difficult questions! After one student has tried to teach, the rest of the class can see how well or badly she did it.

(c) A nutrition teaching outfit. Collect the things you need to make your own nutrition teaching outfit, as shown in Figure 10-3.

(d) Making and using a flannelgraph. Do you remember the Chinese saying from an earlier section? It went like this: what we hear—we forget; what we see—we remember; what we do—we know! Much has been said about how important it is for people to *do* things. If this is not always possible, the next best thing is for them to *see* things. A good way of letting people see things is to use a flannelgraph, which is a special kind of 'picture for teaching'.

Flannel is the name for a special kind of cloth with a fluffy (hairy) surface. The flannelgraph itself is a piece of board, such as a blackboard, or a piece of hardboard, covered with flannel, which you can put up in front of a class and stick pictures to. Pictures of various kinds can be made to stick to this flannel, and put up or taken down as they are needed. Make your flannelgraph like this.

Pin a piece of cloth with a good fluffy surface to your board. Lint, a kind of 'medical flannel' can be used, so can some kinds of blanket. Put the board up in front of the class so that it slopes very slightly backwards.

Get together as many pictures as you can showing the things that you want to teach about. These can be drawings, pictures from the newspapers, photographs, or pictures cut from the charts provided by the Zambian National Food and Nutrition Commission (see Section 11.10). Words or short sentences can be written on pieces of paper or card.

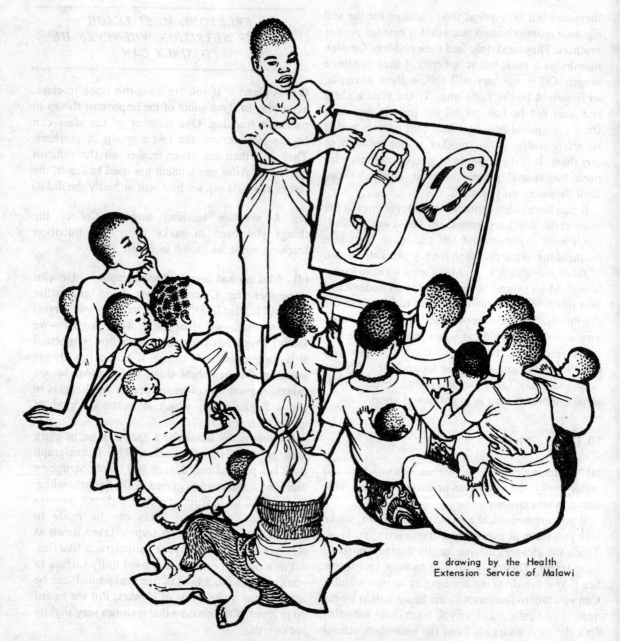

a drawing by the Health
Extension Service of Malawi

10-7, Using a flannelgraph to show that a pregnant mother needs to eat plenty of fish

These pictures will not stick to the flannel as they are, but must have pieces of flannel or sandpaper stuck to the back of them with paste or gum. When these pictures are now placed on the flannelgraph, the sandpaper or flannel will make them stick to it, so that they can be put up and taken down as they are needed.

Always start with your flannelgraph empty. Build up the picture you want to show by asking mothers questions. If you are talking about the foods that a mother should add to her child's porridge, ask the class what foods they would add. When the right answer is given put a picture of that food on the flannelgraph. Build up the picture you want to show by questioning the class in this way. *Always praise a good answer and try to get round a bad one.* A good way of teaching, and especially of using a flannelgraph, is to ask mothers something, to show them something such as a food or a picture of a food, and then to tell them something about what they have been shown: ask—show—tell. Mothers like putting up pictures. Make sure that they can recognize them.

ASK—SHOW—TELL

Whenever you make a flannelgraph, see that it does these things:

It tells a story in which you can see things happen.

It has strong colours that you can see well.

It looks like the things that people are used to seeing.

It has pictures that can be seen from the back of the class.

It makes the people who see it talk about it and ask questions.

It lets some of the people who are seeing it help the teacher to tell the story and so keeps the class interested.

A flannelgraph can be used in many ways. There is a special flannelgraph made which shows the road-to-health graph and which can be used to teach mothers about it. A flannelgraph can also be used to explain the food-path to a class of students. One of the best uses of a flannelgraph is, however, to teach mothers the things that are listed in Section 10.11.

(e) Learning from other people. Whenever you see someone teaching nutrition, think to yourself, is he, or she, doing it well or badly? What can I learn from how I see it being done? How much of what has been said in this chapter is being followed? One way to find this out for a health education talk in a clinic is to make a list (a check list) of all the things that should be part of a health education talk, and to check and see if they are being followed. Is there a health education plan? Is anything being done to evaluate health education? Are any visual aids being used? Are they good ones?

(f) A nutrition lesson for a health centre. Write out a nutrition lesson in the way you have learnt in this chapter. Here is an example. It is taken from a lesson prepared by the Health Extension Service of Malawi.

Behaviour change needed. Families must try to prevent their children getting diarrhoea and look after them properly if they do get it.

Name of lesson. 'Diarrhoea'.

'Want' to be used. Families wanting their children to stay healthy, and not to die from diarrhoea.

Things needed. Cups, spoons, sugar, boiled water, salt.

Lesson. Good afternoon. I am so pleased to see you. Have any of your children had diarrhoea? Do you know of any children who have died of diarrhoea? Do you want your children to get diarrhoea less often, and less seriously, and to be less likely to die when they do get it? If you do the things I am going to show you, your child will be in much less danger from diarrhoea.

Why do children get diarrhoea? A child gets diarrhoea when he has eaten some kinds of food, such as hard beans. This kind of diarrhoea is not serious, and soon stops when a child stops eating foods of this kind.

Diarrhoea is usually caused by a child eating germs. (Try to explain these in a way people will understand. In Malawi they call them *Tizorombo tating'ono tosaonadwe ndi maso*.) Germs live in dirt. A child may drink diarrhoea germs because he has drunk dirty water. How can we make water safe? By boiling it. Always boil your drinking water, especially water for small children.

A child may eat diarrhoea germs because he has eaten food that has been touched by dirty hands, or because it has been on dirty ground, or because flies have been walking on it. Flies carry diarrhoea germs on their legs.

Diarrhoea is serious, because much food and water are lost by a child in his stools. So much water is lost that a child begins to get dry—like a fish being dried! A child with diarrhoea needs water, salt and sugar to put back what he has lost in his diarrhoea. As soon as your child has diarrhoea start to give him back his fluid like this.

Demonstration.   This is how you make salt-and-sugar water. (Mothers are shown how to make it.) Give this to your child slowly, a little at a time, at least every half-hour. Give him as much as he will drink—at least four big cups full a day. Give him food and breast milk as well.

A child with diarrhoea dies easily. Take him to a health centre or hospital if he has any of these things:

If he has a fever;

If there are very many watery stools, or if there is blood in the stools;

If he looks thin and his eyes and his fontanelle sink in. (Explain this. The fontanelle is the soft part of the top of the head of a very young child. When the body loses water it sinks in. It closes and gets harder as he gets older.)

If he starts vomiting or is very weak.

When you are taking your child with diarrhoea to a clinic take some salt-and-sugar water with you, so that he can have a drink on the way.

Things mothers can do.   Let some mothers make salt-and-sugar water for themselves, and let their children taste it.

Evaluation after the lesson.   (Here are some questions to find out if the group has understood what they have been taught.)

Q.   What usually causes diarrhoea?
A.   Eating dirty food or drinking dirty water. Germs live in dirt.

Q.   Why is diarrhoea serious for a young child?
A.   Because it causes him to lose so much water that his body dries up, and he may die.

Q.   How can water from the river be made safe for drinking?
A.   By boiling it to kill the germs.

Q.   What must you give a child with diarrhoea?
A.   A lot to drink.

Q.   How can you make a special drink for a child with diarrhoea?
A.   (Mothers should be able to describe how to make salt-and-sugar water.)

Q.   How often should you give this drink?
A.   At least every half-hour.

Q.   How much should the child get in a day?
A.   At least four cups. More if possible.

Good-bye. Thank you for coming to my lesson. I do hope I will see you again.

Evaluation later and on home visiting.   Are children with diarrhoea coming to the clinic who have already been started on salt-and-sugar water at home? Can mothers make salt-and-sugar water when you visit them at home? Can they answer the questions that have just been listed?

Try to write lessons on other behaviour changes in the same way as this one.

(g)   A nutrition lesson for a primary school.   Can you, from what you have read so far in this book, write a nutrition lesson for a primary class? A lesson for school children needs to be different from a lesson for mothers. Can someone give the lesson and the rest criticize it?

(h)   Running a nutrition quiz.   A quiz is useful for evaluating what you have been teaching. This one was given to us by the Health Extension Service of Malawi. Run a quiz with a group you have already taught a few times. Find questions about the things the group should know. You will need a blackboard and chalk, or small pieces of stick.

Divide your group into two teams. Keep the score by marking points on a blackboard or by using small sticks as points. Start each team with an easy question. Ask a person in the first team a question. If he or she does not know the answer, ask if anyone in the team does. If the answer is right, or nearly right, give the team a point and let everyone clap. Give the right answer, and explain it if necessary, so *everyone* can hear. If nobody in the team knows the answer, tell them and explain it. Then ask the second team a question in the same way.

Don't ask too many questions. Six or ten are enough. Don't laugh if someone does not know the right answer. Put old people in the teams only if they want to join. Clap the winning team at the end.

Here are some questions.

1. Q. How many times should a three-year-old child be fed each day?
   A. At least three times (otherwise he will not be able to eat enough to grow well).

2. Q. Name two foods that make children grow fast.
   A. Any of these: milk, eggs, fish, meat from any animal or bird, insects, beans, peas, groundnuts. (These are protein foods.)

3. Q. What is the best food for a two-month-old baby?
   A. Breast milk—he doesn't need any other food until he is four months old.

4. Q. Why do school children need a good breakfast?
   A. Otherwise they feel tired at school and cannot learn or remember their lessons, or play games well.

5. Q. What is a good breakfast for a school child?
   A. A good porridge containing a protein food, such as porridge and groundnuts, banana and boiled egg. (The answer should include an energy and a protein food.)

6. Q. At what age should a baby start new foods?
   A. At four months. Breast milk is not enough by itself at that age, and if he doesn't learn to eat new foods he will not grow properly and may get sick.

7. Q. How can a mother tell if her baby is growing properly?

8. Q. What should you give a sick child to eat?
   A. A sick child needs soft, clean food like porridge with added protein foods. He needs this food often, four or five times a day. He also needs lots of sweetened boiled water or boiled milk to drink. He should drink every hour.

   A. By taking him to a clinic where he is weighed, and his weight marked on a chart which shows whether he is on the road to health or below it.

9. Q. Does plain porridge make children grow?
   A. Children who eat plain porridge only grow more slowly than they should.

10. Q. Are wild leaves a good food?
    A. Yes, wild leaves help make a good relish.

11. Q. What can you add to plain porridge to make it better for body-building?
    A. Pounded groundnuts, bean flour or mashed beans, egg, fresh or dried milk, pounded fish and minced meat.

12. Q. Small children need food to make them grow. What other people need food for growth?
    A. School-age children, pregnant and nursing mothers.

(i) Secondary school students teaching in the villages. At one secondary school in Zambia groups of four students, two boys and two girls, went to teach in the villages. One of their teachers explained their visits carefully to the headmen first, after which the boys gave talks and the girls cooking demonstrations. They prepared their talks very carefully, visited the villages several times, and took great care to be polite when teaching people older than themselves.

Can you do the same?

Chapter Eleven

HELPING THE COMMUNITY
TO HELP ITSELF

11.1 Community health action. We have just thought about how to teach families to improve their own nutrition. But there are many blocks in the food-path that cannot be taken away by one family alone, and which can only be removed by many people in the community doing things together. To do something is only another way of saying 'to take action'. When, therefore, the people of a community do things together to make their health better, we say that they are taking **'community health action'**. There are some things that the community of people in a village can do to make their nutrition better—there is some action that they can take. There are still more things that the people of a district can do if they work together. There are other things that the people of a province can do, and there are further blocks in the food-path that can only be taken away if the whole country works together. These are the blocks that can only be removed by the national or central government. We can therefore think of community health action for better nutrition as taking place at several steps or levels. These are in the village, in the ward, in the district, in the province and in the country as a whole. This is mostly a book for the people working in villages and districts, or for those who are going to work there; so we will think especially about what **village productivity committees** and **district development committees** can do.

ACTION MEANS **DOING** *SOMETHING*

11.2 Involving the local people. In the last chapter we saw that there are several steps in health education, and that it is no use just telling a mother something, and expecting her to do it. She has first to be shown that she can get something she wants if she feeds her children better. In the same way it is no use just telling the people of a community something, and then expecting them to do it. The whole community have first to understand that malnutrition helps to cause many of their problems, and that they can make their life better by making their nutrition better. The way to begin is to explain the problem of malnutrition to the leaders of the community. See if you can show them figures of how much malnutrition there is in the community. The leaders may be chiefs, headmen, councillors or government officials in the district, especially the district governor or commissioner.

These people lead the community, and if they can be made to think that nutrition is important, and that much can be done to improve it, they may be able to persuade other people in the community to take action—to *do* something! The community have to be made to see that their children need to be well nourished, if they are not to die, and that malnutrition is the cause of many of their problems. They must come to understand not only that nutrition matters, but also that there are many things that can be done to improve it. There are many things they can do themselves, and which ONLY they can do. This is what we mean by 'involving the community'—making people see the problem, care about it and start doing things to get rid of it. The effort needed to involve many people is very hard work—*it is never useless.* It takes a long time to go round and talk to people. The results in the end may be better than you expect.

---

*MALNUTRITION IS A COMMUNITY PROB-
LEM AND NEEDS A COMMUNITY ANSWER*

The first thing a village community should understand is that it must grow most of its own food.

11.3 The community must grow its own food.
Malnutrition can be cured by food, but food has
to come from somewhere. Food can be grown
inside the country, or it can be bought from other
countries, but if it is bought it has to be paid for.
If, for example, Malawi wants to buy food from
New Zealand, she has first to sell things such as
the cotton she grows. With the money she earns
she can then buy food. Many countries do not
have enough things to sell to be able to earn enough
money to buy much of their food. They have
therefore to save the little money they earn to
buy the things they cannot make, such as cars and
machines. They must not waste scarce money
buying food. They must grow what they need to
eat.

Some countries grow too much food and are
able to give it away. America and Canada often
have too much wheat, and America used to have
too much dried skim milk. These gifts of food are
useful, especially when there is a famine. But they
are never enough, and usually only one kind of
food is given. They do not end the problem of
malnutrition, and because they do not help a country to make its agriculture better they may even
make the problem worse. People may come to
think that all food should be given to them and not
try to grow their own. If the gifts of food stop
people might be worse nourished than they were
before.

Food can also be brought by lorry from
one part of the country, where there is plenty, to
another part where there is not enough. But this is
always expensive, and it is often difficult, because
roads may be bad, and there may not be enough
lorries. Every district must thus try to grow as
much as possible of the food it needs. We say it
must look after itself, or be self-supporting.

---

*EVERY DISTRICT MUST GROW ITS
OWN FOOD*

11.4 Everyone must help and someone must start.
It is not easy to start community health action and
to get the community involved. It needs much
patient explaining by whoever tries to start it,
both to individuals and to groups. Someone has
to start, for the community needs a leader—
perhaps that leader is YOU! The leader in community health action need not be one of the ordinary leaders of the community, such as the district
governor, although it is a great help if he is. In
Zambia some of the best community leaders in
nutrition are schoolmasters and priests.

Someone has to start—*and lead*! Perhaps you
have seen cases of marasmus and kwashiorkor
and know that underweight children do not grow
into the clever adults that the country needs.
Perhaps you are keen to drive out malnutrition
from your community. Malnutrition is difficult
to fight, and you will not be able to prevent it
all so that there is not one underweight child left.
If, however, you try hard you may be able to do
something to make nutrition better. There are
several steps that you can take. They start with
your own family and yourself, they go on perhaps
in your job, and end as a volunteer helping the
whole community.

11.5 Beginning with your family and yourself.
Perhaps you are a father or a mother. Are all
your children on the road to health? Are they
immunized against the diseases which help to
cause malnutrition? Are your young children fed
at least three times a day? Do they always have a
protein food added to their porridge? If your
children are at school, do they get breakfast in
the morning and food to take with them for the
middle of the day?

Perhaps you are at school yourself. Can you
help feed your younger brothers and sisters? Can
you cook some food for yourself before you start
walking to school in the morning? Can you take
some food with you to eat in the middle of the
day?

11.6 Fighting malnutrition in your job.   Many
people have jobs in which they can fight malnutrition. It is one of my jobs to write books, so this
is why we have written this one. Doctors, medical
assistants, nurses, midwives, dressers and sweepers
in the clinics can all teach people how to feed
their children. So also can traditional healers

(*ngangas*), who have malnourished children brought to them. Teachers can teach their children about nutrition. Pupils at school can learn about it, because this will help them later on. Priests can tell the people in their churches about it, and may even be able to ask men to clear more land for growing food crops. Farmers and workers in the agricultural department can do much to grow more food. District secretaries, district governors, the 'ten-house chairmen' of Tanzania, and the political workers in UNIP and ANC in Zambia can all make sure that the government fights malnutrition as hard as it can.

But it will be a very long time before there are enough people to fight malnutrition in their jobs, because governments cannot yet train enough nurses, or agricultural assistants, or teachers. But nearly everybody could help in the fight against malnutrition if they would work as volunteers, and much could be done.

11.7 Voluntary nutrition work.   A volunteer is someone who does a job because he thinks it is important, and does not expect to get paid. *Very many things need doing in a community for which there is no pay and no reward.* Nutrition work is only one of them. One of the best things that anyone can do is to work for the good of the people of his district, and to expect no money for it. Most people need to work to earn money to feed their families and so need a paid job. But there are always the evenings, Saturdays, Sundays and the holidays. These are the times in which voluntary work can be done. Some time is needed for resting, *but not all of it!* So much voluntary work needs doing if a country is to develop and go forward, that everyone should make it a rule to do something. Voluntary work in nutrition is a good way to start.

WHAT VOLUNTARY WORK ARE YOU DOING?

Voluntary work is closely tied to *initiative*. This is being able to start something, and keep it going yourself without waiting for other people to do

things. It means getting over difficulties and troubles, and going on and on to the end. Initiative is a great thing to have, and one which needs much practice. Voluntary nutrition work will give you a good chance to practise it.

The kind of voluntary work that you can do depends upon whether you are an adult, or whether you are still at school. If you are an adult, you could join a nutrition group, or some other group doing voluntary nutrition work. A nutrition group is several people who work together to fight malnutrition. If you are still at school, you could join a nutrition club, or even start one yourself.

NUTRITION CLUBS AND NUTRITION GROUPS

11.8 A secondary school nutrition club.   Some secondary schools have many clubs which staff and students join. They may have clubs for sports, or science, or radio or for many other things. A good club to start or join is a 'nutrition club'. The best way to begin is to talk to staff members about the need for a nutrition club, and to see if one of them would join it and be interested in it. It is good to have a staff member in the club, especially if it is going to do useful work in the community.

The first thing that the members of a nutrition club should do is to learn about nutrition, and then they should think about how they can improve it in the district where they are at school. They should start by reading all they can about nutrition, and they may be able to find a doctor, or an agricultural officer, who will come and talk to them about it. The club should try to make the 'community diagnosis of malnutrition' as it is described in Section 9.29, and then think very carefully about how they can remove the blocks in the food-path in their district. The blocks that they can most easily remove will probably be those that can be taken away by health education (see Section 9.24). Club members can teach or give nutrition education in their own school, in the primary schools, in under-fives clinics and in the hospital. But, before anyone can teach, he must know what he is teaching. Club members should thus only teach other people if they themselves have learnt all they can about nutrition first. They should therefore try to set themselves a test on nutrition, and pass it, before they themselves teach other people. It may be possible to have a national exam, with a badge and a certificate for those who pass it.

Club members can also weigh children, and help fill in road-to-health graphs at under-fives clinics. They can teach mothers at the clinics. Most usefully of all, they can visit people in their homes and villages and teach them there. For this they will need nutrition teaching outfits, like the one described in Section 10.10. Sometimes it may be possible for a clinic to be held on a Saturday morning or a free afternoon when there is no school especially so that members can come and help. Senior girls can also be very useful in visiting the mothers of malnourished children at home and teaching them there, particularly if mothers stop coming to the clinics. At one clinic the doctor said he did not know what he would do without the home-visiting that was done by the girls from the school.

Volunteers are needed for many things in hospitals besides nutrition, and senior girls might like to form a club of 'friends of the hospital'. They should start by going with one of their teachers; they should take great care to work with the hospital staff, and they should try to make themselves as useful as they can. The matron will probably be pleased to show them round when they first come, after which they can have a meeting and think about how best they can help. Besides helping to teach mothers from the children's ward and the nutrition rehabilitation unit about nutrition (see Section 11.14), members can be useful in many other ways. They can be interpreters in clinics when a doctor cannot talk the patient's language. They can read to patients, and sell them such things as writing paper and stamps. They can collect newspapers for patients and write letters for them. They can teach patients to read and write, especially children who are going to be in hospital for a long time. If patients learn to read and write about nutrition, they will learn both these things and nutrition at the same time. Members can also

play games, such as rounders and netball or quizzes, with the mental patients.

Pupils from a school are not likely to come to harm in a hospital, except in a tuberculosis ward, where they might catch this disease from the patients. They should therefore either be tested and, if necessary, be given a special vaccine called BCG by the doctor, or they should only talk to the TB patients out of doors. They will be safer there from the TB germs. It is quite safe for members to visit leprosy patients, who may need seeds or help with their gardens or mending their clothes. They will not catch leprosy.

All this work is so much wanted that it must go on from one year to another. At the end of the school year the pupils who are about to leave must therefore show their juniors what to do, for they will have to continue the work next year.

IF YOUR NUTRITION CLUB OR COMMITTEE HAS GIVEN YOU A JOB—DO IT

Members can help to sell food in the local nutrition depots (Section 11.12), and they can make a nutrition stand at the district agricultural show. When there is an open day at the school, club members can take part in it. Clubs can grow their own vegetables and try growing new foods such as soya beans (see Section 3.10). They can make pamphlets (papers) on nutrition in the local language, and they can write nutrition songs, or write and act nutrition plays.

Clubs can also organize a 'nutrition walk' to raise money. In a walk of this kind members ask people in the district to promise to give some money for each kilometre that is walked by club members and their friends, say 5n a kilometre. People who promise to give money in this way are called 'sponsors', and members have often been able to get sponsors for more money than this, and to walk for 30 kilometres and further. If the club tries hard and makes posters to tell people what they are doing, they may be able to make much money to help their nutrition work. In a nutrition walk in Lusaka, President Kaunda himself walked 16 kilometres, and the walk raised K15,000! Perhaps the minister in your province will follow his example.

Another way of getting money is through a 'flag day'. Many small paper flags are made and pins are stuck into them. On the flag is written what the flag is for, and the flags are then sold in the streets to people who pin them on to their shirts. People give whatever sum of money they like for a flag, and the money is carefully collected in a tin. When several members are selling flags for nutrition in a town, many people will soon have flags, and much money will be made. But for both a nutrition walk, and a flag day, there must be people who will either sponsor walkers or buy flags. In poor districts there may not be enough people who have any money to give. Ask police permission before holding a flag day.

EVERYONE SHOULD
DO SOME VOLUNTARY WORK

Schools can do voluntary nutrition work in many ways, and a nutrition club is only one of them. As we have seen, nutrition and agriculture are closely joined together, and if there is no nutrition club in a school it would be very useful for the members of a young farmers club to study nutrition.

As we shall see in Section 11.13, all the nutrition work of a district should be planned together. Nutrition clubs should thus tell the district nutrition committee what they are doing, or hope to do, so that everyone knows what nutrition work is being done in the district.

SECONDARY SCHOOLS SHOULD SERVE
THE COMMUNITY

Secondary school pupils are very fortunate members of the community. They enjoy great benefits while they are at school, and gain much from them after they have left. It is thus only right that they should do what they can for those less fortunate than themselves, and particularly that they help in voluntary work. Perhaps the most useful thing about voluntary nutrition work is

that it takes members of the school into the community, and teaches them about the problems people have. It may give them the habit of doing work of this kind, which they can so usefully continue after they have left school. Nutrition work must therefore be truly *voluntary*, and be done in free time. It should not become just one more subject in the school timetable. Fewer people may do it like this, but then it is often only a few people who do so many of the things that really want doing.

11.9 Nutrition in primary schools.   Primary school children must learn something about nutrition, because they are going to be the mothers and fathers of tomorrow. As yet, only a few of them go on to secondary schools, so they cannot wait till then to learn about nutrition. They are too young to teach themselves in a club, and will have to be taught by their teachers. Some of the 'things to do' at the end of each chapter can be done by primary school children. At one school the children brought a 'picnic' of a balanced meal which they ate one evening by candlelight. A picnic is a meal that people take to eat away from their homes.

TEACH NUTRITION FROM THE EARLY
PRIMARY SCHOOL ONWARDS

Children in a primary school can also grow gardens, and if possible each child should have his own piece of land. Because primary school children are not yet strong enough for much hard work, and because they may anyway have to help on their family gardens at home, these school gardens should be small. Children should be taught better ways of growing food rather than trying to grow very much of it.

11.10 Starting or joining a nutrition group. If you are an adult and have done all that you can in your family and your job, the next thing to do is to talk to many other people about nutrition. In this you are helping other people in the community to know about malnutrition and to fight it. You may find other people who are as keen as you are to prevent it. Talk to everyone you can. Try to

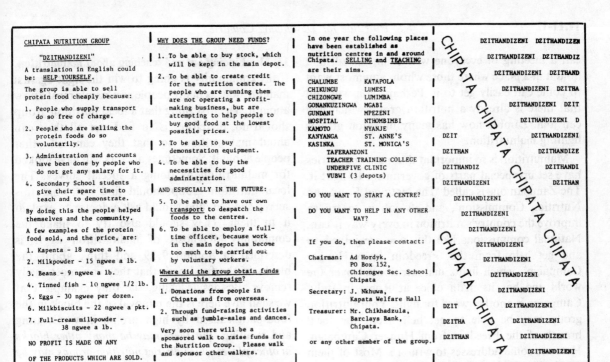

CHIPATA NUTRITION GROUP

"DZITHANDIZENI"

A translation in English could be: HELP YOURSELF.

The group is able to sell protein food cheaply because:

1. People who supply transport do so free of charge.
2. People who are selling the protein foods do so voluntarily.
3. Administration and accounts have been done by people who do not get any salary for it.
4. Secondary School students give their spare time to teach and to demonstrate.

By doing this the people helped themselves and the community.

A few examples of the protein food sold, and the price, are:

1. Kapenta - 18 ngwee a lb.
2. Milkpowder - 15 ngwee a lb.
3. Beans - 9 ngwee a lb.
4. Tinned fish - 10 ngwee a 1/2 lb.
5. Eggs - 30 ngwee per dozen.
6. Milkbiscuits - 22 ngwee a pkt.
7. Full-cream milkpowder - 38 ngwee a lb.

NO PROFIT IS MADE ON ANY

OF THE PRODUCTS WHICH ARE SOLD.

WHY DOES THE GROUP NEED FUNDS?

1. To be able to buy stock, which will be kept in the main depot.
2. To be able to create credit for the nutrition centres. The people who are running them are not operating a profit-making business, but are attempting to help people to buy good food at the lowest possible prices.
3. To be able to buy demonstration equipment.
4. To be able to buy the necessities for good administration.

AND ESPECIALLY IN THE FUTURE:

5. To be able to have our own transport to despatch the foods to the centres.
6. To be able to employ a full-time officer, because work in the main depot has become too much to be carried out by voluntary workers.

Where did the group obtain funds to start this campaign?

1. Donations from people in Chipata and from overseas.
2. Through fund-raising activities such as jumble-sales and dances.

Very soon there will be a sponsored walk to raise funds for the Nutrition Group. Please walk and sponsor other walkers.

In one year the following places have been established as nutrition centres in and around Chipata. SELLING and TEACHING are their aims.

CHALUMBE	KATAPOLA
CHIKUNGU	LUMESI
CHIZONGWE	LUMIMBA
GONANKUZINGWA	MGABI
GUNDANI	MPEZENI
HOSPITAL	NTHOMBIMBI
KAMOTO	NYANJE
KANYANGA	ST. ANNE'S
KASINKA	ST. MONICA'S

TAFERANZONI
TEACHER TRAINING COLLEGE
UNDERFIVE CLINIC
VUBWI (3 depots)

DO YOU WANT TO START A CENTRE?

DO YOU WANT TO HELP IN ANY OTHER WAY?

If you do, then please contact:

Chairman: Ad Hordyk,
PO Box 152,
Chizongwe Sec. School
Chipata

Secretary: J. Nkhuwa,
Kapata Welfare Hall

Treasurer: Mr. Chikhadzula,
Barclays Bank,
Chipata.

or any other member of the group.

DZITHANDIZENI DZITHANDIZEN
DZITHANDIZENI DZITHANDIZ
DZITHANDIZENI DZITHAND
DZITHANDIZENI DZITHA
DZITHANDIZENI DZIT
DZITHANDIZENI D
DZIT DZITHANDIZENI
DZITHAN DZITHANDIZE
DZITHANDIZ DZITHANDI
DZITHANDIZENI DZITHAN
DZITHANDIZENI
DZITHANDIZENI
DZITHANDIZENI
DZITHANDIZENI
DZITHANDIZENI
DZITHANDIZENI
DZIT DZITHANDIZENI
DZITHA DZITHANDIZENI
DZITHAN DZITHANDIZENI
DZITHANDIZENI

CHIPATA CHIPATA CHIPATA CHIPATA CHIPATA CHIPATA CHIPATA CHIPATA CHIPATA CHIPATA CHIPATA

MAKE A PUBLICITY PAMPHLET LIKE THIS FOR YOUR GROUP !

INSIDE

OUTSIDE

— pamphlet folds here —

THE AIM OF THE CHIPATA NUTRITION GROUP

The group has ONE BIG AIM:

TO FIGHT MALNUTRITION

It does that through:

SELLING
AND TEACHING

What does it sell?

PROTEIN FOOD

at very economic prices.

What does it teach?
The relation between

GOOD FOOD
AND
GOOD HEALTH

Who are the members of the group?

EVERYBODY WHO IS
CONVINCED THAT WE
SHOULD FIGHT
MALNUTRITION!!!!!

Contact any member of the group, or

Chipata Nutrition Group,
PO Box 152,
CHIPATA

WHAT IS MALNUTRITION?

A good definition is:

MALNUTRITION IS THE RESULT OF A DIET WHICH DOES NOT PROVIDE THE CORRECT TYPE OF FOOD FOR GOOD HEALTH, FOR THE NORMAL DEVELOPMENT OF CHILDREN AND ADOLESCENTS, NOR FOR NORMAL ACTIVITY AT ALL AGES OF LIFE.
MALNUTRITION is sometimes called

HIDDEN HUNGER

In simple terms:
If children do not get enough protein food they will not grow correctly. Also their brains will not function as well as they could.
If men do not get enough protein food they will not be able to do their work properly. They will get tired easily and will often be ill.
If pregnant women do not get enough protein food their babies will not be very healthy.

IS THERE MALNUTRITION IN ZAMBIA?

YES, VERY MUCH, but people do not realise this enough.

1. Still about 40% of Zambian children die before they are 5 years old, because of malnutrition.
2. A great number of the remaining 60% are mentally or physically damaged because of malnutrition. (i.e. lack of proteins)
3. Many grown-up men cannot do their work as they should do.
4. Many children are not as good at school as they should be.
5. Many women cannot nurse their children well enough.
6. Many pregnant women give birth to weak babies.

THE CAUSE OF THIS

IS

LACK

OF

PROTEIN

IS THERE A SOLUTION TO THE PROBLEM OF MALNUTRITION?

YES, THERE IS!!!!!!!!!!!!!!!!!!!!!!!!
The Government has realised this problem and has established the:

NATIONAL FOOD AND NUTRITION COMMISSION

What are they doing?
They are trying to find out what the causes of malnutrition are and what ways are best to fight malnutrition. They provide informative material and give help to anyone who asks for it.

THE PRESIDENT HIMSELF CALLED UPON THE WHOLE NATION WHEN HE SAID:

"The whole national should participat in this fight against the 'national disease' - malnutrition."

As a response to this call different nutrition groups have been established.

THE CHIPATA NUTRITION GROUP is one of them.

All these groups are voluntary organisations. The members give time or money to fight the 'national disease'.

THE SOLUTION IS THEREFORE DEPENDENT ON ALL THE PEOPLE. IF ALL PEOPLE JOIN AND GIVE THEIR TIME TO HELP OTHERS THEN MALNUTRITION WILL SOON BE WIPED OUT.

11-1, A pamphlet produced by the Chipata Nutrition Group

call a meeting of everyone who is interested, and hold it in a place where those whom you most want to come can easily get to it. Perhaps you will find that there is already a nutrition group which you can join. Zambia now has many nutrition groups fighting malnutrition.

Malnutrition is so important that many countries have set up special parts of government to fight it. The Zambian one is called 'The National Food and Nutrition Commission', and its job is to try to improve the country's nutrition in every way it can. National commissions like this one are joined to and get help from the 'Freedom from Hunger Campaign', which fights malnutrition all over the world and has its main office at Rome in Italy. Campaign is another word for fight. Your nutrition group may be able to get help from the local branch of the Freedom from Hunger Campaign. Here are some addresses to write to. Most of them are the local branches of the Freedom from Hunger Campaign.

BOTSWANA: Officer-in-Charge of Famine Relief/ School Feeding, P.O. Box 96, Gaberone.

KENYA: The National Freedom from Hunger Committee of Kenya, P.O. Box 30762, Nairobi.

MALAWI: District Development Sub-committee, Freedom from Hunger Campaign, c/o Ministry of Development and Planning, P.O. Box 174, Zomba.

RHODESIA: The Organising Secretary, Freedom from Hunger Campaign, Pax House, Union Avenue, Salisbury.

TANZANIA: Tanzanian National Freedom from Hunger Committee, P.O. Box 9192, Dar es Salaam.

UGANDA: The Ugandan Committee for the Freedom from Hunger Campaign, P.O. Box 102, Entebbe.

ZAMBIA: National Food and Nutrition Commission, P.O. Box 2669, Lusaka.

Here are some of the things that local nutrition groups can do. The most useful of them is likely to be teaching about nutrition.

11.11 Finding out and teaching about malnutrition. If the community is going to win the fight against malnutrition, as many people as possible must know about it. The first thing that a local nutrition group should do, therefore, is to find out all they can about malnutrition, so that they can tell other people about it. Sometimes doctors will have looked for malnutrition by doing a special survey. The local nutrition group should find out what this survey showed, and should ask a doctor to explain it to them. They should also try to make the community diagnosis of malnutrition as it is described in Section 9.29 and think about the blocks in the food-path that they can most easily remove. Besides teaching, the only example that we shall give here is the removal of the block in the food-path caused by high profits in wholesaling and retailing. *But there may be many other blocks in other places which district nutrition groups may be able to remove.* They must therefore think very carefully about what these might be, and what they can do about them.

WHAT BLOCKS CAN YOUR CLUB OR GROUP REMOVE?

A group may be able to get posters, pamphlets and papers on nutrition from one of the addresses in Section 11.10. They might also see that this book is on sale and is made as widely available as possible. The group can also organize meetings, in which people are told about malnutrition, and think what can be done about it. This spreading of news and teaching about malnutrition is useful in preparing the way for the district development committee. Some important local person should be asked to open the meeting and to answer questions afterwards.

Many of the things in Section 11.8 that school nutrition clubs can do can also be done by nutrition groups, especially nutrition teaching and helping in under-fives clinics. They can also run nutrition depots as the following section describes.

11.12 Food depots. In some districts the big profits made by wholesalers and retailers are important blocks in the food-path. Nutrition groups can help to remove this block by buying food wholesale and selling it cheaply. In this way poor families can buy more food with their money. In Lusaka volunteers sell this food in special depots called 'nutrition depots'. The groups are called the *Dzithandizeni* groups, which means 'help yourself', and here is an example of what they do. In the smallest shops in the townships of Lusaka groundnuts cost about 95n a kilo, but the Dzithandizeni depots are able to sell them for only 22n a kilo! These depots thus help greatly in fighting malnutrition, and if you are a Zambian and can volunteer to work in them, you will be greatly welcomed, especially by the families whom you can help so much.

'HELP YOURSELF' DOES NOT MEAN HELPING YOURSELF TO THE GROUP'S MONEY

If food is to be sold cheaply, the money that is taken from the mothers must be kept very carefully and used to buy more food for sale. If volunteers sell food and then keep the money themselves— even a little—this greatly harms the work of the group. It means that more food cannot be bought for sale; so volunteers must be honest if their work is to go on. Dishonest volunteers are the greatest danger to the work of Zambia's nutrition depots.

Nutrition clubs and nutrition groups are not the only kinds of voluntary nutrition work, and volunteers of many other kinds can help. In Malawi the Red Cross does much useful work, and in the townships of Lusaka the Zambian Helpers Society is starting to do the same.

Voluntary nutrition work can succeed! Readers may wonder if it is really possible for voluntary nutrition work to do much in a district. It can happen—*and it has happened*—but it requires great dedication (giving of yourself for others), by the people who try to get it going. On a nearby page you will see a pamphlet (a paper) sent round by the Chipata nutrition group. Between them the nutrition group and the nutrition club at the secondary school run 38 nutrition depots, many

of them at rural primary schools. Nearly a hundred boys and girls from the school teach nutrition in the villages on a Saturday afternoon, and the depots between them sell over K 2,000 of food each month.

The next section is about the work of the district nutrition committee. The members of this committee are not volunteers, but are mostly government officers who sit on it as part of their job. This committee can do many things that the groups and clubs cannot do, and they can do some things that it cannot do. All three are needed, and in every district there should be a district nutrition committee, and at least one nutrition club and nutrition group. Each should know what the other is doing, and they should all work together as a team to improve the nutrition of the district. There is more than enough work in most districts for them all to do.

THE DISTRICT NUTRITION PLAN

11.13 The district development committee. Many districts have a district development committee whose job it is to improve and develop the district in every possible way. The district governor may be the chairman or head of the committee, and with him is the top man in the district in every department, such as agriculture, health, education and community development. When there is someone from each department on the committee it is easier for them to work together, and nutrition is only one kind of development in which many departments have a part to play. When several people or departments work together we say that their work is co-ordinated. Nutrition especially needs much carefully co-ordinated hard work. Sometimes it is better if some people from the district development committee make a smaller committee, or **nutrition sub-committee,** which does nutrition only. A smaller committee often works much better than a larger one. It often has much more 'team spirit'. If there is anyone in the district who has been specially trained in nutrition, he should be asked to join it to give his advice.

The first thing the committee will need to know is the community diagnosis of malnutrition in their district, as it is described in Section 9.29. A doctor should be asked to talk about the problems of malnutrition in the district and be helped to make special surveys if necessary. He should tell the committee how much malnutrition there is, and where he thinks the food-path is blocked. The committee must then think about how the blocks in the food-path can be taken away. The food-path is almost always blocked in many places at once, and some blocks will be easier to take away than others.

The committee has to decide which things will make nutrition better most easily with the least money. The things that it decides to do must then be put into a **nutrition plan**, with targets that must be reached for the district. A target is anything which we try to aim for and reach. One target might be to have so many under-fives clinics by a certain time, and another might be to have encouraged villagers to have built so many improved food stores. Because there are likely to be so many blocks, the plan needs to have several parts, and there must be several targets. It may be possible to reach some of the targets quite soon (short-term targets), and others will take much longer (long-term targets).

Targets must also be given priorities. By this we mean that the most urgent targets should be struggled for first, and the lesser ones afterwards. In the last chapter, when we talked about helping the family, we said how necessary it is to teach mothers only the things that are possible for them to do. It is the same with the community. The committee must choose targets which it is possible to reach, not ones which are impossible. Possible targets are those that might be reached with the people and resources (money, materials, etc.) that are available, or could be obtained. The committee should look very carefully at its resources, and make sure that nothing is wasted that might improve the nutrition of the district. It should be especially careful to make the best use of anyone in the district who is skilled in nutrition.

It is not possible to do everything that might be possible everywhere all at once. It is often best to start in one village where the headman and the people are especially interested in improving nutrition, and to do as much as possible in that village. In doing this the committee would be taking **intensive action**—that is a lot of action in one place. At the same time other things, such as better nutrition teaching or planting new crop varieties, can be started at many places in the district. Action which is spread out in this way is **extensive action.** Both kinds are needed, and later on the intensive action can be started in other villages.

The members of the committee must think about how they can remove each of the blocks. Because nutrition is tied up with so many things, there is much for them to think about, and they may get help from reading Chapter 9. In the next sections there are some questions that point to some of the things that a district nutrition committee might do. They have been listed here as questions to which members of the committee must try to find answers. For example, the first one asks, 'Is nutrition being taught in the primary and secondary schools?' The committee have first to find out if it is being taught. If nutrition is not being taught, they have to think about what they might do to see that it will be taught.

Questions like this need answering at different levels. Thus a village, a ward, a district, a province and the nation as a whole, will be able to do different things to answer them. For example, a village might see that a teacher went on a course to learn about nutrition. A ward might arrange for a teacher from every school in the ward to go on such a course. The district or province might run nutrition courses for teachers. The ministry of education for the country could see that nutrition was taught in all teacher-training colleges and that special books were written to help teachers. *In the same way, all the other questions need answering at every level.*

The list of questions is a long one, and some of the things may be most easily done by the national government for the country as a whole. Most of the things in this list are for making nutrition better generally and for improving the supply of protein and joules. If, however, a nutrition survey has been carefully done, it may show that people are especially short of some vitamins or minerals. There may therefore be special things that can be done to improve the supply of these nutrients, such as growing vitamin-containing foods.

So far we have talked as if only districts could make a development committee, but wards and villages can also, and because they are smaller, there are some things that they can do more easily, if they want to. The village productivity committee, especially, can do much to improve nutrition.

A nutrition plan like this can also be made for a whole country, and is called a co-ordinated **Applied Nutrition Programme,** or **ANP.** Our nutrition plan is an ANP at village or district level.

HOW DISTRICT DEVELOPMENT
COMMITTEES CAN REMOVE BLOCKS
ON THE FOOD-PATH

11.14a Making the community aware of the importance of good nutrition. This is the first task of the district development committee, and they must do it in every way they can. A nutrition conference should be held, like that in Section 11.24b, and everyone who might benefit should be able to come to a nutrition course like that in Section 11.24c. This is especially necessary for the ward councillors who may need to be taught in the local language. People who can both teach nutrition and speak the local language are thus very useful for courses of this kind.

Politicians, schoolmasters and priests can play a big part, for they are able to speak to large numbers of people. Newspapers and the radio can also do much, and Zambia is especially fortunate in having a National Food and Nutrition Commission which does all it can to teach everyone in the country the importance of good nutrition.

TEACH NUTRITION AS PART OF OTHER SCHOOL SUBJECTS

11.14b Better nutrition teaching. Lack of nutrition education is often the most important

block on the food-path. It is tied to many other blocks, such as bad ways of farming, bad budgeting and shopping, alcohol, prestige, bottle-feeding and unfair shares of food within the family. There are many sides to education, so here are some questions that the committee should ask itself and try to provide the answers.

Is nutrition being taught in all the upper-primary and secondary schools? Is it being taught in all training schools and colleges, especially those for agriculture and health? Have these schools got the books, posters and all the other things that they need for teaching? Sometimes nutrition can be taught on its own. At other times it is better taught with health science or general science. Both boys and girls must be taught how to budget, and girls especially must be taught how to buy foods by weight. Nutrition cab even be taught in maths classes by teaching children to work out sums like those needed for Section 6.10.

In most districts many of the boys leaving primary schools should be farmers. Most of them will get no more schooling, so they should learn something about farming while they are still in the upper-primary school. Is farming being taught in these schools? Have these schools got gardens? Have these gardens got all the tools, seeds and animals that they need? Are the people who are teaching agriculture in these schools trained to teach it? If not, can they be given at least some training in how to teach it better?

Are there any Young Farmers Clubs? Are these clubs going well? Can they be given any more help? Have they also got all the seeds and tools that they need?

Are mothers at hospitals, clinics and health centres being taught how to feed and look after their children? Is this teaching good enough? Can a local nutrition group be started to help in this teaching? Can the secondary school start a nutrition club to help there also?

Is there a **nutrition rehabilitation unit** at the hospital or health centre? Rehabilitation means making people well again, and a rehabilitation unit is really a small 'hotel' where mothers can stay with their malnourished children. Mothers are

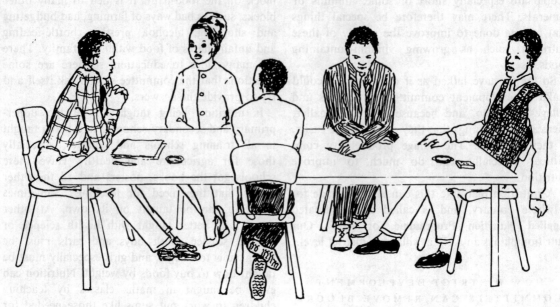

11-2, The village productivity committee

taught how to feed their young children, and can see them getting better on food alone. These units can be cheap buildings like those in the village, and cost little to run. They can do much both to cure malnutrition, and to teach families how to feed their children better. In Kenya, one of the best nutrition rehabilitation units is run by the community development department quite apart from a hospital. Hospitals send malnourished children with their mothers to this unit.

Nutrition education takes a long time to work because it will be some years before the children of today will be the mothers and fathers of tomorrow. This is why it is so important that nutrition education must start in schools *as soon as possible*, if it has not started already.

11.15 Growing more food.   Better agriculture will remove many blocks in the food-path, but it is difficult to make farmers clear more land and farm in a better way. Perhaps the party leaders and especially the ten-house chairmen of Tanzania can help.

Are there enough agricultural assistants, and are they teaching farmers the right things? Perhaps

agricultural assistants should be taught about nutrition? Are there enough of the right seeds? Are the best crop varieties being planted? Are there any new crops, such as soya beans or other legumes, that could be grown in the district? Are enough fertilizers and insecticides being used? Are there enough of them at the right price? Can farmers market their crops, so that they can buy these fertilizers and insecticides? Are there demonstration gardens at the under-fives clinics?

GROWING MORE LEGUMES MAY BE THE EASIEST WAY TO PROVIDE MORE PROTEIN

Can a campaign be organized to plant fruit trees in the district? Can a nursery be started to grow the seedlings?

Is there enough water for the crops and animals? Can the water department dig any more boreholes? Is irrigation (bringing water to the land) possible so that crops can be grown through the dry season?

11.16 Storing and preserving food better.   In Section 9.6 we saw that about one sack of food in every three is eaten by pests. Better food stores are therefore one of the best ways of getting more to eat. Fortunately they are often one of the easiest ways. The agricultural department must therefore find out which is the best kind of food store for the village farmers to make. The things needed to make them must be produced, and the agricultural assistants must then show farmers how to make food stores that will keep pests from spoiling their stored crops.

In many districts it is wise to keep a store of maize from one year to another in case there is not enough rain and the harvest is bad. Has the district got a store of this kind?

In the wet weather washed cassava cannot be dried for pounding into meal. Families may therefore go hungry until the weather gets dry. Can villagers be persuaded to buy and use food bins (big tins) in which to keep their cassava meal so that they can pound meal in dry weather to eat when it is raining?

Preserving food means doing things to try to stop it going bad. Fish and meat and even green leaves are often dried to preserve them. Better ways of preserving foods like these may also help the nutrition of the district.

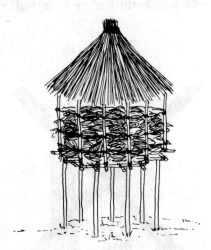

11-3, Can farmers be taught to make better food stores than this one?

11.17 More animal protein.   Even a little animal protein is very good for the nutrition of the young child. Can any more fish be caught? Can they be grown in ponds? Do people keep cows in the best way? Can they keep better cows? Can a good new bull be brought to the district? Can any more chickens, ducks, pigs or goats be kept? Duck eggs are not only useful for preventing malnutrition, but ducks themselves prevent bilharzia by eating the snails that spread this disease. Ducks are thus doubly useful. Are goats milked, and are better varieties of goats needed?

11.18 Better marketing.   District development committees can do much to make food cheaper in the markets. They must try to see that the farmer is paid a good price for the food he grows so that he wants to grow more of it. Food must also be cheap so that mothers can buy it, which means that wholesalers and retailers must make as little profit as possible. Retailers must therefore be large and sell much food, so that they can live on the little profit they make on each kilogram of food they sell. Can food prices in the district be fixed? This means that food has to be sold by weight, and that there must be a right or fixed price for a kilogram of all the common foods. If food is to be sold by weight, every retailer must have scales to weigh food. Food has to come by road to market, and one way to help marketing may be to build better roads.

Fuel for cooking is nearly as important as food; so there must be fixed prices for fuel as well as for food.

11.19 Taking away the block caused by alcohol. In Section 9.11 we found that alcohol is often a bad block in the food-path, and that it is sometimes as if the food-path were blocked by a river of beer! Alcohol is a difficult block to take away, but here are some questions to ask which show some of the things that might be done. Some of them could be done in a district, while others could only be done for the whole country. Some will be easier in town bars than in the villages.

Can the hours of drinking be shortened? Can bars be closed during working hours? Bars may only open if the district secretary gives his permission each year. Can he stop giving permission for new bars? Can he give permission for fewer

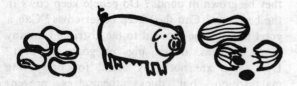

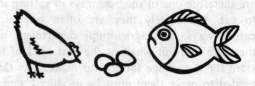

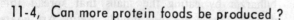

11-4, Can more protein foods be produced ?

bars next year? Can the price of beer be taxed so high that people stop buying so much beer? Can the police stop people making spirits (Malawi gin or *kachasu*)? The most important bars to close are those beside the roads where drivers get drunk so that they crash their lorries. There is one wise district governor who takes away the keys of any lorry driver he finds drinking in a bar! Can anything be done to make beer less easily available during the important times of the year when men should be farming?

Many people drink because there is nothing else to do; so one way to stop them is to give them other ways to spend their time besides drinking. Can amenities like cinemas be provided to keep people out of the bars at the weekends? Can places to eat be provided as well as places to drink? Amenities are things which make a town good to live in, and which provide people with pleasant ways of passing the time.

Mr. Chinyanta, a dresser from Kapata, found that alcohol was a serious block in the food-path. Men were drunk when they should have been in their gardens. Women were drunk when they should have been feeding their children, or weeding their gardens. Fire was thus able to get into the gardens and burn the dry weeds and the crops. He was a member of the village productivity committee and the district development committee, so he explained to these committees about the food-path, and what a serious block alcohol was. He was able to persuade them to give only one bar licence for each village. Bars often run out of beer, so if there is only one bar, people cannot get beer all the time. He talked to the bar owners, and they agreed not to let women with young children into bars.

11.20 Taking away the block caused by people being too sick to work hard. This is not an easy

block to take away, because there are often many people who are slightly sick with malnutrition or other diseases. Even if they are only a little sick it may not be easy to cure them. More health centres can help; so can more medical assistants and nurses to work in them.

Workers who are well fed often work better. Some factories find that their workers work harder if they are given a meal in the middle of the day. If workers can be better fed it may be possible to break the vicious circle that you read about in Sections 7.21 and 9.2.

11.21   Under-fives clinics, bottle-feeding and school feeding.   Bottle-feeding is the worst block in the food-path of the very young child, and it should be one of the easiest to take away. Shopkeepers might be told why bottle-feeding is so bad, and

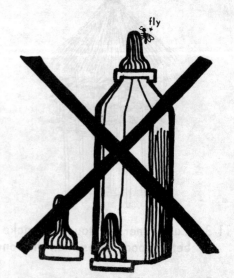

11-5, Can anything be done to take away the block in the food-path caused by bottle-feeding ?

could be asked not to sell bottles unless a mother brings a letter from a doctor or a clinic. This letter would not be given unless a mother had no other way of feeding her child.

As we saw in Sections 2.2 and 7.18, hungry, malnourished school children learn badly, so much of the teaching that they get is wasted. If meals can be given to them at school they may learn much better. Can anything be done to improve school feeding?

Under-fives clinics (Section 1.3) are one of the most important ways of removing the block to the food-path caused by mothers not knowing how to feed their young children. Districts should therefore have enough clinics for *all* children to go to them. Can any more clinics be started? Can volunteers be found to help in them? Are the clinics that there are working in the best way? The most important thing that they do is to teach mothers how to look after their young children. Is this

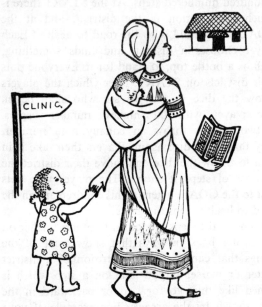

11-6, Are there enough under-fives clinics for every child to go to one ?

teaching being done well? Are children being immunized against the diseases, such as measles, which help to make malnutrition worse? There are so many children and so few health workers that the community must learn to look after its own

children. This is why voluntary work at under-fives clinics is *so* important.

Can a special infant food be made locally, like the one described in Section 7.13?

A COMMUNITY MUST CARE FOR ITS OWN CHILDREN

11.22 Taking away the blocks caused by too short a birth interval, by families having more children than they can feed, and by there being too many people for the land. As you read in Section 9.17, when the children in a family come too quickly they are often malnourished. A child should be at least two and a half years old before his next brother or sister is born. In poor families where there is little food three years or more between children is even better. This gives a child more time for breast-feeding before his mother becomes pregnant again. Also, no family should have more children than they can feed and look after, nor should the number of people in any district grow faster than the food supply.

All this is now quite easy. A mother can have a special piece of plastic called a **loop** put into her womb which stops her having children. When she wants another child her loop can be taken away and she can become pregnant again. She can also be given pills, or an injection, to stop her having children until she wants to have them. This is called family planning, and it is now so useful, safe and cheap that every hospital and health centre should be able to help mothers and fathers plan their families. If people ask for family planning and go on asking they will get it.

11.23a Improved nutrition needs good administration. The government of a district cannot improve nutrition, and remove the blocks in the food-path, unless it works well and the decisions made by the district nutrition committee are followed *by somebody doing something*! This is one of the things that is meant by good administration. The administration of many districts is so bad that almost nothing is done. Too many people spend the time reading the paper when they should be working. Huge piles of fertilizer spoil in the rains because nobody will fill in the forms that enable it to be sold to the farmers. Officials are moved from district to district so frequently that they do not have time to learn about the local problems, and get things going that would improve nutrition. Educational, agricultural and medical officers do not visit, support and care for their staff in the villages as well as they might. In all these ways bad administration prevents the removal of blocks in the food-path—it is itself a very serious block in the food-path.

BAD ADMINISTRATION BLOCKS THE FOOD-PATH

11.23b Evaluation.   Evaluation means seeing if what we have been trying to do is working. One of the most useful things about the road-to-health chart is that we can evaluate what we are doing to improve the nutrition of a child. If he is gaining weight we are succeeding. If he is losing weight we are failing.

In the same way we want to see if our efforts to improve the nutrition of a community are succeeding. This is difficult, because the nutrition of a community is difficult to measure. It is not easy to be sure that there is less malnutrition in a community one year than there was the year before. The easiest way to evaluate the nutrition work that has been done in a district is to look for answers to questions such as these. Are more of the important food crops being grown? Has the price of groundnuts, for example, fallen because there are more of them? Are more children coming to the under-fives clinic? Are they coming more regularly than they did last year? Are more of their immunizations completed?

Another way of evaluating the success of our efforts is to see if fewer cases of malnutrition come to the hospitals and health centres of the district. This again has problems, because malnourished children are not always counted in the same way from one year to another.

In spite of all these difficulties the district nutrition committee should do all it can to evaluate

the success of its efforts. Malnutrition will not be driven out in one year, or in two or three. It will probably take many years, but the battle against it *can be won*! Every few months the committee should meet to see how the fight is going. *Step by step and year by year they will slowly win*!

11.24   T H I N G S   T O   D O

(a) 'The District Nutrition Game'.   It is sometimes possible to learn things by playing a game. Here is one that will help you to learn about the community diagnosis of malnutrition, and the health action that can be taken to improve nutrition. The game is called the District Nutrition Game and can be played by several players.

On a nearby page you will see a picture of the board on which the game is played. There is a START and a GOAL, joined by a long path with a hundred numbered steps. At the START there is 'much malnutrition in the district', and at the GOAL 'every child is on the road to health.' Each player chooses a district, and finds something, such as a bottle top, to stand for it. Everyone puts their districts on START, after which the players throw the dice in turn to see who shall begin. The player with the highest number begins. If two players throw an equally high number, they throw the dice again. Players then take it in turn to throw the dice and move their district the number of steps it shows. The player who gets first to the GOAL, where all his children are on the road to health, wins the game.

Some of the steps are joined to others further on or further back in ways that show some of the things that can make the nutrition of a district better or worse. If you land on a step which is joined like this, go forward or backward in the way shown by the arrows. For example, if your district lands on step 4, go up the path marked 'much voluntary nutrition work' to step 38.

Some steps, such as steps 3 and 6, are marked with wavy lines. These are the 'helps' and 'hindrances' steps. When a player lands on one of these steps there is either a help, or a hindrance, to the nutrition of his district. These helps and hindrances are shown in a list on the next few

New variety of maize is grown by most farmers
in the district
GO FORWARD TEN STEPS

Soil erosion controlled by better farming methods
GO FORWARD FIVE STEPS

The district is given a special vote of money for
nutrition
GO FORWARD SIX STEPS

The president expresses interest in the nutrition
of his people
GO FORWARD TEN STEPS

More land irrigated
GO FORWARD TEN STEPS

Local nutrition groups help in the under-fives
clinics
GO FORWARD SIX STEPS

People learn to look after fish ponds
GO FORWARD THREE STEPS

Marketing co-operative doubles its number of
depots
GO FORWARD FIVE STEPS

Nutrition rehabilitation units opened at all
hospitals and health centres
GO FORWARD FOUR STEPS

Farmers paid for their crops soon enough for
them to buy seed and fertilizer for the next
season
GO FORWARD SEVEN STEPS

Marketing co-operatives under new management
and make increased profit
GO FORWARD THREE STEPS

School feeding scheme started
GO FORWARD FOUR STEPS

Nutrition clubs started in all schools
GO FORWARD THREE STEPS

Improved ways of farming become widely used
GO FORWARD TWELVE STEPS

New primary school curriculum includes nutrition
GO FORWARD TEN STEPS

People stop leaving the land to go to town
GO FORWARD TWENTY STEPS

Most children in the district immunized against
measles
GO FORWARD FOUR STEPS

Family planning started in the district. Families
now need have no more children than they
can feed and look after properly
GO FORWARD TEN STEPS

There are many other helps and hindrances
that you may be able to think of, and if you look at
a newspaper you can often find ideas for them.
The hindrance in the list above about the eggs
that went bad came from a newspaper. Do your
best to make up some of your own help and
hindrance cards.

(b)   Running a nutrition conference.   This section
is mainly for the secretaries of nutrition groups,
who will find that one of the best ways of
generating interest in nutrition in a district or
province is to organize a nutrition conference.
It is aimed at the high level personnel of a district.

Conferences can take many forms, and it is as
well to be quite clear at the outset what its objectives
are to be. Those of the conference described here
are to increase the awareness of malnutrition
among the leaders of the community, *to promote
practical action*, and to encourage the formation
of a provincial or district nutrition committee.

---

*HOLD A CONFERENCE IN EVERY DISTRICT
WHERE THERE IS MALNUTRITION*

Careful attention to detail is essential to the
success of any conference. Start at least three
months ahead by first seeking the support of the
leaders of the province or district. Ask the most
influential person in the community to open the
conference, and do your best to see that he arrives
on time on the day—the programme will be much

put out if he is very late. Try to secure the attendance of the senior officers in health, education, community development and agriculture, as well as the political leaders of the district. Explain carefully to each important person why it is so necessary that he should come. The conference will have lost much of its purpose if most of these people do not come.

Try to obtain the help of outside speakers chosen for their knowledge, authority and lecturing ability. They might be nutritionists or paediatricians working in the country, the MCH (maternity and child health) specialist, or a member of the department of community health at the university. These people are likely to have many engagements and should be written to well in advance.

Choose the time and venue carefully. Try to avoid dates, such as those for elections, when the people you most want may not be able to come. Conferences can often be most conveniently held during the holidays in a secondary school or teacher-training college. A weekend may be the best time if people have jobs they cannot leave in the week. The main room should be large and there should be at least three smaller ones in which groups can meet. See that the main room can be blacked out and encourage your guest speakers to use visual aids. Make sure that meals can be provided, that all participants eat together and that coffee or tea will appear without fail during the morning and afternoon breaks—*it has been well said that if coffee fails a conference fails!* Some participants may need to stay overnight; so see if individual hospitality or, where appropriate, a school dormitory can be made available.

When plans for the conference have been made, prepare an attractive programme, and invite the most influential people working in health, education, agriculture and community development. In making up the number for a conference work from the top downwards, and do not forget the secondary school teachers. Forty participants is a good number, but, as many of those who say they will attend are apt not to turn up on the day, it is wise to invite about sixty. Remind the more important of those who have said that they will attend a week before the conference opens. If funds for mileage, materials, meals, etc., are required, it

may be possible to obtain them from one of the organizations affiliated to the Freedom from Hunger Campaign listed in Section 11.10.

There are many ways of planning the programme. Here is one which has worked well and which is based on the structure of this text. Although the sessions are planned to last an hour or an hour and a half, *it is vital that speakers do not talk for more than twenty minutes, or at the most half an hour, especially immediately after lunch* (!), *so as to leave PLENTY of time for discussion.* If speakers can cut what they say to fifteen minutes, then so much the better. Where, on the programme, sessions follow one another immediately, a five-minute break should be allowed between them.

Saturday

8.00		Conference opened by the District Governor.
8.30–9.30	(1)	The human and economic significance of malnutrition in . . . . district. *First guest speaker.*
9.30–10.30	(2)	What foods are made of. *First guest speaker.*
10.30–11		Break for coffee.
11–12.30	(3)	The growth of children and the consequences of failure. *Second guest speaker.*
12.30–2		Participants lunch together.
2–3.30	(4)	Feeding children. *Second guest speaker.*
3.30–4		Break for tea.
4–5.30	(5)	Why does malnutrition exist? Making the community diagnosis. *First guest speaker.*

Sunday

9–9.30	(6)	How can we prevent malnutrition? *First guest speaker.*
9.30–11	(7)	Conference splits up into groups for agriculture, health, education and community development to discuss PRACTICAL action in the district.
11–11.30		Break for coffee.

11.30–1 (8) Groups meet to discuss their recommendations and put forward proposals.

1.00 Chairman closes the conference.

1.15 Participants have lunch together.

At the beginning of the conference the chairman should ask participants to stand up and introduce themselves. Individual name badges, made if necessary from cardboard, 'Sellotape' and safety pins, are also useful. If possible everyone should be given a cardboard folder to the front of which a duplicated sheet has been stuck describing the conference, some paper and a pencil. If funds are available everyone should also be given a copy of this text, if possible well in advance. See that there are a typewriter, duplicator, stencils and paper available at the conference so that last minute handouts, resolutions, etc., can be prepared. Provide a blackboard, chalk and, if possible, the flannelgraph of the road-to-health chart described in Section 12.3.

It will be seen that the programme suggested for the conference occupies the whole of a Saturday and the following Sunday morning. Although time is short, it is unlikely that participants will be willing to work on Saturday evening, or on Sunday afternoon. The first session should cover the first part of Chapter 2 and expand particularly on Section 2.2. The emphasis should be on the underweight child, and its consequences for the mental development of the individual and the overall development of the nation. Any factual evidence that may be available on the prevalence of malnutrition in the district should be assembled before the conference, and perhaps even collected by the methods suggested in Sections 1.5 and 1.6. It should be presented to the conference in graphic form and later incorporated into the community diagnosis.

The second session should cover some of the more important parts of the second and third chapters. Brief mention should be made of nutrients and food composition, but there will be no time to discuss protein structure, or amino acids, or the NPU. The third session should cover the most important parts of the first chapter and go on to discuss marasmus and kwashiorkor. The fifth session, and the last for Saturday, is particularly important and should cover the food-paths as they are described in Chapter 9. *It should end with members of the conference themselves making the community diagnosis of malnutrition as this is described in Section 9.29.* This should be written on the blackboard as a list of the more important blocks in the food-paths of the district, together with the number of 'plusses' that are to be accorded to them. If participants have copies of this text, the community diagnosis can be recorded in them.

At nine o'clock on Sunday morning one of the guest speakers should quickly go over the community diagnosis of malnutrition, as it was made the previous evening, and suggest some of the things that might be done to remove the blocks in the food-path. After this the conference should break up into four groups, one each for agriculture, health, education, and community development. They should start by electing a chairman and a secretary or *rapporteur*. If one of these can be the senior official locally responsible for that particular sector, then so much the better. Groups should then have plenty of time to discuss the removal of the blocks in the food-path suggested by the community diagnosis, and must try to come up with *a few really practical ideas about what can be done in the district or province. Vague hopes and good intentions are valueless, and the real purpose of the conference should be for influential people in the district to decide what can be done.* One of the most useful things the conference can recommend is the formation of a district nutrition committee.

After coffee, groups should meet in 'plenary session', and the rapporteur of each should *briefly* inform the conference of the action this group considered *practical* in the province or district. When participants have had time to discuss these reports, the chairman should sum up and close the conference; after which everyone should, if possible, have lunch together. As soon as possible afterwards the chairman should prepare a short written report stating what was recommended and who was present.

Because one of the main objectives of such a

conference should be to suggest the formation of a provincial or district nutrition committee, this document could well become their opening brief. It should also be circulated to all participants.

(c) Running a nutrition course.   This section is based on recent Zambian experience. Although designed with specific objectives for medical workers, it could, with minor modification, be adapted for all kinds of field staff who might be able to do anything to promote good nutrition.

Many such staff have been imperfectly trained a long time ago, and their re-training is one of the paramount needs of many ministries. Nutrition is likely to be only one of the fields in which re-training is required, and many re-training courses will not be able to devote much time to it. But, however much nutrition is incorporated in a course, *it is essential that its objectives should include carefully specified improvements in a student's working activity when he returns to his station.* These need to be worked out and stated, and the training course designed to achieve them. Such objectives might include the ability to conduct health education classes, to teach nutrition at the primary school level, or to weigh children and fill in road-to-health charts. More general objectives might be to explain the most important facts of nutrition as they affect health, and to make participants generally better at promoting good nutrition through their jobs.

Those attending such courses can include primary school teachers, agricultural assistants and demonstrators, health assistants and vaccinators, medical assistants and nurses, and, most importantly perhaps, dressers and indoor servants from clinics, because these have great potential influence on the patients. It has been found desirable to make courses as homogeneous as possible, both in the level of basic education of the participants, and in the length of their previous training—if any. Thus it has been found better to have separate re-training courses for dressers and medical assistants. Secondary school teachers are better catered for in the conference described above. However, participants can, and often should, be mixed as far as their field of previous experience is concerned. Thus a course can well contain agricultural assistants, medical assistants and primary schoolmasters.

The course suggested below is for medical staff, such as medical assistants, or, on a different occasion, dressers, its objectives being to enable them to give nutrition education talks and to fill in road-to-health charts. It is designed to last for a week, but if extended over a fortnight to include the general management of under-fives clinics and immunization, it would prepare the participants for the introduction of these clinics in a district. Hold it in an empty residential secondary school during the vacation, and if given suitable notice UNICEF will often provide the funds. Thirty participants is an ideal number, for which a minimum of two staff are needed, but numbers can be scaled up and more staff are welcome. A doctor and a public health nurse make a good combination, but two public health nurses can well run a course of this kind. Particularly careful attention should be paid to the catering arrangements, as these are apt to be the weak point of a course. Make provision for visual aids, particularly transparencies, and also for a duplicator, a typewriter, paper and stencils.

Sunday

8.00 p.m.   *Registration.* The staff and participants are introduced to one another, and the seminar is opened by the District Governor. This is the time for an introductory questionnaire and a multiple choice pre-test of the participants' knowledge.

Monday

9.00 a.m.   *Growth* (first part of Chapter 1).
9.30 a.m.   *Malnutrition and its importance* (Chapter 2).
11.15 a.m.   *Practical.* The age and weight of children (see Section 2.11b).
2.00 p.m.   *Nutrients.* What foods are made of (parts of Chapters 3 and 4).
4.00 p.m.   *Practical.* The food collection (see Section 4.18).
8.00 p.m.   *Slide show.*

Tuesday

8.00 a.m.   *More about protein* (latter part of Chapter 3).

9.30 a.m.   *Food requirements* (Chapter 6).

11.15 a.m.   *Best buys for protein and joules* (Chapter 6).

2.00 p.m.   *Practical.* Class visits a market and either buys food locally or studies its price (see Section 6.10).

4.00 p.m.   *Best buy lists prepared and studied in class.*

8.00 p.m.   *Nutrition film as available.*

Wednesday

8.00 a.m.   *The food-path and the causes of malnutrition* (Chapter 9).

9.30 a.m.   *The community diagnosis of malnutrition* (see Section 9.29).

11.15 a.m.   *Class splits into groups to discuss the ways in which the blocks in the food-path can be removed.*

2.00 p.m.   *Groups report.*
The rest of the afternoon and evening free. The District Nutrition Game might be played on this evening.

Thursday

8.00 a.m.   *Feeding children* (Chapter 7).

9.30 a.m.   *Practical.* Preparing meals for young children (see Section 7.22).

11.15 a.m.   *Teaching better nutrition* (Chapter 10).

2.00 p.m.   *Practical.* Class splits into groups and practises teaching one another.

4.00 p.m.   *The road-to-health chart and how to fill it in* (part of Chapter 1).

8.00 p.m.   *Brains Trust.*

Friday

8.00 a.m.   *Class visits an under-fives clinic.* Participants practise both teaching mothers and filling in the road-to-health charts.

11.30 a.m.   *Test.*

2.00 p.m.   *Course evaluation by students.* Test returned and gone through. Group photograph.

3.00 p.m.   *Groups divide and each prepares a nutrition play.*

8.00 p.m.   *Nutrition plays enacted before an invited audience.*

Saturday

8.00 a.m.   *Participants depart.*

It will be seen that great emphasis has been placed on practical work and that the course contains both a pre-test and a final set of multiple choice questions. These, especially the pre-test, can hardly be too simple. If difficulty is experienced in making them up, a set may be had from the National Food and Nutrition Commission in Lusaka (see Section 11.10). For Monday morning's practical some malnourished children should be brought from the hospital if this can be arranged. At the Brains Trust on Thursday evening, the most knowledgeable people available should answer questions. For the course evaluation on Friday afternoon the participants are asked to send in their comments and suggestions as assistance in planning further courses of a similar kind. The audience for the nutrition plays on the last evening can well be the staff of the school and their families. Both the Brains Trust and the plays have proved surprisingly popular, and the latter have disclosed much unexpected talent.

It is desirable that each participant take away some written material with him for further study and reference, perhaps this manual.

Courses of this kind provide an opportunity, which should not be lost, of letting participants meet their administrative superiors, so that questions can be answered and administrative matters settled.

Courses should be followed up with a visit to staff in the field, and if possible with a further course the following year. One very successful follow-up course started with a day's lectures and discussions after which participants took part in the vernacular instruction of a fresh group of participants, in this case the leaders of women's clubs.

Chapter Twelve

APPENDIX

12.1 The metric system. This book is written in the **metric system.** This means that it uses grams and kilograms, not pounds and ounces. Many countries have already changed from the imperial system of pounds and ounces to grams and kilograms, or will change soon. If you do not understand the metric system, this section may help you.

Because there are 16 ounces in a pound, pounds and ounces are not easy to use. Grams and kilograms are easier to use because there are 1,000 grams in a kilogram. It is easier to change grams into kilograms by dividing by 1,000 than it is to change ounces into pounds by dividing by 16. Just as pounds are shortened to lbs. and ounces to oz., so grams are shortened to g and kilograms to kilo or kg. A gram is a much smaller weight than an ounce. You will understand better what a gram is if you know that a new pencil weighs about five grams or 5 g.

You may want to change pounds into kilos or ounces into grams. If you do, you will find it useful to know that there are 2.2 pounds in a kilo and 28.3 grams in an ounce. Often 28.3 g can be usefully rounded (shortened) to 30 g, but you should not round 2.2 lb. to 2 lb. when you are changing the weight of children from the imperial to the metric system. This is not accurate enough, and a child may be put on the road to health when he is really below it.

Two figures have been drawn to help you make the change more easily and accurately. Figure 12-1 shows you how to change pounds and ounces into grams and kilograms (or the other way around) for any weight from one ounce to 22 pounds. You will see that this figure has a scale which is well spread out for the small weights, but which gets closer together as weights get heavier. A scale of this kind is called a *logarithmic* scale and makes it easier to show a very long scale, such as that shown here, in one figure. It is quite easy to use.

All you have to do is to find the weight you want to change on one side of the scale and then read off what it should be on the other side of the scale. Remember, however, when you are using a scale of this kind, that it is not equally spread out and that each weight is shown by a shorter part of the scale the further up it you go.

Figure 12-2 is a more ordinary scale and is said to be a *linear* rather than a logarithmic scale. It goes from 3 to 20 kilograms, and is for changing the weights of children from the imperial to the metric system, or the other way around. If your under-fives clinic has an imperial weighing scale and you are sent metric road-to-health charts, you will find Figure 12-2 very useful.

12.2 A reading list. Do you want to learn more about nutrition? If you do, here are some books that will help you. They are all in ordinary or standard English, but none of them is particularly difficult.

Human nutrition in tropical Africa, Latham, M., United Nations Food and Agriculture Organization, Rome, 1965.

Child nutrition in developing countries, Jelliffe, D. B., United States Department of Health, Education and Welfare, sold by the Superintendent of Documents, U.S. Government Printing Office, Washington D.C., 20402, U.S.A.

Visual aids in nutrition education, Holmes, A.C., United Nations Food and Agriculture Organization, Rome, 1968.

Learning better nutrition, Ritchie, Jean A. S., United Nations Food and Agriculture Organization, Rome, 1967.

The next section is for the people who may use this book to teach with.

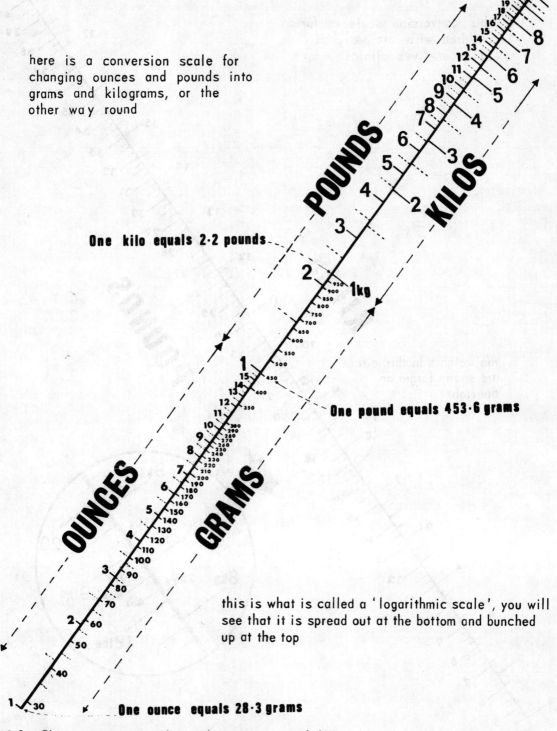

here is a conversion scale for
changing ounces and pounds into
grams and kilograms, or the
other way round

POUNDS

KILOS

One kilo equals 2·2 pounds

1kg

One pound equals 453·6 grams

this is what is called a 'logarithmic scale', you will
see that it is spread out at the bottom and bunched
up at the top

OUNCES

GRAMS

One ounce equals 28·3 grams

12-1, Changing ounces and pounds to grams and kilos

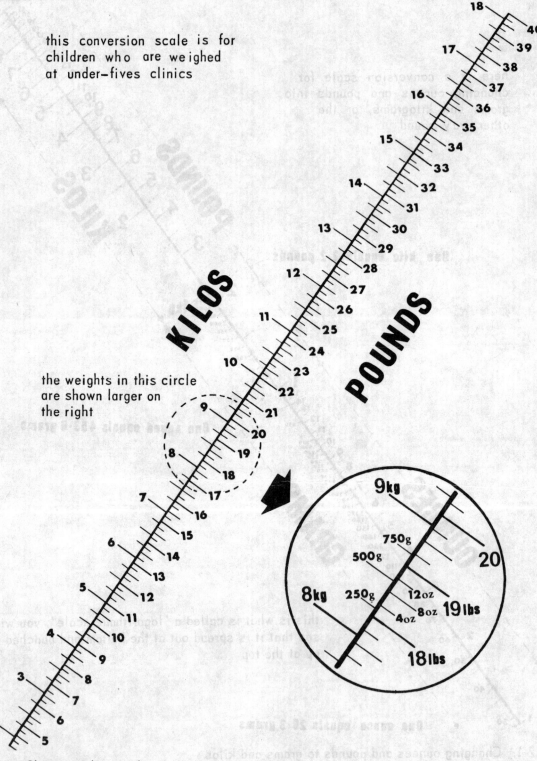

this conversion scale is for children who are weighed at under-fives clinics

KILOS

POUNDS

the weights in this circle are shown larger on the right

9kg
750g
500g
8kg
250g
12oz
8oz
4oz
18lbs
19lbs
20

12-2, Changing the weight of children from pounds to kilos

12.3 Some notes for teachers. This book has been written to cover most of the content of a course on nutrition suitable for the staff listed in the introduction, and also as a 'teach yourself' text for voluntary nutrition workers. It may require modification for teaching in schools, and only some of the material it covers is likely to be suitable for primary schools. It is suggested that, where possible, a course in nutrition should follow the general sequence of its chapters, but it may on occasion be convenient to put Chapter 9 on the food-paths, and particularly its practical work, after Chapter 2 on the failure of growth.

The ultimate purpose of learning nutrition is to provide practical help to those who need it. Thus, any instruction in nutrition, no matter how brief or how humble, must prepare students to do this. They will be prepared to give this help, both through their skills and their attitude, if their course can be made as practical as possible. This means that *nutrition has to be learnt in homes and markets* as well as in the classroom. Any nutrition course which does not plan to provide active practical instruction can be said to have failed before it has begun.

Practical work has been provided for here as 'things to do' at the end of each chapter. Most of them have been tried out on many occasions and found to work well with the students for whom this book is intended. The equipment required is minimal, students like visiting people's homes, and most families like being visited. It is worth making considerable effort to work out the best protein and joule buys in Section 6.6, since all practical advice in shopping depends upon it. The simplest kind of metric balance is all that is needed, and if students are sent with a letter, it has been found that many shopkeepers will let them weigh food without buying it. The mathematics needed is much less formidable than it looks, the most difficult operation being long division by a two-figure number. *When examples are required for teaching mathematics, see if some of them can be taken from the field of nutrition.*

One of the best ways of organizing practical work is to do it in the form of projects, pairs of students choosing different 'things to do' and presenting their results to the assembled class. This may be particularly valuable if time is short.

Teaching materials come second only to practical work. Teachers within Zambia should write to the National Food and Nutrition Commission (NFNC), Box 2669, Lusaka. Those outside it should write to Teaching Aids at Low Cost (TALC), 30 Guildford Street, London W.C.1. The following may be available, either free or at minimal charge.

Three sets of multiple choice questions. 300 multiple choice questions were composed and allocated at random into sets A, B and C, which thus cover the same material and are of the same complexity. They are intended for use as a pre-test to see what is known before a course starts, a test at the end of the course, and a test some months later to see what has been retained. (TALC) (NFNC)

A variety of posters and other visual materials forming a teaching kit. (NFNC)

A flannelgraph of the road-to-health chart. This depicts the chart used in Zambia. State whether the pounds or kilos version is required. (TALC) (NFNC)

A stencil for the road-to-health chart. This is a quarto size electric stencil of the standard Zambian metric chart. It enables many cheap copies of the chart to be run off for practice teaching purposes with the aid of an ordinary duplicator. (NFNC)

12.4 References. Most of this book is the outcome of the nutrition activity that was going on in Zambia while it was being written, and of conversations with those involved in it, many of whose contributions are gratefully acknowledged in the introduction. Much further assistance was also obtained from the following:

FAO (1968), *Food Composition Tables for Use in Africa.*

FAO *Nutritional Studies*, No. 15 (1957), 'Calorie Requirements'.

WHO/FAO *Nutrition Meetings Report Series*, No. 37 (1965), 'Protein Requirements'.

Holmes, A. C., (1968), *Visual Aids in Nutrition Education*, FAO, Rome.

Jelliffe, D. B., (1966), *The Assessment of the Nutritional Status of the Community*, WHO, Geneva.

Jelliffe, D. B., (1968), *Child Nutrition in Developing Countries*, U.S. Department of Health, Education and Welfare.

Jelliffe, Patrice F. E., and D. B., (1969), *Supplement to the Journal of Tropical Paediatrics*, **15,** 4, 'The Arm Circumference as a Public Health Index of Protein-Calorie Malnutrition of Early Childhood'.

Latham, M., (1965), *Human Nutrition in Tropical Africa*, FAO, Rome.

PAHO *Scientific Publication* No. 217 (1970), 'Guidelines to Young Child Feeding in the Contemporary Caribbean'.

Ritchie, Jean A. S., (1967), *Learning Better Nutrition* FAO, Rome.

Stanfield, J. P., (1971), *Supplement to the Journal of Tropical Paediatrics and Environmental Child Health*, **17,** 1, 'Recent Approaches to Malnutrition in Uganda'.

Use has also been made of the WHO/FAO publication on energy and protein requirements due for release in 1973, which was seen in draft form, and its recommendations incorporated in the text.

·VOCABULARY-INDEX

absorption When digested food is taken through the wall of our intestines into our body we absorb it, 3.7

action Doing. To take action is to do something, 11.1

acute An acute disease is a short and often severe one, 7.20

adult A grown-up man or woman, 1.1

arm circumference The distance round the upper mid-arm, 1.5

aflatoxin A poison that is found in mouldy foods, 5.5

alcohol When we drink beer it is the alcohol in it that makes us drunk, 4.15, 9.11, 11.19

amino acids Proteins are made by joining together a hundred or more much smaller things called amino acids, 3.7

anaemia A disease in which the blood gets too pale and thin, 4.7, 4.10

antiseptic A substance used for killing micro-organisms (germs) *outside* the body on the skin, 8.11

artificial The opposite to natural. Something which is artificial is made by man, 8.1

basic wage The lowest wage that anyone with a full-time paid job should get. This is usually fixed by the government, 6.8, 6.10d

best buy The best way to buy certain things, such as protein and joules, 6.4, 6.5, 6.10a

bilharziasis A disease caused by worms which live in the veins of the bladder or large bowel. Also called schistosomiasis, 9.2

birth interval The time or space between a child's birth and that of his next brother or sister, 7.6, 9.17a

block on the food-path Something which cuts or blocks the path which food takes from the fields, where it is grown, to the body of the child who eats it, Chapter 9.

boss Your boss is the person you work for, 7.17

bottle-feeding, Chapter 8.

brand name Special names that some factories use for the things they make. 'Coca-Cola',

'Castle' beer and 'Lactogen' are brand names, 4.15

breakfast The first meal of the day, 4.3, 7.18

breast-feeding 7.1, 7.2

budgeting Planning to spend money in the best way, 6.8, 9.9

bulk The space or volume that something of a given weight takes up. When a small weight of maize meal is boiled with water it makes a large bulk of porridge. Cooking oil or margarine have many joules of energy in a small bulk, 7.8

bull A male or man cow, 11.17

calcium A mineral from which bones are made, 4.12

calorie An old way of measuring energy. 1 calorie =4.18 joules, 4.1b and footnote.

canteen A place where workers can eat, 7.21

carbohydrate A starchy, sugary, or floury nutrient in food that provides the body with energy, 3.4, 4.2

carbon dioxide A gas made of oxygen and carbon which is formed when food is 'burnt' in the body, or fuel is burnt in a fire, 3.7, 4.1

caries Holes in the teeth, or dental decay, 4.13, 4.15, 5.4

cash crop A crop that is grown specially for sale, 9.5

cassava A common plant with thick white roots that can be dried and pounded into a flour which is almost pure carbohydrate, 4.2

caterpillar This is a caterpillar: 3.6, 9.12

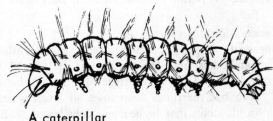

A caterpillar

cells The small pieces or 'bricks' from which the body is made, 3.7

chain Things make a chain when they are joined together in a line. A necklace is a chain of beads, 3.7

chlorine One of the elements in common salt. Chlorine gas is used to kill micro-organisms in water, 4.17b

chronic A chronic disease is a long lasting one, 7.20

colostrum The first milk that comes to a mother's breast when her child is born, 7.2

community The people who work and live together in the same place. The people who live in the same district form a community, so do the pupils and teachers living in a secondary school, Introduction, Chapter 11.

community diagnosis A measure of how sick a community of people are, what diseases make them sick and why they get these diseases, 9.25, 11.11

community health action The things a community do (the action they take) to make their health better, 11.1

condensed milk A kind of thick, sticky, tinned milk containing much sugar, 5.3, 8.4

consonants All the letters of the alphabet except A, E, I, O and U, 3.7

cream The top part of milk containing the fat and many of the joules, 4.2, 5.3

crèche A place where children can be left for a few hours and where there is someone to look after them, 7.17

crops Plants that are grown for eating or selling, 9.1, 9.5

custom Something we do because everyone else in our community does it, 9.4

cyanide A poison in some kinds of cassava root, 5.5

damp Slightly wet, 5.5

decimal A way of writing fractions as tenths, hundredths and thousandths, etc., 1.1, 12.1

dehydration Lack or shortage of water. A baby with bad diarrhoea soon loses so much water in his stools that he becomes dehydrated, 7.20

depot A store or shop, 11.12

detergent A kind of strong soap. 'Tide', 'Surf', 'Dreft', etc., all contain detergents, 8.11

develop A country is said to develop when the people in it get richer and when there are more paid jobs, factories, schools, hospitals, clinics, roads, houses, etc., 2.2

diagnosis When a doctor diagnoses a patient he finds out which diseases he has, 9.25

digestion The breaking down of food into smaller, simpler parts. When protein is digested in our stomach and intestines it is split (cut) into amino acids from which it was made, 3.7

diarrhoea A disease in which there are many liquid stools, 7.20

disease Something, such as malnutrition, malaria, or measles, which stops a person being healthy and makes him sick, 2.3

district development committee A special committee for developing a district, 11.13

District Nutrition Game A game for learning about the causes of malnutrition, 11.24a

divorce The separation or going away of a man from his wife, 9.16, 9.23

Dzithandizeni movement A group of unpaid nutrition workers in Zambia, 11.12

ecology This is the study of something in relation to the community in which it is, 9.29

educational diagnosis The health education that a community need to improve their health, 10.1

elements The simplest things from which everything is made, 3.7, 4.4, 4.9, 4.10, 4.11, 4.12, 4.13

energy The ability to do work, 4.1

energy food Food which makes a person able to do work, 4.2

enzymes Digestive enzymes are substances in the gut that digest food by breaking it down into small pieces, 3.7, 7.20

essential Something which is necessary and which we cannot do without, 3.7

evaporated milk A kind of liquid tinned milk without added sugar, which has been made concentrated by taking away some of the water, 5.3

faeces The waste from the bowel. Also called stools, 4.17a

family planning By family planning methods we mean the methods that parents use so that they shall have children only when they want them, 9.17a, 11.22

famine There is a famine in a district when there is no food to eat, 4.3, 11.3

fizzy drink A bottled drink with bubbles of gas (carbon dioxide) in it, 4.15

flannelgraph A kind of 'teaching picture' using a cloth called flannel, 10.16d

fluid Something which flows, such as water, tea, milk or beer, 7.20

fluorine A mineral element found in water which helps to make strong teeth, 4.13

folic acid A vitamin found in green leaves that the body needs to make blood, 4.7

food collection A collection of foods used for teaching, 4.18a

food depot A shop or store where food is sold without profit, 11.12

food-path A path that we picture food going along from the fields where it is grown to the body of the person who uses it, Introduction, 9.1

food table A table showing the amounts of the different nutrients in various foods, Table 19, 6.5

fuel The wood, paraffin or charcoal, gas or electricity used for cooking, 9.15

full cream milk Milk straight from the cow from which the cream (fat) has not been removed, 5.3

fungi Small white or coloured plants that grow on damp food or vegetable matter. Most fungi are very small. The word mould is often used instead of fungus, 5.5, 9.5

fungicide A poisonous substance for killing fungi, 9.5

germ This word has at least two meanings. (1) It can mean the part of a seed from which the young plant grows, 4.3. (2) A germ can also mean a very small living thing that can grow in the body and cause disease. The word micro-organism is often used instead of germ, 7.20, 8.11

goitre A swelling of the thyroid gland. This gland is in the lower part of the front of the neck, 4.11

grain The seed of such plants as maize, wheat or rice, 4.3

gram A small weight. There are about 28 grams in an ounce. Gram is written g, 12.1

graph A special kind of 'picture' which shows you how things are related to one another, such as a child's age and his weight, 1.2

groundnut A legume which has fruit underneath the ground. It is also called a monkey-nut or a peanut, 3.10, 7.11

group Several of the same things together, 11.7

growth curve The line of dots that a child's weight makes on his road-to-health chart, 1.2, 2.9

gums The parts of our mouths which hold our teeth, 4.8

gut The stomach and intestines, 3.7, 4.5, 7.20

harvesting Gathering crops from the fields when they are ready, 9.1

health centre A kind of very good clinic or dispensary, which does everything to make a family's health better except the things that can only be done by a hospital, 11.14

health education Education which tries to change a person's behaviour in a way which will improve his health, 9.24, Chapter 10.

human A man, woman or child, 5.3

hunger The feeling of not having had enough to eat, 5.1

hypochlorite An antiseptic containing chlorine that is useful for killing the micro-organisms (germs) in feeding bottles, 8.11

immunization Preventing someone getting a disease by giving him a special 'medicine' called a vaccine, 1.3

infant A young child under one year old, 7.14

insecticide A poisonous substance for killing insects, 9.5, 11.15

iodine One of the mineral elements the body needs, 4.11

iron A mineral element which the body needs to make blood, 4.10

IR-8 A specially good variety of rice, 9.5

'Jik' A brand of hypochlorite antiseptic used for sterilizing feeding bottles, 8.11

joule A unit used for measuring energy. It has replaced the calorie in nutrition, 4.1b and footnote (4.18 joules=1 calorie).

kapenta The Zambian name for a common kind of small lake fish. It is often dried, 6.3

keratomalacia An eye disease, 4.5

kilogram A weight of 1,000 g. A kilogram is equal to 2.2 pounds. Kilogram is often shortened to kilo or kg, 12.1

kilojoule, kJ A thousand joules, 4.1b

kwacha The larger kind of Zambian money. A hundred ngwee (100 n) make one kwacha (K1). The kwacha is a little larger than the USA dollar. K1 = $1.4

kwashiorkor A serious disease caused by lack of protein and joules in which a child is usually underweight and has swollen feet, 2.5

lactose The special sugar found in milk, 5.3

lard A soft white cooking fat made from the fat of animals, 4.2

latrine A small room or house where people go to pass the waste from their bodies. In a pit latrine the waste goes into a deep hole in the ground, 4.17, 9.20

legumes The family of plants to which peas, beans and groundnuts belong, 3.10

Likuni phala An infant food made in Malawi by grinding together maize, beans and groundnuts, 7.13

local Belonging to that place, 5.6, 11.10

local-events calendar A list of the dates on which things which have happened in a district that can be used for telling a child's age, 1.3, 1.6e

locust A kind of jumping insect which eats green plants, 3.6

lunch The meal eaten in the middle of the day, 7.18

lysine One of the essential amino acids which is scarce in maize, 3.7

malnutrition Disease caused by not getting enough of the right food to eat, Introduction.

marasmus A disease of children caused by lack of food (both protein and joules) in which a child becomes very thin indeed, 2.6

matoke The Ugandan word for a food made by steaming a variety of green bananas, 4.3

meal (1) Flour, such as that made from powdered grain or cassava. (2) The word is also used to mean the food that is eaten at any one time. Breakfast, lunch and supper are meals, 4.3

measles A serious disease of young children, 1.3, 2.3, 7.20

megajoule, MJ A million joules, 4.1b

methionine One of the essential amino acids that is scarce in peas, 3.7

micro-organisms Germs. Micro means small. Micro-organisms are very small living things which we cannot see with our eyes. Most of them are harmless. Some grow in our bodies and cause disease, 7.20, 8.1

midwife A nurse who is specially trained to help mothers have their babies, 10.1

'Milton' A kind of hypochlorite antiseptic used for killing the harmful micro-organisms in feeding bottles, 8.11

minced Cut into small pieces, 7.15

minerals Substances like salt and the elements iron, calcium, fluorine and iodine which are found in the ground, 4.4

minimum family food budget The least amount of money that an average or ordinary-sized family in the district needs to spend on food each month. Minimum means least, 6.8, 6.10d

mould A small white or coloured plant which grows on damp food, 5.5

mortar A strong wooden pot in which grain is pounded into flour. It is used with a heavy wooden stick called a pestle, 7.11

necklace A string of beads put round the neck, 3.7

net protein utilization The same as NPU, 3.8

ngwee A small coin used in Zambia. 100 ngwee or 100 n equals one kwacha or K1, Introduction.

nicotinic acid A group B vitamin found in groundnuts that prevents the disease called pellagra, 4.6

non-essential amino acid An amino acid that the body can make for itself out of other amino acids, 3.7

non-foods Things we eat or drink that are no use to our bodies as foods, 4.15

normal This word can be used in several ways to mean healthy, usual, ordinary or average, 7.1

NPU This stands for Net Protein Utilization and is given in per cent (%). It is a way of saying how good a protein is for body-building, 3.8

nourished A well-nourished child is a well-fed child, Introduction.

nshima The stiff, solid food made by boiling maize or cassava flour in water, 5.7

nutrients The things that foods are made of. Proteins, carbohydrates, oils, fats, vitamins, minerals and water are nutrients, 3.1

nutrition The study of food, and how our bodies use food.

nutrition club A club formed by people who are interested in nutrition, 11.8

nutrition conference A group of people who come together for a short time to study nutrition, 11.24b

nutrition course, 11.24c

nutrition group A group of people interested in doing nutrition work, 11.8

nutrition rehabilitation unit A small 'hotel' or hostel where malnourished children can stay with their mothers and be cured by being properly fed, 11.14b

offal The inside parts of an animal, such as the heart, liver, lungs, etc., 3.6

ounce A measure of weight equal to 28.3 grams. 16 ounces make 1 pound, 12.1

pellagra A disease caused from having too little of the B vitamin called nicotinic acid, 4.6

PEM or Protein Energy Malnutrition This used to be called PCM, or Protein Calorie Malnutrition, 2.8

pestle The heavy stick that is used to pound grain into flour. It is used with a strong wooden pot called a mortar, 7.11

pesticide Poisonous substances for killing some kinds of pests, 9.5

pests Animals, insects or plants which harm food and crops. Termites, rats and monkeys are pests, 9.5

placenta The placenta or afterbirth is the part of the inside of the womb where a child joins his mother's body, 2.2a

plantain A kind of banana which stays green and has to be cooked, 4.3

porridge A thin food made of maize, millet, cassava or other staple that is given to children, 5.6, 7.3

poster A big picture for teaching or telling people something, 10.10

pounded Made into a powder, 7.11

pregnant A woman is said to be pregnant when there is a child inside her, 3.2, 7.6

preserve To keep food so that it does not go bad, 11.16

prestige, prestigious Respect or admiration for something, or a way of doing something, 9.12

prevent To prevent something is to stop it happening, 11.4

printer Someone who makes or prints books, 3.7

profit The money that a shopkeeper makes when he sells something for more than he has spent on it, 6.3, 9.8a

proportion Part of something compared to the whole of it.

protective foods Foods containing vitamins or minerals which stop the body getting some diseases. Protection means guarding or keeping harm away, 3.1, 4.14

proteins The most important nutrient from which our bodies are made, Chapter 3.

puberty The time when a boy becomes a man and a girl becomes a woman, 7.18

reference Something to which other things can be compared or referred, 3.7

reference protein A reference protein is a specially good kind of protein which is 100 per cent used for body-building (it has an NPU of 100%) and to which other proteins can be compared. Egg and mother's milk are reference proteins, 3.7

refined Refined flour is made from grain from which the outer parts have been removed, 4.3

relish The vegetables, meat and fish that are eaten with the staple, 5.6

repair To repair something is to mend it, 3.3

retailer A person who buys and sells in small amounts, 9.1, 11.12

road to health The path between the upper and lower lines on a child's weight-for-age graph, 1.3

road-to-health chart This is a special weight-for-age graph that is used at an under-fives clinic, 1.3

safety belt A strong belt that helps to stop someone in a car from hurting himself if the car has an accident, 9.24

salt-and-sugar water A home-made medicine for diarrhoea, 7.20

scale A machine for weighing, 1.3 and footnote

scarce Something is scarce when there is only a little of it and it is hard to get.

scurvy A disease due to lack of vitamin C in which the gums swell up and bleed, 4.8

secretary A woman who types in an office, 7.17

shanty-town A community of people living close together without proper houses, water, drains or roads, and usually also without clinics or schools, 1.3, 9.23

shopping guide A list of the best shops to go to for each kind of food, 6.10b

skim To take away the top part of a liquid. To skim milk is to take the cream away from it, 5.3

skimmed milk Milk from which all the cream has been taken away and in which all the protein has been left, 5.3

soya bean A special bean containing much protein, 3.10, 11.15

staple The main food of a country. Cassava and maize are staple foods, 4.3

sterilize To kill all the micro-organisms in something. This is usually done by heating it, 8.10

stool The waste from the bowel, 7.20

substance Anything which is the same all through.

suckling Sucking at the breast. A breast-feeding child, 7.1

surplus crop The extra food that a family grows for selling, 9.5

survey A search for something. A nutrition survey is a search to see what the nutrition of a community is like, and how much malnutrition there is, 1.5, 1.6, 9.25, 11.13

tablespoon A large spoon used for serving food from a big dish to a plate. A dessertspoon is smaller and is used by adults for eating with, 8.6

teaspoon A small spoon used for stirring tea, 8.6

ten-house chairman The lowest party leader in Tanzania. He is in charge of ten households, 11.6

tortoise An animal with four legs and a hard shell that walks very slowly along the ground, 3.6

turtle An animal with four legs and a hard shell that swims in lakes or the sea, 3.6

umbilical cord The cord which joins a baby to the inside of his mother's womb, 2.2, 3.2

underweight A child is underweight if he is malnourished and not as heavy as he should be for his age, 1.1, 2.1

vaccine A special medicine which is given to people to stop them getting some diseases, 1.3

visual aid Something which can be seen and which helps in teaching, such as a picture, or a flannelgraph, 10.10

vitamin A nutrient which is only needed in very small amounts and which the body cannot make for itself, 3.1, 4.4

vitamin A A vitamin needed to keep the eyes healthy, 4.5

vitamin B A group of vitamins, one of which is nicotinic acid, that prevents the disease called pellagra, 4.6

vitamin C A vitamin needed to keep the gums and small blood vessels healthy, 4.8

volunteer Someone who works for no money or for very little money, 11.7

vomit To bring up the food in your stomach, or be sick, 7.20

vowels The letters A, E, I, O and U, 3.7

wholesaler A person who buys and sells in large amounts, 9.8, 11.12

womb The place where a child grows inside his mother, 3.2

yolk The yellow part of an egg.

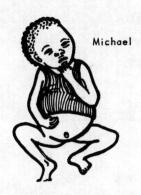

Michael

The battle against malnutrition CAN be won !

Published by Oxford University Press, Eastern Africa, Oxford House, P.O. Box 72532, Mfangano Street, Nairobi, Kenya . . . and printed . . . P.O. Box 1064, Ltd. P.O. Box 30615 Singapore . . . Oxford University Press, Nairobi, by photo reproduction by Paramount Photo Litho, P.O. Box 571, Wilson Airport.

Published by Oxford University Press, Eastern Africa Branch, P.O. Box 72532,
Monrovia Street, Science House, Nairobi and printed by Kenya Litho Ltd.,
P.O. Box 40775, Changamwe Road, Nairobi, on paper manufactured by
Panafrican Paper Mills, P.O. Box 535, Webuye Kenya.